The Management of Metastatic Triple-Negative Breast Cancer: An Integrated and Expeditionary Approach

Authored by

Katarzyna Rygiel
Department of Family Practice
Medical University of Silesia (SUM)
3 Maja St., 41-800, Zabrze
Poland

The Management of Metastatic Triple-Negative Breast Cancer: An Integrated and Expeditionary Approach

Author: Katarzyna Rygiel

ISBN (Online): 978-981-5196-02-3

ISBN (Print): 978-981-5196-03-0

ISBN (Paperback): 978-981-5196-04-7

need for a court order if at any point you breach any terms of this License Agreement. In no event will any delay or failure by Bentham Science Publishers in enforcing your compliance with this License Agreement constitute a waiver of any of its rights.

3. You acknowledge that you have read this License Agreement, and agree to be bound by its terms and conditions. To the extent that any other terms and conditions presented on any website of Bentham Science Publishers conflict with, or are inconsistent with, the terms and conditions set out in this License Agreement, you acknowledge that the terms and conditions set out in this License Agreement shall prevail.

Bentham Science Publishers Pte. Ltd.
80 Robinson Road #02-00
Singapore 068898
Singapore
Email: subscriptions@benthamscience.net

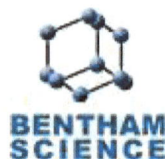

BENTHAM SCIENCE

CONTENTS

FOREWORD i

PREFACE iii

PART 1

CHAPTER 1 UNRAVELING ETHNIC DISPARITIES IN TRIPLE-NEGATIVE BREAST
CANCER (TNBC): EXPLORING THE IMPACT OF METABOLIC, REPRODUCTIVE,
ENVIRONMENTAL, AND SOCIAL FACTORS ON THE DISEASE COURSE IN AFRICAN-
AMERICAN (AA) WOMEN POPULATION 1
    INTRODUCTION 1
    HOW CAN WE APPROACH ETHNIC DISPARITIES IN TNBC SURVIVAL? – A
    ROADMAP OF POSSIBLE UNDERLYING BIOLOGIC AND NON-BIOLOGIC RISK
    FACTORS OR CAUSES OF TNBC IN AA VS. EA (OR NHW) WOMEN 3
    A SPOTLIGHT ON THE FAMILY HISTORY AND GENETIC MUTATIONS: THE
    IMPACT OF ETHNICITY ON MOLECULAR MAKE-UP IN TNBC 7
    SOCIOECONOMIC DISPARITIES IN BC – A LINK BETWEEN THE ECONOMIC
    DEPRIVATION AND DYSFUNCTIONAL HEALTHCARE PATH 8
    BEHAVIORAL AND CULTURAL FACTORS ACCOUNTING FOR BC DISPARITIES IN
    AA WOMEN 9
    THE UNDERESTIMATED ROLE OF INSUFFICIENT PHYSICAL ACTIVITY AS A
    RISK FACTOR IN BC DISPARITIES – REFLECTIONS FROM THE SELECTED
    CLINICAL STUDIES 12
    IMPACT OF INADEQUATE NUTRITION ON BC DISPARITIES –INSIGHTS FROM
    MAJOR CLINICAL STUDIES 13
    CONCLUSION 14
    REFERENCES 16

CHAPTER 2 A CLOSER LOOK AT THE ANDROGEN RECEPTOR (AR)-POSITIVE AND
AR-NEGATIVE METASTATIC TRIPLE-NEGATIVE BREAST CANCER: CAN WE APPLY
NOVEL TARGETED THERAPEUTICS? 22
    INTRODUCTION 22
        Various Molecular Subtypes of TNBC 23
    THE UNDETERMINED PROGNOSTIC VALUE OF ANDROGEN RECEPTOR (AR) IN
    WOMEN WITH TNBC 24
    THE INFLUENCE OF ANDROGEN RECEPTOR (AR) ON POTENTIAL
    THERAPEUTIC CHOICES IN PATIENTS WITH TNBC 25
    DIFFICULTIES WITH STANDARDIZATION OF ANDROGEN RECEPTOR (AR)
    TESTING 27
    TARGETED APPROACHES TO TNBC RESISTANT TO THERAPY: FOCUSING ON
    "WEAK POINTS" OF AGGRESSIVE CANCERS 27
        Immune Checkpoint Inhibitors (ICI) (Atezolizumab and Pembrolizumab) 28
    POLY-ADP-RIBOSE POLYMERASE (PARP) INHIBITORS (OLAPARIB AND
    TALAZOPARIB) 32
        Anti-Trop-2 Antibody-drug Conjugate (ADC) (Sacituzumab Govitecan-hziy) 33
    SELECTED ACTIONABLE PHARMACOLOGIC TARGETS AND EMERGING
    THERAPIES ON THE HORIZON 33
    CONCLUSION 34
    REFERENCES 35

CHAPTER 3 LIQUID BIOPSY: INSIGHTS INTO MONITORING TUMOR DYNAMICS AND
RESPONSE TO THERAPY IN PATIENTS WITH BREAST CANCER 39

INTRODUCTION 40

HOW LIQUID BIOPSY CAN BE USED IN MONITORING METASTATIC BC
PROGRESSION AND TREATMENT? 41

TRANSLATING A LEARNING EXPERIENCE FROM THE SOLAR-1 TRIAL INTO
CLINICAL PRACTICE: THE APPROVAL OF ALPELISIB AND THERASCREEN 42

AN IMPORTANCE OF CTDNA MUTATIONAL ANALYSIS IN THE MANAGEMENT
OF PATIENTS WITH METASTATIC BC 43

CIRCULATING TUMOR DNA ANALYSIS TO HELP DIRECT THERAPY IN
ADVANCED BC (PLASMAMATCH): THE UNIQUE TOOL TO IDENTIFY
SENSITIVITY 44

AN IMPACT OF THE LIQUID BIOPSY ON THE PERSONALIZED TREATMENT OF
WOMEN WITH METASTATIC BC 45

    Useful Ways of Predicting the Patients' Survival and BC Recurrence 45

    Can the Circulating Tumor Cell (CTC) Count be Used for a Selection of the First-line
    Therapy (CHT or ET) in Women with HR–positive, HER2-negative Metastatic BC? 47

    Can ctDNA Monitoring During the Neoadjuvant Chemotherapy (CHT) Course Reveal a
    Patient's Risk for Distant BC Metastases? 47

    Can Lack of ctDNA Clearance in Early Period of Neoadjuvant Chemotherapy (NAC) be a
    Predictor of Poor Response to Treatment? 47

    How to Predict the BC Metastatic Relapse Before the Clinical Recurrence? 48

CONCLUSION 49

REFERENCES 50

CHAPTER 4 IMPORTANCE OF BIOMARKER CONVERSIONS AS "ROAD SIGNS" TO
MANAGE WOMEN WITH METASTATIC BREAST CANCER: HOW TO USE THEM FOR
PERSONALIZED CARE OF THESE PATIENTS? 53

    INTRODUCTION 53

    COMMON CONVERSIONS OF BIOMARKER'S STATUS IN METASTATIC BREAST
    CANCER 54

    ALTERATIONS OF THE BIOMARKER'S STATUS IN METASTATIC BREAST
    CANCER AND THEIR POTENTIAL ROLE IN THE PROGNOSIS AND THERAPY 55

    COMMON BIOMARKERS OR THEIR COMBINATIONS MATCHED WITH
    TARGETED TREATMENTS FOR BREAST CANCER 57

    BIOMARKERS' SHIFTS IN METASTATIC BREAST CANCER AND THEIR
    REASSESSMENT: A POTENTIAL ROLE IN THE PROGNOSIS AND TREATMENT 57

    CONSIDERATIONS OF INTERTUMOR AND INTRATUMOR HETEROGENEITY:
    CHALLENGES AND OPPORTUNITIES 59

        Tumor Evolution and Its Connections with Changing of the Biomarker's Status in
        Metastatic Breast Cancer 60

    CONCLUSION 61

    REFERENCES 63

CHAPTER 5 PUTTING IT ALL TOGETHER: CLINICAL PEARLS OF RECENTLY
APPROVED THERAPIES FOR TRIPLE-NEGATIVE BREAST CANCER 65

    INTRODUCTION 66

    A SPECIAL TASK OF PARP INHIBITORS: TARGETING ENZYMES THAT REPAIR
    DNA DAMAGE 67

    WHO CAN BENEFIT THE MOST FROM PARP INHIBITORS? - GOOD NEWS FROM
    THE OLYMPIAD AND THE EMBRACA TRIALS FOR WOMEN WITH METASTATIC
    BRCA-POSITIVE TNBC 67

        Shifting Gears to Immunotherapy: Who Can Be A Winner? 68

        The Role of Ventana and Dako Assay in PD-L1 Testing 70

Sacituzumab Govitecan - An Antibody Drug Conjugate (ADC) Starting the "Optimistic Wave" of Therapy for Patients with Metastatic TNBC 71
A Spotlight on HER2-low BC: Diagnostic Challenges to HER2 Status Interpretation 71
The Remarkable Place of ADCs for Patients with Metastatic TNBC and HER2-low BC 73
How to Put Immune Checkpoint Inhibitors and PARP Inhibitors Into Perspective? Considerations of Targeted Therapeutic Options and Their Sequence in Patients with TNBC Associated With the BRCA Mutation and PD-L1 Positivity 73
CONCLUSION 73
REFERENCES 75

CHAPTER 6 THE WAY OUT FROM THE LABYRINTH OF ANTICANCER THERAPIES FOR PATIENTS WITH BREAST CANCER: HOW CAN WE IMPROVE THEIR CARDIAC SAFETY AND QUALITY OF LIFE? 77
INTRODUCTION 77
FREQUENT SIDE EFFECTS OF ANTICANCER TREATMENTS AND THEIR PERCEPTION IN PATIENTS WITH BREAST CANCER 79
A SPOTLIGHT ON TWO "FACES" OF PAIN SECONDARY TO ANTICANCER THERAPIES IN PATIENTS WITH BREAST CANCER: PERIPHERAL NEUROPATHY AND LYMPHEDEMA 80
HOW CAN WE APPROACH DEPRESSION AND COGNITIVE IMPAIRMENT IN PATIENTS WITH BREAST CANCER FROM DIFFERENT PERSPECTIVES? 81
HOW CAN WE ADDRESS THE MANAGEMENT OF MENOPAUSAL SYMPTOMS IN YOUNGER WOMEN UNDERGOING CHEMOTHERAPY FOR BREAST CANCER? 82
HOW TO ASSESS CARDIOTOXICITY RELATED TO TREATMENTS FOR BREAST CANCER? 82
MAY STANDARD PHARMACOTHERAPY FOR HEART FAILURE PROVIDE CARDIOPROTECTIVE EFFECTS FOR WOMEN WITH BREAST CANCER? 85
HOW TO REDUCE CARDIOTOXICITY RELATED TO TREATMENTS FOR BREAST CANCER? FOCUS ON CARDIO-ONCOLOGY, REHABILITATION, AND INTEGRATIVE INTERVENTIONS 89
FURTHER DIRECTIONS: EFFORTS TO DEVELOP THE "KNOWLEDGE NETWORK" FOR PERSONALIZED MEDICINE GOALS 90
CONCLUSION 91
REFERENCES 93

CHAPTER 7 CAN WE FIND A NONINVASIVE TOOL OF PRECISION MEDICINE THAT CAN ALWAYS BE USED FOR THE INDIVIDUALIZED TREATMENT OF WOMEN WITH BREAST CANCER? 96
INTRODUCTION 96
The Goals and Tools of Precision Medicine 97
AN EMERGING P4 MODEL: TRANSFORMATION FOR A NEW HEALTHCARE SYSTEM 97
A Role of Personomics as A Tool to Fulfill the Unmet Healthcare Needs 99
The Aliki Initiative: Teaching Personomics In The Academic Setting 100
Unique Values of the Patient-centered, "Humanistic" Approach to Medical Management ... 100
Current Possibilities of Personalized Medical Care for Women with Breast Cancer 101
COMMON LIMITATIONS OF PERSONALIZED MEDICAL CARE FOR WOMEN WITH BREAST CANCER 102
Selected Therapeutic Targets in Advanced or Metastatic TNBC 103
CONCLUSION 104
REFERENCES 105

PART 2

CHAPTER 8 DISTRESS – OUR "INTERNAL ENEMY": HOW TO "DISARM" OR LESSEN ITS NEGATIVE IMPACT ON THE PSYCHOPHYSICAL CONDITION OF WOMEN WITH TRIPLE-NEGATIVE BREAST CANCER? 108
    INTRODUCTION 108
    WHAT CAN PATIENTS WITH CANCER, CANCER CARE TEAMS, AND CAREGIVERS DO WHEN THE DISTRESS BECOMES VERY SERIOUS? 110
        Simple Tools to Help Measure Distress 111
    HOW TO TAKE AN ACTIVE ROLE IN PERSONAL MANAGEMENT OF THE CANCER-RELATED DISTRESS AND COOPERATE WITH THE CANCER CARE TEAM? – THE ART OF "DO'S" AND "DON'TS" 111
    HELPFUL OPTIONS TO MANAGE CANCER-RELATED DISTRESS AND ITS COMPLICATIONS 114
    CONCLUSION 115
    REFERENCES 117

CHAPTER 9 TEACHING THE BRAIN HOW TO COUNTERACT DISTRESS: PRACTICAL LESSONS ABOUT THE STRESS AND RELAXATION RESPONSES FOR WOMEN WITH TRIPLE-NEGATIVE BREAST CANCER 118
    INTRODUCTION 118
    OPPOSITE PHYSIOLOGIC ACTIONS OF TWO PARTS OF THE AUTONOMIC NERVOUS SYSTEM (ANS) – THE SYMPATHETIC NERVOUS SYSTEM (SNS) AND THE PARASYMPATHETIC NERVOUS SYSTEM (PNS) 120
    HOW THE PARASYMPATHETIC NERVOUS SYSTEM (PNS) ACTIVATION CAN BE APPLIED TO BENEFIT WOMEN WITH TNBC? 121
    COMBINING THE AWARENESS ABOUT AUTONOMIC NERVOUS SYSTEM (ANS) SIGNALS WITH INFORMAL APPLICATIONS OF COGNITIVE AND BEHAVIORAL INTERVENTIONS: HOW TO MAKE A POSITIVE TRANSFORMATION? 122
    ELICITING RELAXATION RESPONSE TO RESTORE A CALMING BALANCE OF THE MIND AND A HEALING POTENTIAL OF THE BODY 122
    HOW TO TEACH THE BRAIN TO REENGAGE IN THE REPAIR OF SOME STRESS-RELATED DAMAGES? – A THERAPEUTIC "MENU" TO CHOOSE FROM, FOR WOMEN WITH TNBC 124
    CONCLUSION 125
    REFERENCES 127

CHAPTER 10 AN INTERSECTIONAL NEUROSCIENCE APPROACH FOR DISADVANTAGEOUS POPULATIONS: MEDITATION PRACTICE AS A POSSIBLE SUPPORT OPTION FOR WOMEN WITH BREAST CANCER? 129
    INTRODUCTION 129
        Intersectional Neuroscience (IN) - A Novel Research Model That Can Help Determine Mental States during Meditation in Diverse Populations of Participants 131
    EVALUATING MULTIVARIATE MAPS OF BODY AWARENESS (EMBODY) - THE INNOVATIVE TASK TO "DECIPHER" MENTAL STATES DURING THE BREATH-FOCUSED MEDITATION 131
    A POSSIBLE APPLICATION OF THE COMMUNITY-BASED PARTICIPATORY RESEARCH (CBPR) TO INTRODUCE INTERSECTIONAL METHODOLOGY TO BRIDGE THE GAP BETWEEN RESEARCH AND PRACTICE 132
    HOW THE DIFFERENT ATTENTIONAL STATES DURING THE BREATH-FOCUSED MEDITATION CAN BE MEASURED? 133

EMPLOYING AN INTERSECTIONAL NEUROSCIENCE APPROACH TO DEVELOP
METRICS OF MEDITATION PRACTICE IN DISADVANTAGEOUS GROUPS OF
PARTICIPANTS: A POSSIBLE FUTURE STRATEGY FOR WOMEN WITH BREAST
CANCER 133
CONCLUSION 135
REFERENCES 137

CHAPTER 11 MAY WE ADJUST THE "THIRD WAVE" OF COGNITIVE AND
BEHAVIORAL THERAPIES (CBT) AND PSYCHOLOGICAL PROCESSES OF CHANGE
FOR WOMEN WITH BREAST CANCER? 139
INTRODUCTION 139
AN ADVENT OF THE "THIRD-WAVE" COGNITIVE AND BEHAVIORAL
THERAPIES AND PROCESS-BASED APPROACHES TO PATIENTS WITH BREAST
CANCER 140
A FOCUS ON CONTEXT AND FUNCTION: A COMBINED APPROACH FROM THE
COGNITIVE AND BEHAVIORAL DIRECTIONS 142
HOW CAN WE ACCOMMODATE THE KEY PSYCHOLOGICAL PROCESSES OF
CHANGE TO HELP ACHIEVE THE PATIENT'S PERSONALIZED GOALS MORE
EFFECTIVELY? 143
PSYCHOLOGICAL PROCESSES OF CHANGE IN SIX BASIC DOMAINS: A FOCUS
ON FLEXIBLE THERAPEUTIC OPTIONS VS. TRADITIONAL SIGNS OR SYMPTOMS
ANALYSIS IN THE SCOPE OF THEIR APPLICATIONS 144
Cognition 145
Affect 146
Attention 146
Self 148
Motivation 148
Behavior 149
PSYCHOLOGICAL FLEXIBILITY – THE COURAGE OF OVERCOMING BARRIERS
BY USING CROSS-DIMENSIONAL CONCEPTS 149
FUNCTIONAL ANALYTIC PSYCHOTHERAPY (FAP) – POTENTIAL VALUES TO
THE PATIENTS AND THEIR CLINICAL/CANCER CARE TEAMS 150
CONCLUSION 151
REFERENCES 152

CHAPTER 12 EXCEPTIONAL RESPONDERS: EXPLORING THE MOLECULAR "MAKE-
UP" OF PATIENTS WITH CANCER WHO EXPERIENCED RECOVERY 154
INTRODUCTION 154
The Exceptional Responders Initiative (ERI) – New Hopes and Challenges Uncovered by a
Pilot Study 155
AN IMPACT OF PRECISION ONCOLOGY ON THE EXCEPTIONAL RESPONDERS
INITIATIVE (ERI) 157
SELECTED TOOLS OF PRECISION ONCOLOGY APPLIED IN THE EXCEPTIONAL
RESPONDERS INITIATIVE (ERI) 157
THE NCI-MATCH TRIAL - A MOLECULAR ANALYSIS FACILITATING THE
CHOICE OF OPTIMAL ONCOLOGIC THERAPY 158
CHALLENGES IN INVESTIGATING THE EXCEPTIONAL RESPONDERS AND
EXCEPTIONAL RESPONSES 159
FUTURE STEPS TO UNLOCK THE DOOR TO NOVEL ANTICANCER TREATMENTS 159
THE POWER OF INTEGRATED STUDIES – THE INTERFACE BETWEEN THE
PATIENTS, TUMORS, AND SOCIO-EPIDEMIOLOGICAL RISK FACTORS FOR
MALIGNANCIES 161

A SPOTLIGHT ON THE NETWORK OF ENIGMATIC EXCEPTIONAL RESPONDERS (NEER) 162

    CONCLUSION 164

    REFERENCES 165

CHAPTER 13 RADICAL REMISSIONS: UNIQUE LESSONS FROM PATIENTS WITH CANCER WHO WERE ABLE TO DEFY THE ODDS AND RECOVER 166

    INTRODUCTION 167

        "The Radical Remission Project"-Directions for Future Research and Navigation Through the Labyrinth of False Hope 168

    INDIVIDUAL PATTERNS USED BY SOME PATIENTS WHO EXPERIENCED UNUSUAL RECOVERY FROM CANCER AND TYPICAL REASONS FOR REFUSING CONVENTIONAL ONCOLOGY TREATMENTS 170

    BASIC EXPECTATIONS OF "EXCEPTIONAL" PATIENTS WITH CANCER AND "REVERSIBLE" OBSTACLES FROM THEIR HEALTHCARE PROFESSIONALS 172

    THE PILLARS OF EFFECTIVE COMMUNICATION BETWEEN ONCOLOGY PATIENTS AND THEIR PHYSICIANS 173

    COMPLEMENTARY AND INTEGRATIVE MEDICINE (CIM) AND INTEGRATIVE ONCOLOGY: BENEFICIAL "LINKS" IN THE CARE OF PATIENTS WITH CANCER 174

    THE INTEGRATIVE ONCOLOGY SCHOLARS (IOS) PROGRAM – BRIDGING THE GAP IN THE COMPREHENSIVE CANCER CARE 174

    CONCLUSION 176

    REFERENCES 179

CHAPTER 14 HOW CAN WE REDEFINE HOPE AND GRATITUDE TO HELP PATIENTS WITH BREAST CANCER BUILD THEIR "NEW LIFE"? 181

    INTRODUCTION 181

    PRECIOUS "SECRETS" OF LONG-TERM SURVIVORS OF BREAST CANCER 182

    A "FRESH LOOK" AT HOPE, GRATITUDE, AND SPIRITUALITY CONCEPTS IN THE CONTEXT OF PATIENTS WITH BREAST CANCER 183

        Gratitude in the Brain: Cerebral Representation of the Gratitude Model 184

    HOW TO DISCOVER A NEW MEANING IN LIFE? – SIMPLE "TAKEAWAYS" FOR PATIENTS WITH BREAST CANCER 185

    PSYCHOSOMATIC AND SOCIAL EXPERIENCES OF YOUNGER AND OLDER WOMEN WITH BREAST CANCER: A UNIQUE LEARNING OPPORTUNITY 185

    COMMON DIFFERENCES IN THE PSYCHOSOCIAL PERCEPTIONS OF BREAST CANCER DIAGNOSIS AND THERAPY BETWEEN YOUNGER AND OLDER WOMEN 186

    IMPACT OF THE DIAGNOSIS AND TREATMENT OF BREAST CANCER ON PERSONAL RELATIONSHIPS WITH THE SPOUSE, CHILDREN, AND OLDER PARENTS 188

    INVISIBLE "ENEMY" - FEAR OF CANCER RECURRENCE (FCR) AND FEASIBLE INTERVENTIONS TO CONTROL FCR IN THE CARE FOR SURVIVORS OF BREAST CANCER 188

    CONCLUSION 189

    REFERENCES 190

CHAPTER 15 THE SELF-KINDNESS COMPONENT OF MINDFULNESS MEDITATION: A HELPFUL STRATEGY TO ENHANCE EMOTION REGULATION AND REDUCE THE DEPRESSION AND DISTRESS SYMPTOMS IN WOMEN WITH BREAST CANCER 191

    INTRODUCTION 191

THE SELF-KINDNESS – A BASIC COMPONENT OF MINDFULNESS MEDITATION THAT CAN IMPROVE EMOTION REGULATION, DECREASE DISTRESS PERCEPTION AND INCREASE RESILIENCE 192

TWO OPPOSITE DIRECTIONS OF THE EMOTION REGULATION - SELF-KINDNESS STRATEGY AND RUMINATION PROCESS 193

THE COMBINATION OF ATTENTION, SENSE OF SELF, BEHAVIOR, AND MOTIVATION – A BUSY "INTERSECTION" WHERE THE "TRAFFIC" CAN BE CONTROLLED BY THE SELF-KINDNESS APPROACH 194

CONCLUSION 195

REFERENCES 196

CHAPTER 16 COMPASSION-FOCUSED THERAPY (CFT): INTRODUCING A PROCESS-BASED SYSTEM OF PSYCHOTHERAPY TO HELP PATIENTS WITH BREAST CANCER   198

INTRODUCTION 198

A CONCEPT OF COMPASSION AS AN INNOVATIVE THERAPEUTIC MODALITY USING BEHAVIORAL APPROACHES - POSSIBLE BENEFITS OF CFT FOR THE PATIENTS WITH BREAST CANCER 199

ACCESSIBLE TECHNIQUES FOR ENHANCING THE BIDIRECTIONAL MIND AND BODY CONNECTIONS 200

A DIFFERENT PERSPECTIVE ON POSSIBLE "REPROGRAMMING" NEGATIVE EMOTIONS: A PSYCHOEDUCATION AND BEHAVIORAL PRACTICES FOR IMPROVEMENT OF THE PATIENTS' FUNCTIONING 201

CHALLENGES IN INTRODUCING NOVEL INTEGRATED CARE MODELS - CONSIDERING THE USE OF HORIZON SCANNING METHODOLOGIES 203

ENABLING AND CONSTRAINING FACTORS TO THE HORIZON SCANNING FOR NOVEL INTEGRATED HEALTHCARE MODELS 203

CONCLUSION 204

REFERENCES 205

CHAPTER 17 HOW CAN MEDICAL PROFESSIONALS MAINTAIN COMPASSION FOR THEIR PATIENTS WITH BREAST CANCER? 206

INTRODUCTION 206

WHY COMPASSION AND EMPATHY ARE SO CRUCIAL TO DELIVERING THE HIGH-QUALITY HEALTHCARE? 207

HOW THE HEALTHCARE PROFESSIONALS COULD MAINTAIN THEIR COMPASSION OR EMPATHY IN A DAILY PRACTICE? 208

LESSONS LEARNED FROM STUDIES OF MEDICAL PROFESSIONALS ABOUT THEIR STRATEGIES FOR MAINTAINING COMPASSION AND EMPATHY FOR PATIENTS 209

THE TRANSACTIONAL MODEL OF COMPASSION (TMC): AN IMPORTANT PROCESS TO ENHANCE COMPASSION SKILLS 209

SUSTAINABLE COMPASSION TRAINING (SCT): A POTENTIAL STRATEGY TO BE USED BY MEDICAL PRACTITIONERS 210

NAVIGATING THROUGH THE MAIN STRATEGIES FOR COMPASSION IN THE PATIENT CARE – HELPFUL DIRECTIONS TO CONSIDER FOR MEDICAL PROFESSIONALS 212

THE IMPORTANCE OF APPLYING PROCESS-BASED INTERVENTIONS TO THE CLINICAL/CANCER CARE TEAMS FIRST, AND THEN, TO THEIR PATIENTS 213

CONCLUSION 214

REFERENCES 216

APPENDIX 218

METASTATIC BREAST CANCER 218
HIGHLIGHTS FOR PATIENTS WITH BREAST CANCER TO REMEMBER &
PRACTICAL QUESTIONS TO ASK 218
    Where does Breast Cancer (BC) Start? 218
    How does BC Spread in the Body? 218
HOW DO YOU CHOOSE AN OPTIMAL TREATMENT PLAN FOR A WOMAN WITH
TRIPLE-NEGATIVE BREAST CANCER (TNBC)? 220
    What is the Role of Monitoring in Patients with TNBC? 220
    What are some Recommended or Preferred Options in the Systemic Therapy for HER2-
    negative BC? 221
    How BC Progression can be Manifested? 222
WHAT ARE THE MAIN TOPICS THAT A PATIENT WITH BC AND HER PHYSICIAN
NEED TO DISCUSS BEFORE CONSIDERING AN APPLICATION OF THE NEW LINE
OF SYSTEMIC THERAPY? 223
    What are the most Important Steps in Shared Decision-making? 224
WHICH FACTORS USUALLY PLAY A ROLE IN THE PERSONAL OR SHARED
DECISION-MAKING OF PATIENTS WITH BC? 225
IN WHICH WAY A SECOND OPINION CAN BE HELPFUL FOR A WOMAN
DIAGNOSED WITH BC? 225
WHAT ARE THE MAIN BENEFITS OF ATTENDING SUPPORT GROUPS? 227
POSSIBLE QUESTIONS TO ASK DOCTORS ABOUT BC DIAGNOSIS, PROGNOSIS,
AND TREATMENT OPTIONS 227
REFERENCES & RESOURCES 232
HELPFUL MEDICAL TERMINOLOGY 233

SUBJECT INDEX 237

FOREWORD

Nowadays, several women with breast cancer (BC) experience positive therapeutic effects and longer survival. However, certain BC subtypes, like triple-negative breast cancer (TNBC) (in the advanced or metastatic stages) remain the major challenge, because of their aggressive behavior, heterogeneity, high recurrence rates, and resistance to traditional therapies. One important reason why TNBC is so difficult to treat is the lack of targetable receptors (such as estrogen receptor (ER), progesterone receptor (PR), and human epidermal growth factor receptor 2 (HER 2)) on the malignant cell's surface. This feature, together with a propensity for visceral metastases, presents an unmet medical need.

Although the latest research advances in the BC area have resulted in some innovative therapeutic strategies, many of these novel agents have certain toxic effects, and therefore, careful patient selection, monitoring, and prompt treatment of side effects are required. To yield the benefits of new targeted therapies and to counteract their possible toxicities, both sides that are involved in TNBC care, the healthcare professionals and the patients must be well-prepared for long-term cooperation. Such collaborative efforts demand clinician's updated knowledge about novel therapeutic strategies and clinical trials in the TNBC area. Also, building professional relationships and communication networks with the patients and their caregivers is very important.

At the same time, the patients themselves need to be adequately informed about some basic principles of TNBC, and they should be personally engaged in the therapeutic course of their disease. For instance, the patients need to learn some skills, such as self-observation and self-care, as well as precise communication with the treatment team members. It appears that pharmaceutical care would be a perfect avenue to accomplish the objectives of safe and effective BC care. However, in the reality of typical, busy oncology centers, these necessities are often difficult to fulfill, due to various reasons (*e.g.*, lack of time, incentives, and organizational support). In the face of these demands, the book titled: "**The Management of Metastatic Triple-Negative Breast Cancer: An Integrated and Expeditionary Approach**" offers a possible solution.

One of the remarkable features of this book is a reader-friendly presentation of topics in form of the well-structured graphs and tables, which contain helpful, multidisciplinary information. A brought thematic spectrum of this book, contained in separate chapters (organized in the form of two, conveniently overlapping parts), provides a clear, comprehensive, and updated knowledge base for medical care teams in Breast Care Units and other oncology settings. It should be noted that this is another book of this author, in which she responds to the challenge of combining the efforts of members of medical care teams, with various areas of expertise (*e.g.*, physicians, pharmacists, diagnosticians, physical therapists, psychologists, and nurses) to work together, to achieve improvement in health condition and the quality of life of the patients with TNBC, and other subtypes of BC.

The author very insightfully analyses many therapeutic aspects of BC and emphasizes the crucial role of education and overcoming barriers of fear or uncertainty. Moreover, she highlights the necessity of embarking on a difficult path that leads to accomplishing beneficial effects (not only in terms of clinical parameters but also in the psychological domains of a patient's life). This is particularly important since in patients with TNBC, receiving multiple medications is often related to an adverse phenomenon of polypharmacy, often observed in multi-morbidity, associated with poly-therapy. Therefore, limiting the adverse effects of recommended therapies to a necessary minimum would be extremely beneficial (*e.g.*, with regard to many new targeted therapies). This demanding task is primarily addressed to both physicians and pharmacists, who should create two integrated "pillars" of patient management. In addition, this book promotes the concept of patient-centered, personalized care. It encourages clinicians to be open-minded, adequately trained, and ready to constantly exchange their expertise to serve the afflicted patients with BC to improve their outcomes.

Finally, this book provides many useful, easily accessible tools to attain these goals. It would be very important for medical and pharmacy students or residents to be introduced to these integrative concepts of care from the early stages of their professional education. As an academic teacher with many years of experience, I would definitely recommend this book as a practical reference in many educational environments, for teaching multidisciplinary teams of medical professionals and students, as well as patient advocates, caregivers, and women suffering from BC.

Lucyna Bułaś
Department of Pharmaceutical Technology
Faculty of Pharmaceutical Sciences in Sosnowiec
Kasztanowa 3, 41-200 Sosnowiec
Poland

PREFACE

Despite recent therapeutic advances in **metastatic triple-negative breast cancer (TNBC),** it still remains an incurable disease. The latest progress in the TNBC research has resulted in some **innovative therapeutic options**, such as **immunotherapy, antibody-drug conjugates (ADC), and inhibitors of poly (ADP-ribose) polymerase (PARP)**, which can be applied in combination (or in sequence) with standard chemotherapy (CHT) regimens. Such **targeted therapies** bring some hope with regard to the prognosis for many women suffering from metastatic TNBC. However many of these novel agents have some serious **adverse effects**, and thus, the right patient selection, careful monitoring, and rapid delivery of medical therapies to relieve side effects are imperative.

To address these issues, a book titled: **"The Management of Metastatic Triple-Negative Breast Cancer: An Integrated and Expeditionary Approach"** integrates multidisciplinary knowledge and experience from the perspective of medical professionals and researchers in the TNBC area, and combines it with the patient's point of view. This book is composed of two parts.

PART 1

An Overview of the Ethnic Disparities and Current or Emerging Targeted Therapies for Patients with Advanced or Metastatic Triple-Negative Breast Cancer (TNBC).

PART 2

The Role of Patient Education, Empowerment, and Communication with Medical Teams, and Psychological or Supportive Approaches in Advanced or Metastatic Breast Cancer (BC).

The first chapter of Part 1 introduces some important aspects of ethnicity, obesity associated with metabolic syndrome and chronic inflammation, as well as reproductive, social, and environmental factors, which can greatly influence TNBC outcomes. This is critically important for an understanding of the risk, development, and progression of TNBC in various ethnic groups, such as African American (AA) and European American (EA) women. Moreover, considerations of predisposing and aggravating environmental, socioeconomic, and behavioral factors, which may have a major impact on BC prevention, course, and survival are briefly presented.

Consecutive chapters of **Part 1** discuss current and emerging targeted therapies for patients with advanced or metastatic TNBC, based on recent, major clinical trial results. Recommendations for clinicians and patients are briefly summarized at the end of each chapter. The last chapter of Part 1 describes a noninvasive "tool" of Precision Medicine that may be considered for the individualized treatment of women with BC. This tool attempts to link the main clinical objectives with the personal goals of the patients suffering from advanced or metastatic TNBC or other difficult-to-treat BC subtypes.

The initial chapters of **Part 2** provide focused psychoeducational information for patients with advanced or metastatic stages of BC (*e.g.*, TNBC subtype). This information is designed to facilitate clear communication between the patients and the treatment team members. Subsequent chapters of Part 2 contain different cognitive and behavioral concepts and examples of the relevant therapeutic strategies. They include easily available techniques for coping with stress, which accompanies women with BC, during multiple diagnostic and therapeutic stages, and often aggravates their health conditions.

Traditionally, in the majority of publications concerning BC, the medical and psychological topics are usually presented as two separate groups of problems, while in reality, such a division is rather artificial, since these issues are always interrelated. To properly address this need, the book highlights an **integrative approach** to these deeply interconnected areas. Also, the added value of this book consists of **blending the latest evidence from research trials in the TNBC area with clinical practice and feasible psycho-educational approaches**, which can be suitable **for individual patients and their caregivers**. Combining targeted treatments for TNBC with effective coping with distress (commonly associated with uncertain or poor prognosis and overwhelming adverse effects of different targeted therapies) as well as simple lifestyle modifications represent the key elements, that can substantially ameliorate outcomes, even in the most vulnerable patients with metastatic TNBC.

Importantly, this book **bridges the gap between the strictly clinical or research-related aspects of BC management and the personal needs and expectations of patients with BC**. It also invites medical professionals who are physicians, psychologists, pharmacists, and researchers in the field of BC to conduct open **dialogues with patients, aimed at their practical education and support**. It also includes helpful **resources for the support of both the patients and their medical caregivers**, as "partners" and "co-passengers" of their joint "expedition" to conquer BC and reclaim the necessary balance or comfort in life.

In addition, this book presents a **novel concept of a challenging journey for patients with TNBC** (or other aggressive subtypes of BC, especially in advanced or metastatic stages), which can be perceived or interpreted as a series of stimulating "adventures" and meaningful educational events. This, in turn, can shed some bright light on a serious, chronic disease, like BC, and its interconnected risk factors. Such an approach may **positively influence the attitude of many women suffering from BC**. Hopefully, instead of approaching a diagnosis and therapy of TN BC as a terrifying "war", composed of devastating "battles", the patients may **change their perspective on this life-threatening disease**, and view it as a real **opportunity to use the modern armamentarium of current pharmacologic therapies and noninvasive, cost-effective, feasible psychological, and supportive modalities to improve their outcomes.**

Finally, the **purposely changed narration**, used in many chapters, is **intended to re-direct many suboptimal cognitive and emotional stereotypes**, which are often perpetuated by numerous patients with BC. To accomplish these long-term goals, it is necessary **to teach the medical team members to positively "re-orient" women with BC,** so that they can stay **motivated, and engaged in active participation in their oncology care**. It requires a lot of time, effort, initiative, expertise, and cooperation within multidisciplinary teams of medical providers. However, in the long run, this may **beneficially transform the approach to BC, its management, and prevention**. Simultaneously, well-educated and empowe- red patients may be able to communicate and integrate their efforts with the professional actions of the medical teams, in charge of their care.

Katarzyna Rygiel
Department of Family Practice
Medical University of Silesia (SUM)
3 Maja St., 41-800, Zabrze
Poland

Part 1

An Overview of the Ethnic Disparities and Current or Emerging Targeted Therapies for Patients with Advanced or Metastatic Triple-Negative Breast Cancer (TNBC).

"What lies behind us and what lies before us are tiny matters compared to what lies within us."

Oliver Wendell Holmes

CHAPTER 1

Unraveling Ethnic Disparities in Triple-Negative Breast Cancer (TNBC): Exploring The Impact of Metabolic, Reproductive, Environmental, and Social Factors on the Disease Course in African-American (AA) Women Population

Abstract: Triple-negative breast cancer (TNBC) is a particularly **aggressive subtype** of **breast cancer (BC)** in which the expression of the **estrogen receptor (ER), progesterone receptor (PR)** and **human epidermal growth factor receptor (HER2)** is absent or very low. TNBC consists of approximately 15-30% of the invasive BC cases in the United States (US) Women with TNBC represent a heterogeneous population with regard to their ethnicity and biology including the genetic make-up metabolic or hormonal profile as well as the socioeconomic status (SES) cultural behavioral educational levels. Notably **African-American (AA)** women usually have a **higher prevalence of TNBC and a worse prognosis** compared to **European-American (EA)** or Non-Hispanic White (NHW) women. The goal of this chapter is to elucidate the possible interplay of inherited and acquired, often lifestyle-related risk factors which can stimulate the initiation and development of the most aggressive subtypes of TNBC in AA women compared to their EA (or NHW) counterparts. In particular this chapter explores some ethnic disparities in TNBC mainly in the example of the US where such disparities have been studied in clinical research. This chapter also focuses on differences in TNBC risk factors healthcare patterns clinical outcomes between AA and EA (or NHW) women. It briefly discusses the multi-factorial etiology of these disparities *e.g* genetic, hormonal, metabolic, behavioral, cultural, socio-economical and environmental. Presented short analysis of a dynamic blend of inherited and acquired variables also provides some directions for the reduction of these disparities, to improve TNBC outcomes, among women from ethnic groups, such as AA.

Keywords: Acquired, Ethnic groups, Healthcare disparities, Inherited, Risk factors, Triple-negative breast cancer (TNBC).

INTRODUCTION

Triple-negative breast cancer (TNBC) is a particularly aggressive subtype of breast cancer (BC), in which the expression of the **estrogen receptor (ER),**

progesterone receptor (PR), and **human epidermal growth factor receptor (HER2)** is absent or very low [1]. TNBC consists of approximately 15-30% of the invasive BC cases in the United States (US) [1]. In general, **African-American (AA) women** have a **higher incidence of TNBC, worse outcomes**, and higher mortality rates compared to European-American (EA) (or non-Hispanic White (NHW)) women [2]. In addition, TNBC is more prevalent in western sub-Saharan African patients compared to their EA (or NHW) counterparts [2]. TNBC risk factors and possible causes can be divided into inherited (or biologic) and acquired (or non-biologic) categories [3]. An inherited or genetically determined ancestry and acquired or socio-environmental factors can considerably influence the outcomes of patients with TNBC [3]. This is a complicated network that is very difficult to untangle and classify into separate domains. However, there are some distinctive patterns that can be recognized. For instance, the genes that women inherit, affect the way how they metabolize certain medications, what adverse effects they may experience from specific pharmaceutic agents, and what kind of therapies could be the most suitable or contraindicated for them.

A recent study has indicated certain similarities in TNBC, especially with regard to genetics, tumor biology, and environmental risk factors, which were noted in African and AA patients with BC [4]. Also, various observations suggest that the West African origin of women afflicted with BC could have been related to their inherited susceptibility to TNBC [5, 6]. Moreover, some changes in the expression of many genes, connected with the cell's growth, differentiation, invasion, and metastasis, have been revealed in BC tumors of AA females, to a higher degree than in the EA (or NHW) women [7]. In addition to genetic or molecular differences, an advanced BC presentation at diagnosis, and a higher burden of metabolic comorbidities, certain unequal socioeconomic standards (*e.g.*, residential, occupational, or educational) can contribute to poor survival rates, especially among AA women [8]. Similarly, various socio-environmental determinants widely influence how the surrounding world interacts with women with BC, from different ethnic populations [9]. In this dynamic exchange process, both conscious and unconscious biases may, to some degree, have an important impact on shaping bilateral relationships between women with BC (or at high risk for BC) and the medical systems or local community services, where they live, work or go to school.

The aim of this chapter is to elucidate the potential interplay of biological and non-biological risk factors, which can stimulate the initiation and development of the most aggressive subtypes of TNBC. In particular, this chapter explores ethnic disparities in TNBC between AA women and their EA counterparts (mainly in the example of the US, where such disparities have been studied in clinical research). It focuses on some differences in TNBC risk factors, healthcare patterns, and clinical outcomes, between AA and EA (or NHW) women. It briefly discusses the multi-factorial etiology of these disparities (*e.g.*, genetic, hormonal, reproductive, metabolic, behavioral, cultural, socioeconomic, and environmental). This chapter also indicates some clear directions, on how to reduce the above-mentioned disparities, in order to improve TNBC outcomes, especially among AA women.

HOW CAN WE APPROACH ETHNIC DISPARITIES IN TNBC SURVIVAL? – A ROADMAP OF POSSIBLE UNDERLYING BIOLOGIC AND NON-BIOLOGIC RISK FACTORS OR CAUSES OF TNBC IN AA *VS.* EA (OR NHW) WOMEN

It should be highlighted that certain differences in the genetic makeup and the tumor biology of BC exist between AA women and their EA (or NHW) counterparts.

Although it has been reported that BC incidence rates are similar for AA and EA (or NHW) women, the TNBC incidence rates in the younger group (*e.g.*, before 45 years of age) are higher among AA, compared to EA (or NHW) females [9]. In contrast, in the older group (*e.g.*, between 60 and 84 years of age), the BC incidence rates are higher in EA (or NHW) women than in their AA counterparts. Nevertheless, AA women have a higher probability of dying from BC at any age [9, 10]. In light of such ethnic disparities in BC survival, some specific BC risk factors and possible causes have been proposed (*e.g.*, relevant to the hormonal, metabolic, and reproductive processes) [11].

In general, BC subtypes include the ER-positive and HER2-positive, the ER-positive and HER2-negative, and the basal-like (BL) BC, which is considered to be synonymous with the triple-negative (TNBC) (characterized by an absent or very low expression of the ER, PR, and HER2). In fact, TNBC usually represents the most aggressive BC subtype [1, 9, 11]. Notably, the incidence of TNBC in AA, predominantly in younger females, is two times higher than the one in EA (or NHW) women [9, 10]. Also, it has been noted that pregnancy and multi-parity augment the risk of TNBC (while these reproductive factors decrease the risk of HR-positive BC) [12]. Since AA usually have more children at a younger age, and they engage in short breastfeeding periods, their risk of TNBC increases, compared to EA (or NHW) women [12]. Moreover, according to a recent study, it has been shown that TNBC in women of African ancestry was characterized by a more common loss of androgen receptor (AR) expression, and worse overall survival (OS) compared to those of European ancestry [13]. Notably, AA women with an AR-negative TNBC have expressed a specific molecular signature, and predominance of BL1, BL2, and immunomodulatory (IM) subtypes of TNBC (Fig. **1**) [13].

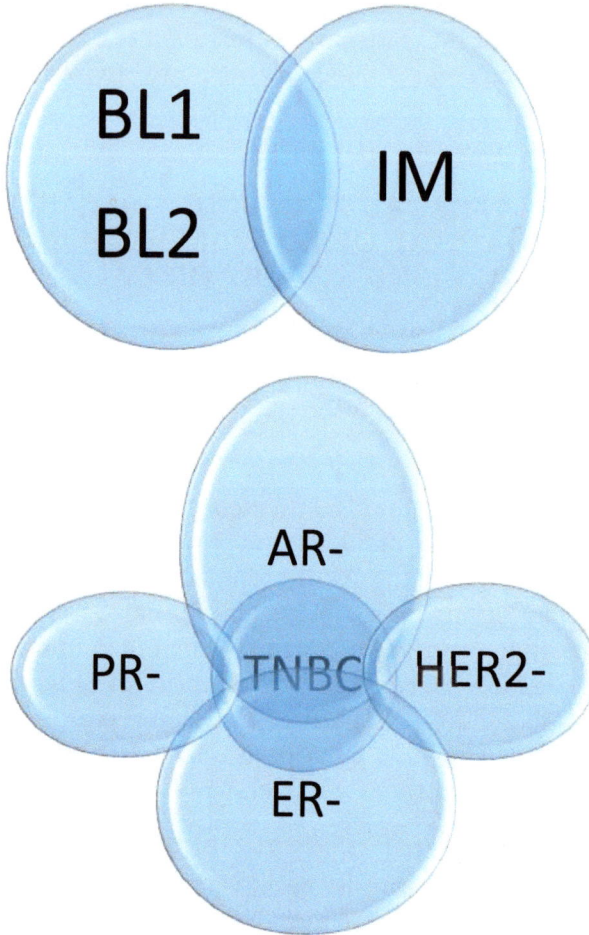

Fig. (1). TNBC in women of African ancestry - a frequent loss of AR expression, common BL1, BL2 or IM subtypes, and poor outcomes. TNBC, triple-negative breast cancer; AR, androgen receptor; ER, estrogen receptor; PR, progesterone receptor; HER2, human epidermal growth factor receptor2; BL, basal-like; IM, immunomodulatory.

Also, AA patients with AR-negative TNBC usually have a more aggressive disease course and worse prognosis, compared to those with AR-positive TNBC [13, 14]. In addition, some other differences between AA and EA (or NHW) women include the blood levels of **sex** hormones, growth factors, and the expression of steroid hormones or growth factor receptors, tumor suppressor genes, or chromosomal abnormalities [15 - 18]. Such biological discrepancies among AA and EA (or NHW) women may have an impact on therapeutic recommendations and clinical outcomes in patients with from these ethnic groups (Fig. **2**).

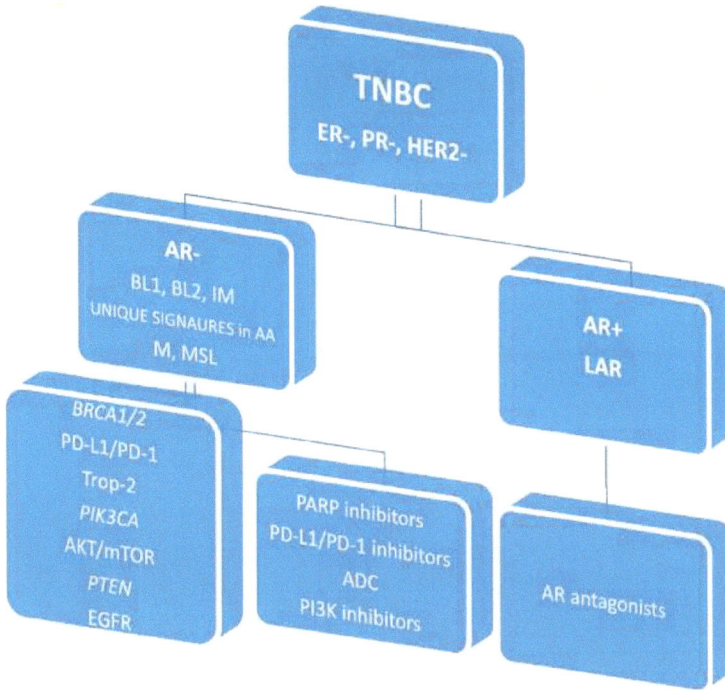

Fig. (2). TNBC heterogeneity and new or emerging therapeutic targets. TNBC, triple-negative breast cancer; ER, estrogen receptor; PR, progesterone receptor; HER2, human epidermal growth factor receptor2; AR, androgen receptor; BL, basal-like; IM, immunomodulatory; M, mesenchymal; MSL, mesenchymal stem-like; LAR, luminal androgen receptor; *BRCA*, breast cancer gene; PD-1, programmed cell death-1; PD-L1, programmed death-ligand 1; Trop-2, trophoblast cell surface antigen 2; *PIK3CA*, phosphatidylinositol-4, 5-bisphosphate 3-kinase catalytic subunit alpha PI3K, phosphoinositide 3-kinase; AKT, protein kinase B; mTOR, mechanistic (mammalian) target of rapamycin; PTEN, phosphatase and tensin; EGFR, epidermal growth factor receptor; PARP, poly (ADP-ribose) polymerase; ADC, antibody-drug conjugate; AA, African-American.

Furthermore, many non-biological issues, such as socioeconomic disadvantages (*e.g.*, related to low income and lack of medical insurance), limited access to healthcare facilities (*e.g.*, causing significant delays in BC screening, diagnostic tests, or modern therapies), unsafe neighborhood, deprivation of nutritious food, lack of comfortable zones for physical exercises or recreation, as well as uncontrolled daily stress (*e.g.*, due to violence, injustice, poverty, uncertainty, or insecurity) are often superimposed on genetic, hormonal, and metabolic components, especially in AA women [9, 19, 20]. Such a combination of biological and non-biologic variables, associated with TNBC can deteriorate outcomes in AA women (Fig. **3**) [9, 19, 20].

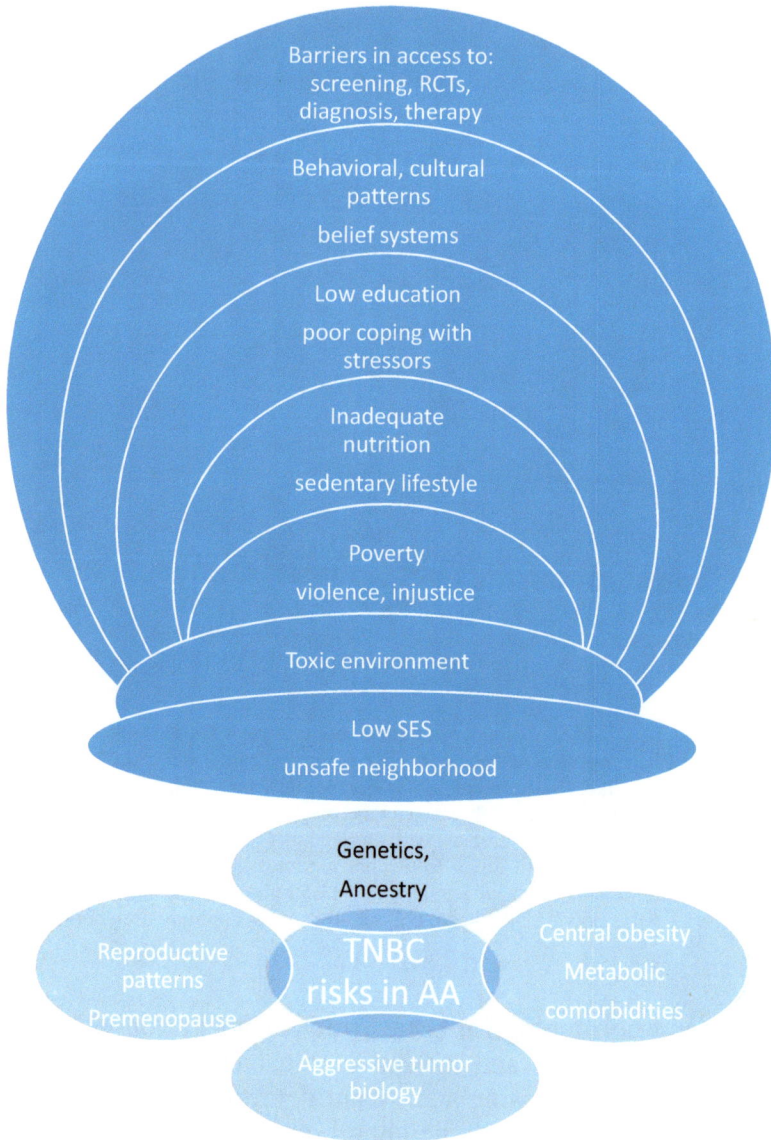

Fig. (3). Multifactorial risk factors and possible causes that influence adverse prognosis in AA women with TNBC. TNBC, triple-negative breast cancer; AA, African-American; RCTs, Randomized Controlled Trials; SES, socioeconomic status.

In general, early BC detection (*via* screening), prompt diagnosis, and comprehensive treatment, as well as reduction of tobacco smoking, have improved the health condition of numerous women with BC [21]. However, in spite of these efforts, several AA women still have a lover probability to receive a state of the art diagnostic workup and therapy, compared to their EA (or NHW) counterparts [22]. To rectify this situation, innovative approaches, beyond the current standards, will be necessary to actively promote BC prevention, improve healthcare path, augment survival, and reduce BC mortality.

A SPOTLIGHT ON THE FAMILY HISTORY AND GENETIC MUTATIONS: THE IMPACT OF ETHNICITY ON MOLECULAR MAKE-UP IN TNBC

Family history (FH) of BC depends on the number of family members affected, the age at diagnosis, and the number of unaffected women in the pedigree [23]. A woman's BC risk is increased if she has a first-degree relative with BC at a young age or if she has multiple relatives with BC [23]. Approximately 5–10% of BCs have been attributed to heredity [24]. In particular, the *BRCA* (breast cancer gene) *1* and *BRCA 2* gene mutations, which are located on chromosomes 17 and 13, respectively, are responsible for the majority of autosomal dominant inherited BCs. *BRCA1* and *BRCA2* genes produce tumor suppressor proteins, which allow to repair DNA damages and reinforce the stability of cellular genetic material [24]. If *BRCA1* and *BRCA2* are mutated, cells may create genetic abnormalities, often leading to cancer development.

Such mutations are related to some degree to the woman's ethnic background. In particular, *BRCA1* mutations, are encountered mostly in Ashkenazi Jewish women (8.3%). In contrast, they are less prevalent in Hispanic women (3.5%), NHW women (2.2%), AA women (1.3%), and Asian women (0.5%) [25]. In addition, over a half of women with inherited harmful *BRCA1* mutation, and slightly less than a half of those with the inherited *BRCA2* mutation, will develop BC by the age of 70 [14, 26].

Also, about 40% of females with inherited a *BRCA1* mutation and 11–17% of women with inherited a harmful *BRCA2* mutation will develop ovarian cancer by the age of 70 [26].

Likewise, women diagnosed with BC, associated with harmful *BRCA1/2* mutations have a higher probability for developing a second BC (*e.g.*, in the ipsilateral or the contralateral breast) compared to those, without *BRCA1/2* mutations [14, 26].

Notably, many patients with BCs, who carry a *BRCA1* mutation, may have a TNBC subtype that frequently has a worse outcome, than other BC subtypes [14, 26]. Therefore, it has been recommended that women with early-onset BC and women with a positive FH for *BRCA1/2* mutations should undergo genetic testing, at the time of BC diagnosis [14, 26].

It should be highlighted that the *BRCA1/2* mutations are responsible for BC in almost 50% of families with several cases of BC, while some other mutations, which are linked to a smaller increase in BC risk include *PALB2, PTEN, TP53, ATM, CDH1, CHEK2,* and *STK11* genes [14, 26, 27]. In particular, mutations in the *PALB2* tumor suppressor gene are associated with a risk of BC similar to the one related with *BRCA1/2* mutations, since the PALB2 protein collaborates with the BRCA1/2 proteins in repairing DNA breaks [28]. Notably, more than one-third of women with the *PALB2* mutation will develop BC by age 70, and this risk is doubled in women with the FH of BC and the *PALB2* mutation [28].

SOCIOECONOMIC DISPARITIES IN BC – A LINK BETWEEN THE ECONOMIC DEPRIVATION AND DYSFUNCTIONAL HEALTHCARE PATH

BC risk factors, incidence, prevalence, survival, and mortality rates that are different in particular ethnic groups, can also vary, depending on socioeconomic conditions [9, 29]. For instance, the key socioeconomic parameters that influence disparities in BC mortality, include poverty, social injustice, and disadvantaged educational or occupational aspects of life [30]. In particular, poverty has been linked with decreased rates of BC screening, late-stage diagnosis, inadequate therapy, or incomplete follow up care, as well as increased death rate from BC [9, 31, 32]. A cascade of challenges that economically disadvantaged AA women often experience include lack of health insurance, difficulties in access to well-trained healthcare practitioners, modern medical equipment and infrastructures, as well as insufficient education and support [3, 9, 33].

This, in turn, often leads to lower rates of mammography screening and greater probability of advanced-stage BC at diagnosis, and delayed or substandard therapy [9, 34]. Moreover, common metabolic comorbidities, such as obesity, diabetes mellitus type 2 (T2DM), arterial hypertension (HTN), and cardiovascular disease (CVD)) are more prevalent in economically deprived women (*e.g.*, AA) [35]. Also, in the underserved populations, there is limited access to fresh and healthy alimentary products, and lack of safe space for physical exercises [2, 5, 36]. This, in turn, often contributes to central (abdominal) obesity with an abnormal carbohydrate and lipid metabolism, which can be linked with subsequent worse prognosis of BC [2, 5, 19, 36, 37]. In essence, poverty and related to it cluster of factors, including lack of primary care physician, untreated comorbidities, lack or limited health insurance, unhealthy lifestyle (*e.g.*, tobacco smoking, inadequate nutrition, and lack of regular physical activity), insufficient health information or lower literacy level, as well as maladaptive responses to overwhelming daily stressors contribute to BC disparities among women. A cluster of these conditions is commonly seen in AA women (Fig. **3**) [9, 19, 38].

Furthermore, long-term exposures to many environmental toxic agents, including endocrine-disrupting chemicals (EDC), which are present in several commercial, industrial, and personal care products are almost unavoidable, especially for women with the low socioeconomic status (SES) [39]. The most hazardous EDC involve polycyclic aromatic hydrocarbons (PAH), organochlorines (*e.g.*, polychlorinated biphenyls (PCBs) and dioxins), phenols (*e.g.*, bisphenol A (BPA)), phthalates, parabens, benzene, ethylene oxide, pesticides (*e.g.*, organo-halogenated agents, and dichlorodiphenyltrichloroethane (DDT) that was withdrawn from the market), and certain metals (*e.g.*, cadmium) [40, 41]. Notably, EDC, and different forms of hormone replacement therapy, which act upon breast tissue, have an impact on BC risk or development (Table 1) [40, 41].

Regretfully, certain attitudes of medical personnel may also aggravate disparities in BC mortality rates (*e.g.*, negative perceptions or manners exhibited towards AA or low SES women *vs.* positive or neutral attitudes, displayed towards EA (or NHW) and high SES women) [42]. In particular, the Carolina Breast Cancer study has shown that the aggressive subtypes of BCs, which are less responsive to standard treatments and characterized by poor survival (*e.g.*, TNBC), are more prevalent in younger AA, and Hispanic women living in low SES areas [43]. In addition, many AA women rely more on their breast self-examination, as an effective method for BC detection, compared to EA (or NHW) women [44]. Unfortunately, such a habit can decrease the rates of mammography testing among AA women, and may lead to overlooking some underlying pathologies of breast tissue [44].

BEHAVIORAL AND CULTURAL FACTORS ACCOUNTING FOR BC DISPARITIES IN AA WOMEN

Behavioral Patterns and Belief Systems differ considerably among AA and EA (or NHW) women, with relation to their attitudes toward BC screening procedures. In particular, AA women may be prone to avoiding mammography, since they can be afraid of pain, discomfort, embarrassment, and unknown consequences of exposure to radiation (during this procedure) [45, 46]. Since many AA women can experience anxiety about the findings of the test, it is crucial to provide clear and practical educational information that will be well-adjusted to a woman's belief system [47, 48].

Table 1. An interplay between inherited and acquired risk factors or causes, which can affect outcomes of the TNBC in AA compared to EA (or NHW) patients.

INHERITED/BIOLOGIC RISK FACTORS FOR TNBC	**Genetics** Women born with *BRCA* mutation are > to develop TNBC; 70% of all BCs diagnoses in women with the *BRCA* mutation are TNBCs	**Ancestry** TNBC is more likely to be diagnosed in AA & Hispanic women (vs. NHW & Asians)	**Obesity & its comorbidities** Insulin resistance dysglycemia, dyslipidemia, diabetes mellitus type 2 (T2DM), hypertension (HTN), cardiovascular disease (CVD)	**Hormonal imbalance due to reproductive cycle & pre-menopause in** younger women (< 50 years of age)
ACQUIRED/BEHAVIORAL ENVIRONMENTAL/NON-BIOLOGIC RISK FACTORS FOR TNBC	**Socioeconomic status (SES)** Unemployment, or insecure workplace, low income, lack of medical insurance, scarcity of nutritious food, unsafe neighborhood lack of places for exercises	**Access to healthcare services** Limited (or none) access leading to delays in BC screening, diagnosis, therapy	**Behavioral, educational, and cultural issues** Low education & specific behaviors or beliefs influence decision-making about BC prevention, diagnosis & treatment, or participation in RCTs	**Environmental toxicity** The elevated burden of exposure to chemical & physical toxins in the air/water, soil pollutions, and heavy metals: cadmium, lead & arsenic)
OVERLAPPING AREAS OF COMMON BIOLOGIC & NON-BIOLOGIC RISK FACTORS FOR TNBC	**Genetics, ancestry & low SES:** sub-standard living/working conditions dysfunctional healthcare path	**Reproductive issues** very young age at 1st childbirth, short breast –feeding period, multi-parity, use of oral contra-ceptives for >1 year	**Metabolic complications of central obesity** metabolic syndrome, prediabetes, a combination of hormonal, metabolic & pro-inflammatory dysfunctions	**Uncontrolled stress response** poverty, injustice, violence, insecurity, processed food (< quality, > quantity), sedentary lifestyle
STAGES OF TNBC	**Stage 0** isolated in one part of the breast (*e.g.*, a duct or lobule), no signs of spreading	**Stage 1** is typically localized, **Stage 2** local growth or spread	**Stage 3** larger tumor, affecting lymph nodes	**Stage 4** spreads beyond the breast, and local lymph nodes to other tissues & organs

(Table 1) cont.....

COMMON BIOLOGIC FEATURES OF TNBC	TNBC is more aggressive, has a worse prognosis & > recurrence rates (post treatment) than other types of BC	TNBC often has a higher grade than other BC types	TNBC usually is a "basal-like" (BL) subtype (the cells resemble the basal cells that line the breast ducts)	TNBC is often grade 3 BL cancers are usually more aggressive & higher grade
TREATMENT OPTIONS FOR TNBC	**Neoadjuvant CHT** - when TNBC is treated with CHT before surgery, a pCR, DFS & OS are better; pCR (absence of active cancer cells) allows judging the effectiveness of neoadjuvant treatment by looking at the tissue removed during surgery, to detect if any active cancer cells are present	**PARP inhibitors** PARP inhibitors (olaparib = Lynparza & talazoparib = Talzenna) are approved to treat advanced HER2-negative BC in women with a *BRCA1* or *BRCA2* mutations; PARP enzymes repair DNA damage in healthy & cancer cells; PARP inhibitors block the PARP enzyme, so that cancer cells with a *BRCA1/2* mutation cannot repair DNA damage	**Immunotherapy** Atezolizumab (Tecentriq) in combination with the CHT, nab-paclitaxel or albumin-bound paclitaxel (Abraxane) is approved to treat unresectable locally advanced or metastatic TNBC, PD-L--positive BC; Atezolizumab is an immune checkpoint inhibitor (ICI); ICIs target specific proteins, which help cancer cells hide from the immune system (the PD-L1 protein). By inhibiting PD-L1, Atezolizumab allows immune system cells to detect & kill the cancer cells	TNBC is usually treated with a combination of surgery, CHT, & radiation therapy (RT); **PARP inhibitors & ICIs** are now added to treat the selected pts with TNBC

BC, breast cancer; TNBC, triple-negative breast cancer; AA, African-American; EA, European-American; NHW, non-Hispanic White; RCT, Randomized controlled trial; PARP, poly (ADP-ribose) polymerase; BRCA, breast cancer gene; ICI, immune checkpoint inhibitors; CHT, chemotherapy; RT, radiation therapy; pCR, pathologic complete response; DFS, disease-free survival; OS, overall survival; T2DM, diabetes mellitus type 2; HTN, arterial hypertension; CVD, cardiovascular disease; pts, patients.

Social Injustice or Racial Discrimination in Health Care can also account for
BC disparities between AA and EA (or NHW) women (*e.g.*, a history of unethical experiments, violence and abuse, endured by AA in the past could have led to the mistrust into medical authorities and services) [3, 49]. This can play a certain role

in the style, in which AA manage their medical care needs [49]. Furthermore, various forms of racial prejudice may account for the differences in mammography referrals between AA and EA (or NHW) women (*e.g.*, AA were more likely than EA (or NHW) women to mention lack of recommendation of mammography screening by their physician, as a reason for not having undergone BC screening) [50].

Spirituality often plays a key role in managing the health-related needs of AA women [51, 52]. For instance, numerous AA are more likely than their EA (or NHW) counterparts to rely on divine interventions for BC management rather than on the indicated medical therapies [52, 53]. Spirituality may also be beneficial for many AA women, since certain spiritual beliefs may be powerful drivers, determining health-related behaviors in AA women with BC (*e.g.*, motivation to regular BC screening and necessary treatments) [54]. In addition, an evaluation of cancer knowledge, attitudes, beliefs, and practices among AA and Hispanic women, by their medical providers can be instrumental for creating feasible interventions in different ethnic groups women with BC [55]. In summary, a constellation of **poverty, belief system,** and **social injustice** accounts directly or indirectly to BC disparities, in various ethnic populations of women. Notably, AA are influenced by those factors to a larger degree than EA (or NHW) women. In reality, such factors can contribute to lower BC survival rates among AA, in comparison to their EA (or NHW) counterparts.

THE UNDERESTIMATED ROLE OF INSUFFICIENT PHYSICAL ACTIVITY AS A RISK FACTOR IN BC DISPARITIES – REFLECTIONS FROM THE SELECTED CLINICAL STUDIES

Many studies have demonstrated that women who are physically active have a lower risk of BC than inactive ones [56]. This reduced risk of BC has been seen in both premenopausal and postmenopausal women; however, the evidence for the association is stronger for postmenopausal BC [57]. Moreover, postmenopausal women who increase their physical activity level may reduce the risk of BC, contrary to those, who do not exercise after menopause [58]. According to a report from the retrospective study, it was shown that women who were 40 years old or younger, who engaged in four or more hours of physical activity per week, were able to lower their BC risk by more than 50%, as compared to those, who were less active, in the same age group [59]. Moreover, based on a meta-analysis of prospective studies, BC risk was decreased by an average of 12%, due to performing physical activity [60]. It has been estimated that approximately one-fourth to one-third of BC cases are associated with elevated body weight and inadequate physical activity [61]. In particular, AA women are often overweight or obese and have higher body mass index (BMI; weight in kilograms divided by height in meters, squared) and waist-to-hip ratios (WHR) compared to EA (or NHW) females [2, 5, 62]. The lack of regular physical exercises, frequently associated with unhealthy eating and inefficient coping skills in the face of overwhelming stressors, in AA women, may explain why they have much higher rates of obesity, which represents a major risk factor for BC [2, 3, 5, 9, 63, 64].

The Carolina Breast Cancer Study has revealed significant racial differences in physical activity among BC survivors, according to which, AA women compared to EA (or NHW) women were less likely to meet national physical activity guidelines, after BC diagnosis [65].

Similarly, a study by the Northeast Ohio Breast Cancer Survivors has found a gradual decline in physical activity levels after high school completion, in AA females compared to EA (or NHW) women [66]. It should be highlighted that physical exercises lower the levels of estrogen and regulate the blood levels of insulin-like growth factors that have been associated with BC development [67]. In addition, exercises control blood glucose and lipid levels, and thus, women who are physically active tend to be healthier and are more likely to maintain a normal body weight, compared to those, who do not exercise [67]. In a proposed surveillance model for rehabilitation for patients with BC, it has been recommended that such patients should be educated about the importance of physical exercises at the time of their BC diagnosis. In addition, they need to be provided with the necessary support to stay reasonably active, during the consecutive stages of BC diagnosis, treatment, and rehabilitation [68].

IMPACT OF INADEQUATE NUTRITION ON BC DISPARITIES –INSIGHTS FROM MAJOR CLINICAL STUDIES

A nutritional style widely contributes to health disparities in BC. For instance, the American Cancer Society (ACS) recommends mostly plant-based meals (*e.g.*, vegetables, fruits, and grains, rich in antioxidants and dietary fiber), significant reduction of animal-based products (*e.g.*, pork, beef, lamb, bacon, sausage, hot dogs), and elimination of artificial sweets, or highly processed food or beverages (*e.g.*, rich in carbohydrates with a high glycemic index, saturated fats or trans-fats) [2, 3, 9, 69].

The Women's Intervention Nutrition Study (WINS) concluded that modest weight loss associated with randomization to a low-fat diet improved relapse-free survival in early-stage BC; however, the significance of these associations was not maintained in the long-term follow-up [70]. Paradoxically, the intervention that included fat reduction and a diet high in vegetables, fruits, and fiber did not lead to the reduction of body mass, according to the *Women's Healthy Eating and Living (WHEL)* study [71]. Furthermore, the WHEL trial has reported no association with recurrence or better disease prognosis in women with BC [71]. These contradicting results may be a result of weight loss in the WINS, but not in the WHEL trial [69 - 71]. Notably, several studies have demonstrated that a diet rich in vegetables, fruit, poultry, fish, and low-fat dairy products has been associated with a reduced risk of BC; however, it is unclear if any specific vegetables, fruits, or other foods can specifically decrease BC risk [69].

It should be highlighted that the HEAL study recruited AA and Hispanic women from the US (California, Washington, and New Mexico states) and reported that women with early-stage BC, who consumed diets low in calories, added sugar, alcohol and saturated fats (a quality diet) had a 60% reduced risk of all-cause mortality and an 88% lower risk of BC-related mortality [72]. Another report from the HEAL study revealed that a quality diet was correlated with reduced levels of circulating inflammatory biomarkers [73]. The HEAL study is very unique, since it is one of only a few large studies, which is comprised of an ethnically diverse patient population, recruited from different geographic locations [73]. Importantly, ethnically diverse BC survivors differ in their levels of long-term adherence to dietary interventions, physical activity and obesity rates [74 - 76]. Overall, the role of several dietary factors in BC risk is inconclusive; however, there is much evidence from epidemiologic studies that indicate that dietary style (*e.g.*, a woman's food intake, in both the qualitative and quantitative aspects) may be linked with promotion or inhibition of the development of BC. In particular, a higher consumption of dietary fiber and vitamin D along with a lower intake of saturated fat and red meat may reduce BC risk and improve metabolic parameters [69, 76]. Further epidemiological studies are warranted to investigate the association between dietary quality and quantity and BC risk.

CONCLUSION

Women with triple-negative breast cancer (TNBC) represent a heterogeneous population, with regard to ancestry, ethnicity and biological background (including genetic make-up, and tumor metabolic or hormonal profile), as well as socioeconomic status (SES), cultural, educational, and behavioral patterns. Significant disparities exist between AA and EA (or NHW) women, particularly in relation to TNBC incidence, prevalence, disease course, and survival rates.

Notably, TNBC is an aggressive BC subtype that disproportionately affects *BRCA1* mutation carriers and young women of African origin (*e.g.*, western sub-Saharan Africa). In addition, women of African origin with TNBC have usually worse clinical outcomes than those of European descent. In general, insufficient access to health care services often due to socioeconomic, educational, or cultural barriers results in delays and lack of proper medical care or follow-up for BC screening, diagnosis, and treatment. This, in turn, contributes to many cases of patients, who present with BC at advanced stages, with poor prognosis (*e.g.*, since their low income may result in a lack of health insurance and no access to indicated genetic testing and breast magnetic resonance imaging (MRI)) for TNBC.

However, it still remains unclear whether or not the differences in outcomes will persist after making adjustments for uneven availability of medical care (*e.g.*, timely BC screening, diagnostic work-up, comprehensive treatment, management of comorbidities, and participation in clinical studies), as well as for the financial status, education level, and various aspects of social and community support.

Certainly, unsafe neighborhoods and an excessive burden of toxic environmental exposures (*e.g.*, air, water, or soil pollution, and heavy metals, like cadmium, lead, and arsenic) unavailability of healthy food, and lack of regular physical exercises, often combined with daily stressful circumstances, can perpetuate a vicious circle of obesity, metabolic derangements, tissue inflammation, and aggressive TNBC biology. It should be highlighted that despite lower BC incidence rates, AA and Hispanic women have usually a worse prognosis and lower survival rates, compared to their EA (or NHW) counterparts. AA women also tend to suffer from many comorbidities, psychological, and socioeconomic issues. All of these factors are relevant to their unfavorable TNBC outcomes.

Due to the heterogeneity and very aggressive behavior of metastatic TNBC, it is crucial to have various treatment targets and easily accessible therapeutic options. Therefore, a deep insight into the interplay of the genetic, metabolic, hormonal, socioeconomic, and environmental components will allow us to more accurately predict and affect TNBC outcomes, especially in disadvantageous ethnic populations of women.

Hopefully, in the future, this will help the afflicted patients, and their doctors to find novel, multi-level, and at the same time, feasible strategies to overcome disparities in this devastating female cancer. In addition, the health-related decision-making process, during which patients communicate with their healthcare personnel, should be focused on a reasonable control of modifiable TNBC risk factors.

• Assessing the **impact of biological & non-biological risk factors** is crucial to outlining the most urgent **unmet needs of women with TNBC**;

• Having such directions will facilitate making small, but concrete **steps for the reduction of the disparities in women from various ethnic populations**, like AA, to improve their TNBC outcomes;

• Fortunately, several of the **acquired BC risk factors are modifiable,** and thus, amenable to interventions, which would **help ameliorate** many of the unacceptable **disparities** in this area;

• New strategies for the **care coordination and delivery** of indicated, modern, **targeted therapies**, across various healthcare settings, are necessary to achieve real equity in access to the recommended, more personalized medical care path.

REFERENCES

[1]   Gupta GK, Collier AL, Lee D, *et al.* Perspectives on triple-negative breast cancer: current treatment strategies, unmet needs, and potential targets for future therapies. Cancers 2020; 12(9): 2392.
[http://dx.doi.org/10.3390/cancers12092392] [PMID: 32846967]

[2]   Siddharth S, Sharma D. Racial disparity and triple-negative breast cancer in African-American women: A multifaceted affair between obesity, biology, and socioeconomic determinants. Cancers 2018; 10(12): 514.
[http://dx.doi.org/10.3390/cancers10120514] [PMID: 30558195]

[3]   Yedjou CG, Sims JN, Miele L, *et al.* Health and racial disparity in breast cancer. Adv Exp Med Biol 2019; 1152: 31-49.
[http://dx.doi.org/10.1007/978-3-030-20301-6_3] [PMID: 31456178]

[4]   Scott LC, Mobley LR, Kuo TM, Il'yasova D. Update on triple-negative breast cancer disparities for the United States: A population-based study from the united states cancer statistics database, 2010 through 2014. cancer 2019; 125(19): 3412-7.
[http://dx.doi.org/10.1002/cncr.32207] [PMID: 31282032]

[5]   Dietze EC, Sistrunk C, Miranda-Carboni G, O'Regan R, Seewaldt VL. Triple-negative breast cancer in African-American women: Disparities versus biology. Nat Rev Cancer 2015; 15(4): 248-54.
[http://dx.doi.org/10.1038/nrc3896] [PMID: 25673085]

[6]   Williams DR, Mohammed SA, Shields AE. Understanding and effectively addressing breast cancer in african american women: Unpacking the social context. Cancer 2016; 122(14): 2138-49.
[http://dx.doi.org/10.1002/cncr.29935] [PMID: 26930024]

[7]   Stewart PA, Luks J, Roycik MD, Sang QXA, Zhang J. Differentially expressed transcripts and dysregulated signaling pathways and networks in African American breast cancer. PLoS One 2013; 8(12): e82460.
[http://dx.doi.org/10.1371/journal.pone.0082460] [PMID: 24324792]

[8]   Vona-Davis L, Rose DP. The influence of socioeconomic disparities on breast cancer tumor biology and prognosis: A review. J Womens Health 2009; 18(6): 883-93.
[http://dx.doi.org/10.1089/jwh.2008.1127] [PMID: 19514831]

[9]   Prakash O, Hossain F, Danos D, Lassak A, Scribner R, Miele L. Racial disparities in triple negative breast cancer: A review of the role of biologic and non-biologic factors. Front Public Health 2020; 8: 576964.
[http://dx.doi.org/10.3389/fpubh.2020.576964] [PMID: 33415093]

[10]   Nishi A, Milner DA Jr, Giovannucci EL, *et al.* Integration of molecular pathology, epidemiology and social science for global precision medicine. Expert Rev Mol Diagn 2016; 16(1): 11-23.
[http://dx.doi.org/10.1586/14737159.2016.1115346] [PMID: 26636627]

[11]   Chlebowski RT, Chen Z, Anderson GL, *et al.* Ethnicity and breast cancer: Factors influencing differences in incidence and outcome. J Natl Cancer Inst 2005; 97(6): 439-48.
[http://dx.doi.org/10.1093/jnci/dji064] [PMID: 15770008]

[12]   Palmer JR, Boggs DA, Wise LA, Ambrosone CB, Adams-Campbell LL, Rosenberg L. Parity and

lactation in relation to estrogen receptor negative breast cancer in african american women. Cancer Epidemiol Biomarkers Prev 2011; 20(9): 1883-91.
[http://dx.doi.org/10.1158/1055-9965.EPI-11-0465] [PMID: 21846820]

[13]   Davis M, Tripathi S, Hughley R. AR negative triple negative or *quadruple negative* breast cancers in African American women have an enriched basal and immune signature. PLoS One 2018; 13(6): e0196909.
[http://dx.doi.org/10.1371/journal.pone.0196909] [PMID: 29912871]

[14]   Garrido-Castro AC, Lin NU, Polyak K. Insights into molecular classifications of triple-negative breast cancer: Improving patient selection for treatment. Cancer Discov 2019; 9(2): 176-98.
[http://dx.doi.org/10.1158/2159-8290.CD-18-1177] [PMID: 30679171]

[15]   Dunnwald LK, Rossing MA, Li CI. Hormone receptor status, tumor characteristics, and prognosis: A prospective cohort of breast cancer patients. Breast Cancer Res 2007; 9(1): R6.
[http://dx.doi.org/10.1186/bcr1639] [PMID: 17239243]

[16]   Mehrotra J, Ganpat MM, Kanaan Y, *et al.* Estrogen receptor/progesterone receptor-negative breast cancers of young African-American women have a higher frequency of methylation of multiple genes than those of caucasian women. Clin Cancer Res 2004; 10(6): 2052-7.
[http://dx.doi.org/10.1158/1078-0432.CCR-03-0514] [PMID: 15041725]

[17]   Dookeran KA, Dignam JJ, Ferrer K, Sekosan M, McCaskill-Stevens W, Gehlert S. p53 as a marker of prognosis in African-American women with breast cancer. Ann Surg Oncol 2010; 17(5): 1398-405.
[http://dx.doi.org/10.1245/s10434-009-0889-3] [PMID: 20049641]

[18]   Loo LWM, Wang Y, Flynn EM, *et al.* Genome-wide copy number alterations in subtypes of invasive breast cancers in young white and african american women. Breast Cancer Res Treat 2011; 127(1): 297-308.
[http://dx.doi.org/10.1007/s10549-010-1297-x] [PMID: 21264507]

[19]   Dietze EC, Chavez TA, Seewaldt VL. Obesity and triple-negative breast cancer. Am J Pathol 2018; 188(2): 280-90.
[http://dx.doi.org/10.1016/j.ajpath.2017.09.018] [PMID: 29128565]

[20]   Bradley CJ, Given CW, Roberts C. Race, socioeconomic status, and breast cancer treatment and survival. J Natl Cancer Inst 2002; 94(7): 490-6.
[http://dx.doi.org/10.1093/jnci/94.7.490] [PMID: 11929949]

[21]   McWhorter WP, Mayer WJ. Black/white differences in type of initial breast cancer treatment and implications for survival. Am J Public Health 1987; 77(12): 1515-7.
[http://dx.doi.org/10.2105/AJPH.77.12.1515] [PMID: 2823619]

[22]   Servick K. Breast cancer. Breast cancer: A world of differences. Sci 2014; 343(6178): 1452-3.
[http://dx.doi.org/10.1126/science.343.6178.1452] [PMID: 24675948]

[23]   Claus EB, Risch NJ, Thompson WD. Using age of onset to distinguish between subforms of breast cancer. Ann Hum Genet 1990; 54(2): 169-77.
[http://dx.doi.org/10.1111/j.1469-1809.1990.tb00373.x] [PMID: 2382970]

[24]   Ye F, He M, Huang L, *et al.* Insights into the impacts of brca mutations on clinicopathology and management of early-onset triple-negative breast cancer. Front Oncol 2021; 10: 574813.
[http://dx.doi.org/10.3389/fonc.2020.574813] [PMID: 33505905]

[25]   Malone KE, Daling JR, Doody DR, *et al.* Prevalence and predictors of BRCA1 and BRCA2 mutations in a population-based study of breast cancer in white and black American women ages 35 to 64 years. Cancer Res 2006; 66(16): 8297-308.
[http://dx.doi.org/10.1158/0008-5472.CAN-06-0503] [PMID: 16912212]

[26]   Parmigiani G, Chen S, Iversen ES Jr, *et al.* Validity of models for predicting BRCA1 and BRCA2 mutations. Ann Intern Med 2007; 147(7): 441-50.
[http://dx.doi.org/10.7326/0003-4819-147-7-200710020-00002] [PMID: 17909205]

[27]   PDQ Cancer Genetics Editorial Board. Genetics of Breast and Gynecologic Cancers (PDQ®): Health Professional Version.PDQ Cancer Information Summaries. Bethesda, MD: National Cancer Institute (US) 2021.

[28]   Antoniou AC, Casadei S, Heikkinen T, *et al.* Breast-cancer risk in families with mutations in PALB2. N Engl J Med 2014; 371(6): 497-506.
[http://dx.doi.org/10.1056/NEJMoa1400382] [PMID: 25099575]

[29]   Newman LA, Martin IK. Disparities in breast cancer. Curr Probl Cancer 2007; 31(3): 134-56.
[http://dx.doi.org/10.1016/j.currproblcancer.2007.01.003] [PMID: 17543945]

[30]   Freeman HP. Poverty, culture, and social injustice: Determinants of cancer disparities. CA Cancer J Clin 2004; 54(2): 72-7.
[http://dx.doi.org/10.3322/canjclin.54.2.72] [PMID: 15061597]

[31]   Lacey L, Whitfield J, Dewhite W, *et al.* Referral adherence in an inner city breast and cervical cancer screening program. Cancer 1993; 72(3): 950-5.
[http://dx.doi.org/10.1002/1097-0142(19930801)72:3<950::AID-CNCR2820720347>3.0.CO;2-S] [PMID: 8334648]

[32]   Hirschman J, Whitman S, Ansell D. The black:White disparity in breast cancer mortality: The example of Chicago. Cancer Caus Contro 2007; 18(3): 323-33.
[http://dx.doi.org/10.1007/s10552-006-0102-y] [PMID: 17285262]

[33]   Doose M, Sanchez JI, Cantor JC, *et al.* Fragmentation of care among black women with breast cancer and comorbidities: The role of health systems. JCO Oncol Pract 2021; 17(5): e637-44.
[http://dx.doi.org/10.1200/OP.20.01089] [PMID: 33974834]

[34]   Freeman HP, Chu KC. Determinants of cancer disparities: Barriers to cancer screening, diagnosis, and treatment. Surg Oncol Clin N Am 2005; 14(4): 655-69.
[http://dx.doi.org/10.1016/j.soc.2005.06.002] [PMID: 16226685]

[35]   Doose M, Tsui J, Steinberg MB, *et al.* Patterns of chronic disease management and health outcomes in a population-based cohort of black women with breast cancer. Cancer Causes Control 2021; 32(2): 157-68.
[http://dx.doi.org/10.1007/s10552-020-01370-5] [PMID: 33404907]

[36]   Orman A, Johnson DL, Comander A, Brockton N. Breast Cancer: A lifestyle medicine approach. Am J Lifestyle Med 2020; 14(5): 483-94.
[http://dx.doi.org/10.1177/1559827620913263] [PMID: 32922233]

[37]   Ferrini K, Ghelfi F, Mannucci R, Titta L. Lifestyle, nutrition and breast cancer: Facts and presumptions for consideration. Ecancermedicalscience 2015; 9: 557.
[http://dx.doi.org/10.3332/ecancer.2015.557] [PMID: 26284121]

[38]   Silber JH, Rosenbaum PR, Ross RN, *et al.* Disparities in breast cancer survival by socioeconomic status despite medicare and medicaid insurance. Milbank Q 2018; 96(4): 706-54.
[http://dx.doi.org/10.1111/1468-0009.12355] [PMID: 30537364]

[39]   Rudel RA, Fenton SE, Ackerman JM, Euling SY, Makris SL. Environmental exposures and mammary gland development: state of the science, public health implications, and research recommendations. Environ Health Perspect 2011; 119(8): 1053-61.
[http://dx.doi.org/10.1289/ehp.1002864] [PMID: 21697028]

[40]   Terry MB, Michels KB, Brody JG, *et al.* Environmental exposures during windows of susceptibility for breast cancer: A framework for prevention research. Breast Cancer Res 2019; 21(1): 96.
[http://dx.doi.org/10.1186/s13058-019-1168-2] [PMID: 31429809]

[41]   Rodgers KM, Udesky JO, Rudel RA, Brody JG. Environmental chemicals and breast cancer: An updated review of epidemiological literature informed by biological mechanisms. Environ Res 2018; 160: 152-82.
[http://dx.doi.org/10.1016/j.envres.2017.08.045] [PMID: 28987728]

[42]　Van Ryn M, Burke J. The effect of patient race and socio-economic status on physicians' perceptions of patients. Soc Sci Med 2000; 50(6): 813-28.
[http://dx.doi.org/10.1016/S0277-9536(99)00338-X] [PMID: 10695979]

[43]　Carey LA, Perou CM, Livasy CA, *et al.* Race, breast cancer subtypes, and survival in the carolina breast cancer study. JAMA 2006; 295(21): 2492-502.
[http://dx.doi.org/10.1001/jama.295.21.2492] [PMID: 16757721]

[44]　Powe BD, Daniels EC, Finnie R, Thompson A. Perceptions about breast cancer among African American women: Do selected educational materials challenge them? Patient Educ Couns 2005; 56(2): 197-204.
[http://dx.doi.org/10.1016/j.pec.2004.02.009] [PMID: 15653249]

[45]　Miller AM, Champion VL. Attitudes about breast cancer and mammography: Racial, income, and educational differences. Women Health 1997; 26(1): 41-63.
[http://dx.doi.org/10.1300/J013v26n01_04] [PMID: 9311099]

[46]　Skinner CS, Arfken CL, Sykes RK. Knowledge, perceptions, and mammography stage of adoption among older urban women. Am J Prev Med 1998; 14(1): 54-63.
[http://dx.doi.org/10.1016/S0749-3797(97)00008-1] [PMID: 9476836]

[47]　Russell KM, Monahan P, Wagle A, Champion V. Differences in health and cultural beliefs by stage of mammography screening adoption in African American women. Cancer 2007; 109(S2) (Suppl.): 386-95.
[http://dx.doi.org/10.1002/cncr.22359] [PMID: 17133417]

[48]　Mascara M, Constantinou C. Global perceptions of women on breast cancer and barriers to screening. Curr Oncol Rep 2021; 23(7): 74.
[http://dx.doi.org/10.1007/s11912-021-01069-z] [PMID: 33937940]

[49]　Chen FM, Fryer GE Jr, Phillips RL Jr, Wilson E, Pathman DE. Patients' beliefs about racism, preferences for physician race, and satisfaction with care. Ann Fam Med 2005; 3(2): 138-43.
[http://dx.doi.org/10.1370/afm.282] [PMID: 15798040]

[50]　Vernon SW, Vogel VG, Halabi S, Bondy ML. Factors associated with perceived risk of breast cancer among women attending a screening program. Breast Cancer Res Treat 1993; 28(2): 137-44.
[http://dx.doi.org/10.1007/BF00666426] [PMID: 8173066]

[51]　Gibson LM, Hendricks CS. Integrative review of spirituality in African American breast cancer survivors. ABNF J 2006; 17(2): 67-72.
[PMID: 18402346]

[52]　Johnson KS, Elbert-Avila KI, Tulsky JA. The influence of spiritual beliefs and practices on the treatment preferences of African Americans: A review of the literature. J Am Geriatr Soc 2005; 53(4): 711-9.
[http://dx.doi.org/10.1111/j.1532-5415.2005.53224.x] [PMID: 15817022]

[53]　Lannin DR, Mathews HF, Mitchell J, Swanson MS. Impacting cultural attitudes in African-American women to decrease breast cancer mortality. Am J Surg 2002; 184(5): 418-23.
[http://dx.doi.org/10.1016/S0002-9610(02)01009-7] [PMID: 12433605]

[54]　Mansfield CJ, Mitchell J, King DE. The doctor as God's mechanic? Beliefs in the southeastern United States. Soc Sci Med 2002; 54(3): 399-409.
[http://dx.doi.org/10.1016/S0277-9536(01)00038-7] [PMID: 11824916]

[55]　Carter J, Park ER, Moadel A, Cleary SD, Morgan C. Cancer knowledge, attitudes, beliefs, and practices (KABP) of disadvantaged women in the South Bronx. J Cancer Educ 2002; 17(3): 142-9.
[PMID: 12243219]

[56]　Neilson HK, Farris MS, Stone CR, Vaska MM, Brenner DR, Friedenreich CM. Moderate-vigorous recreational physical activity and breast cancer risk, stratified by menopause status: A systematic review and meta-analysis. Menopause 2017; 24(3): 322-44.

[http://dx.doi.org/10.1097/GME.0000000000000745] [PMID: 27779567]

[57] Hildebrand JS, Gapstur SM, Campbell PT, Gaudet MM, Patel AV. Recreational physical activity and leisure-time sitting in relation to postmenopausal breast cancer risk. Cancer Epidemiol Biomarkers Prev 2013; 22(10): 1906-12.
[http://dx.doi.org/10.1158/1055-9965.EPI-13-0407] [PMID: 24097200]

[58] Eliassen AH, Hankinson SE, Rosner B, Holmes MD, Willett WC. Physical activity and risk of breast cancer among postmenopausal women. Arch Intern Med 2010; 170(19): 1758-64.
[http://dx.doi.org/10.1001/archinternmed.2010.363] [PMID: 20975025]

[59] Fintor L. Exercise and breast cancer risk: Lacking consensus. J Natl Cancer Inst 1999; 91(10): 825-7.
[http://dx.doi.org/10.1093/jnci/91.10.825] [PMID: 10340899]

[60] Wu Y, Zhang D, Kang S. Physical activity and risk of breast cancer: A meta-analysis of prospective studies. Breast Cancer Res Treat 2013; 137(3): 869-82.
[http://dx.doi.org/10.1007/s10549-012-2396-7] [PMID: 23274845]

[61] Rose DP, Komninou D, Stephenson GD. Obesity, adipocytokines, and insulin resistance in breast cancer. Obes Rev 2004; 5(3): 153-65.
[http://dx.doi.org/10.1111/j.1467-789X.2004.00142.x] [PMID: 15245384]

[62] Agurs-Collins T, Ross SA, Dunn BK. The many faces of obesity and its influence on breast cancer risk. Front Oncol 2019; 9: 765.
[http://dx.doi.org/10.3389/fonc.2019.00765] [PMID: 31555578]

[63] Sephton SE, Sapolsky RM, Kraemer HC, Spiegel D. Diurnal cortisol rhythm as a predictor of breast cancer survival. J Natl Cancer Inst 2000; 92(12): 994-1000.
[http://dx.doi.org/10.1093/jnci/92.12.994] [PMID: 10861311]

[64] Zhao P, Xia N, Zhang H, Deng T. The Metabolic syndrome is a risk factor for breast cancer: A systematic review and meta-analysis. Obes Facts 2020; 13(4): 384-96.
[http://dx.doi.org/10.1159/000507554] [PMID: 32698183]

[65] Hair BY, Hayes S, Tse CK, Bell MB, Olshan AF. Racial differences in physical activity among breast cancer survivors: Implications for breast cancer care. Cancer 2014; 120(14): 2174-82.
[http://dx.doi.org/10.1002/cncr.28630] [PMID: 24911404]

[66] Thompson CL, Owusu C, Nock NL, Li L, Berger NA. Race, age, and obesity disparities in adult physical activity levels in breast cancer patients and controls. Front Public Health 2014; 2: 150.
[http://dx.doi.org/10.3389/fpubh.2014.00150] [PMID: 25285306]

[67] Winzer BM, Whiteman DC, Reeves MM, Paratz JD. Physical activity and cancer prevention: A systematic review of clinical trials. Cancer Caus Contr 2011; 22(6): 811-26.
[http://dx.doi.org/10.1007/s10552-011-9761-4] [PMID: 21461921]

[68] Stout NL, Binkley JM, Schmitz KH, *et al.* A prospective surveillance model for rehabilitation for women with breast cancer. Cancer 2012; 118(S8): 2191-200.
[http://dx.doi.org/10.1002/cncr.27476] [PMID: 22488693]

[69] Kotepui M. Diet and risk of breast cancer. Contemp Oncol 2016; 1(1): 13-9.
[http://dx.doi.org/10.5114/wo.2014.40560] [PMID: 27095934]

[70] Chlebowski RT, Blackburn GL, Thomson CA, *et al.* Dietary fat reduction and breast cancer outcome: Interim efficacy results from the women's intervention nutrition study. J Natl Cancer Inst 2006; 98(24): 1767-76.
[http://dx.doi.org/10.1093/jnci/djj494] [PMID: 17179478]

[71] Pierce JP, Natarajan L, Caan BJ, *et al.* Influence of a diet very high in vegetables, fruit, and fiber and low in fat on prognosis following treatment for breast cancer: The women's healthy eating and living (WHEL) randomized trial. JAMA 2007; 298(3): 289-98.
[http://dx.doi.org/10.1001/jama.298.3.289] [PMID: 17635889]

[72]   George SM, Irwin ML, Smith AW, *et al.* Postdiagnosis diet quality, the combination of diet quality and recreational physical activity, and prognosis after early-stage breast cancer. Cancer Caus Contr 2011; 22(4): 589-98.
[http://dx.doi.org/10.1007/s10552-011-9732-9] [PMID: 21340493]

[73]   Kang DW, Lee J, Suh SH, Ligibel J, Courneya KS, Jeon JY. Effects of exercise on insulin, igf axis, adipocytokines, and inflammatory markers in breast cancer survivors: A systematic review and meta-analysis. Cancer Epidemiol Biomarkers Prev 2017; 26(3): 355-65.
[http://dx.doi.org/10.1158/1055-9965.EPI-16-0602] [PMID: 27742668]

[74]   Paxton RJ, Jones LA, Chang S, *et al.* Was race a factor in the outcomes of the women's health eating and living study? Cancer 2011; 117(16): 3805-13.
[http://dx.doi.org/10.1002/cncr.25957] [PMID: 21319157]

[75]   Paxton RJ, Phillips KL, Jones LA, *et al.* Associations among physical activity, body mass index, and health-related quality of life by race/ethnicity in a diverse sample of breast cancer survivors. Cancer 2012; 118(16): 4024-31.
[http://dx.doi.org/10.1002/cncr.27389] [PMID: 22252966]

[76]   Lu Shin KN, Mun CY, Shariff ZM. Nutrition indicators, physical function, and health-related quality of life in breast cancer patients. Asian Pac J Cancer Prev 2020; 21(7): 1939-50.
[http://dx.doi.org/10.31557/APJCP.2020.21.7.1939] [PMID: 32711419]

A Closer Look at the Androgen Receptor (AR)-positive and AR-negative Metastatic Triple-Negative Breast Cancer: Can We Apply Novel Targeted Therapeutics?

Abstract: Based on the **androgen receptor (AR)** expression, **triple-negative breast cancer (TNBC)** (that is estrogen receptor (ER), progesterone receptor (PR), and human epidermal growth factor receptor 2 (HER2) negative), can further be divided into **AR-negative TNBC** (also known as **quadruple-negative breast cancer (QNBC)**, a more frequent TNBC subtype) and AR-positive TNBC.

The paucity of treatment targets makes QNBC very difficult to manage. Moreover, in the absence of AR expression, many breast cancers (BCs) often display aggressive behavior, leading to negative outcomes in afflicted women. At present, some novel therapeutic targets have emerged, and hopefully, the relevant targeted strategies will improve the survival of patients with QNBC.

This chapter briefly outlines the main TNBC subtypes and focuses on the AR expression (its presence *vs.* absence), and potential treatment approaches, including **AR antagonists (ARA)**. In addition, this chapter overviews certain molecular characteristics of TNBC and presents recently approved targeted therapies.

Keywords: Androgen receptor (AR), AR antagonists (ARA), Antibody drug conjugate (ADC), Immune checkpoint inhibitors (ICI), Poly ADP-ribose polymerase (PARP) inhibitors, Quadruple-negative breast cancer (QNBC), Triple-negative breast cancer (TNBC).

INTRODUCTION

Triple-negative breast cancer (TNBC), characterized by the negative **estrogen receptor (ER), progesterone receptor (PR)**, and **human epidermal growth factor receptor 2 (HER2)** expression, usually demonstrates higher rates of relapse, greater metastatic potential, and shorter overall survival (OS), compared to other **breast cancer (BC)** subtypes [1]. It has been suggested that TNBC could be sub-divided into a more prevalent, **androgen receptor (AR)-negative subtype**, also known as **quadruple-negative breast cancer (QNBC)** subtype, and a **"classical", AR-positive TNBC subtype** (Fig. **1**) [1]. It appears that multiple, interrelated genetic and environmental factors can influence the incidence, course, and prognosis of this devastating malignancy, across different ethnic and socioeconomic populations of women [2]. In comparison to other BC subtypes, TNBC and QNBC are characterized by a more invasive tumor behavior (*e.g.*, frequent local recurrences and distant metastases) and resistance to treatment, leading to negative outcomes [3]. Also, these aggressive BC subtypes have been more prevalent among women of African origin, and in the pre-menopausal group (*e.g.*, below 50 years of age) [2]. In addition, some major factors related to the augmented risk of TNBC and QNBC involve metabolic disorders (*e.g.*, obesity, metabolic syndrome (MS), pre-diabetes, and type 2 diabetes mellitus (T2DM), reproductive factors (*e.g.*, short breastfeeding period, high parity, oral contraceptive usage for over one year, and gestational diabetes), inappropriate nutrition (*e.g.*, the predominance of highly caloric and processed food, rich in saturated fats, trans-fats, and refined carbohydrates), physical inactivity, and low socioeconomic status or educational level. In particular, **obesity, accompanied by metabolic dysfunctions and pro-inflammatory conditions, a sedentary lifestyle, and a brief lactation** period has been associated with **abnormal secretion of androgens** [4]. The heterogeneous nature of TNBC and QNBC, as well as the diversity of the afflicted patient populations, require individualized and comprehensive management strategies. Recently, some innovative therapeutic targets have emerged, which could possibly improve the survival of many women suffering from this malignancy [5].

This chapter briefly outlines the main TNBC and QNBC subtypes and describes the current and future research directions in this area. It focuses on the AR expression (its presence *vs.* absence), and potential treatment approaches, including **AR antagonists (ARA)** and some recently approved molecular targeted therapies.

Various Molecular Subtypes of TNBC

TNBC has been divided into the following molecular subtypes: **basal-like subtypes (BL1** and **BL2), mesenchymal (M), mesenchymal stem-like (MSL), immunomodulatory (IM), and luminal androgen receptor (LAR)** (Fig. **2**) [3, 5, 6]. According to a similar categorization, the BL1 and BL2 can also be presented as **basal-like immunosuppressed (BLIS)**, and **basal-like immune activated (BLIA)** subtypes [7]. It has been reported that different TNBC subtypes revealed significant variability in response to neoadjuvant or adjuvant **chemotherapy (CHT)**. It should be underscored that **BL1** has shown a more beneficial response to CHT than the LAR subtype [8]. Conversely, TNBC presents a greater sensitivity to CHT than the non-TNBC subtypes. On the other hand, however, several women with advanced or metastatic TNBC have been resistant to standard CHT regimens (*e.g.*, anthracycline and taxanes) [3, 4]. This unmet need is one of the driving forces behind searching for innovative treatment targets and compatible diagnostic tests or biomarkers [3, 9].

THE UNDETERMINED PROGNOSTIC VALUE OF ANDROGEN RECEPTOR (AR) IN WOMEN WITH TNBC

Androgen receptor (AR) may serve as the prognostic biomarker in BC [10]. Based on a recent multi-institutional study, it has been shown that AR-positive status was consistent with a more favorable prognosis among groups of women from the US and Nigeria [10]. In contrast, a worse prognosis was reported among their counterparts from Ireland, Norway, and India [10]. In addition, no prognostic value was noted in the group of women from the UK [10]. Interestingly, it has been reported that the ER status affects the prognostic value of AR. For instance, the AR expression suggests a good prognosis in the ER-positive BC, but the significance of AR expression in the ER-negative BC is still unclear [11].

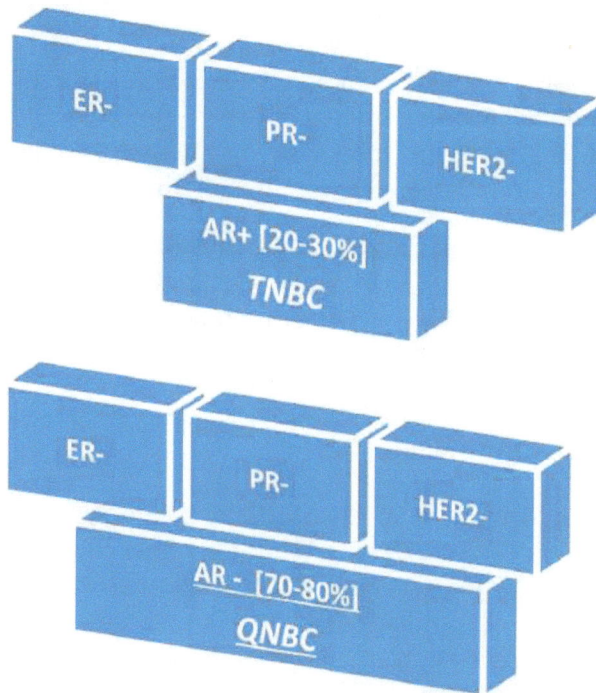

Fig. (1). A receptor profile of the Triple-negative breast cancer (TNBCs) and Quadruple-negative breast cancer (QNBC) [1, 5]. Abbreviations: AR, Androgen receptor; ER, Estrogen receptor; HER2, Human epidermal growth factor receptor 2; PR; Progesterone receptor.

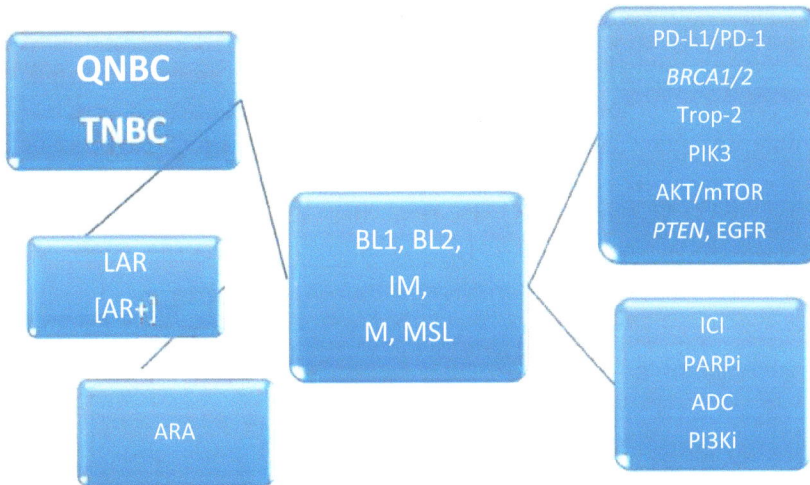

Fig. (2). Molecular subtypes, therapeutic targets, and treatment strategies for patients with Triple-negative breast cancer (TNBCs) and Quadruple-negative breast cancer (QNBC) AR, Androgen receptor; Molecular subtypes: BL, Basal-like; IM, Immunomodulatory; LAR, Luminal androgen receptor; M, Mesenchymal; MSL, Mesenchymal stem-like; Therapeutic targets: PD-L1, programmed death ligand 1; PD-1, programmed cell death protein-1; BRCA1/2, tumor suppressor genes;Trop-2, Trophoblast cell-surface antigen; PI3K, phosphoinositide-3 kinase; AKT/mTOR, protein kinase B/the mammalian target of rapamycin; PTEN, phosphatase and tensin; EGFR, epidermal growth factor receptor; Treatment strategies: ICI, immune checkpoint inhibitors; PARPi, Poly ADP-ribose polymerase (PARP) inhibitors; ADC, Antibody drug conjugate; PI3Ki, PI3K inhibitors; ARA, AR antagonists.

Nevertheless, due to several methodological differences, and small samples examined in different studies in this area, the prognostic value of AR in TNBC still remains undetermined, and thus, further research in this area is certainly needed, before drawing any definite conclusions.

THE INFLUENCE OF ANDROGEN RECEPTOR (AR) ON POTENTIAL THERAPEUTIC CHOICES IN PATIENTS WITH TNBC

AR is a transcription factor (TF), participating in the natural development of the breast gland (*via* signaling at the level of steroid hormone receptor, in the cell nucleus), and also, it can contribute to BC initiation and progression [12]. However, the exact influence of AR signaling on TNBC development is still not completely known. AR is expressed in about one-third of TNBCs [13], and it has been noted that **AR antagonists (ARA)** (*e.g.*, **bicalutamide** and **enzalutamide)**, have shown some beneficial effects among patients with AR-positive TNBC [14, 15].

In reality, a positive AR expression in the LAR TNBC subtype has been related to a greater sensitivity to ARA, while the BL1 subtype achieved the highest

pathological complete response (pCR) rate, after an application of **neoadjuvant chemotherapy (NAC)** [6]. In contrast, the BL2 and LAR revealed the lowest pCR rates, after using NAC [6, 16]. In addition, recent clinical trials that examined the ARA therapies (*e.g.*, bicalutamide, enzalutamide, and abiraterone acetate plus prednisone) with CHT, among women with TNBC, have shown some beneficial effects of such treatment combinations [14, 15, 17]. Also, a neoadjuvant **MDACC ARTEMIS** trial has been addressing a population of patients with TNBC (in stages I–III), in whom the treatment has been adjusted, according to BC molecular profiling results [18]. For instance, in case of positive AR expression, the participants have been receiving enzalutamide and paclitaxel (a component of the standard NAC) [18].

Notably, various AR splice variants (AR-Vs) are products of rearranging or alternative splicing of the AR transcript [19]. Importantly, the AR-Vs are characterized by an absence of the ligand-binding domain (LBD), which serves as a target for enzalutamide, and can activate target genes [19, 20]. In fact, the AR and AR-V7 can differentially regulate target gene expression, depending on the recruitment of AR or its splice variant. Since it has been noted that the AR-V7 expression is related to adverse prognosis in many patients with BC, there is a growing interest in the exploration of the AR-V7, as a potential novel therapeutic target in patients with TNBC [13, 21].

Importantly, AR can also govern tumor growth in some TNBC subtypes, which express low levels of AR. For instance, the AR-positive tumor cell subpopulation may stimulate the growth of **cancer stem cell (CSC)**-like cells, promoting resistance to CHT and recurrence of malignancy [22]. Therefore, the AR-targeting agents can be beneficial for patients with TNBC, even if their AR expression levels remain low (*e.g.*, below 1%) [22]. In fact, the use of a combination of enzalutamide (ARA) and paclitaxel (CHT) can be more effective in preventing cancer recurrence (*e.g.*, *via* targeting the CSC-like cells) than the application of paclitaxel alone [22].

In addition, low AR levels have been related to higher pCR rates in a clinical study assessing neoadjuvant cisplatin plus paclitaxel with or without everolimus in patients with TNBC [23]. Another study has shown that the AR expression can predict the effects of therapy with tamoxifen in patients with TNBC [24]. For instance, in women with TNBC, the AR-positive status corresponded with a favorable response to tamoxifen, while the AR-negative status was consistent with a failure of tamoxifen therapy [24].

DIFFICULTIES WITH STANDARDIZATION OF ANDROGEN RECEPTOR (AR) TESTING

In contrast to the ER, PR, and HER2 testing, which represent standard clinical practice, AR testing has not been standardized due to the lack of consensus regarding its prognostic value. Since women with AR-negative TNBC (QNBC) usually suffer from a more aggressive malignancy course and worse prognosis, compared to those with AR-positive TNBC, a standardization of AR testing merits a formal resolution. The QNBC has its own specific molecular make-up, and thus, it would be beneficial to "formally" recognize it as a clinically relevant BC subtype, which is different from a "classical" TNBC [25]. At this point, immunohistochemistry (IHC) analysis of AR seems to be a feasible test to be applied for this purpose [25]. In order to develop innovative, targeted treatments for patients with AR-negative TNBC (QNBC) and AR-positive TNBC, the specific differences between these BC subtypes need to be explored, and then translated into targeted therapies. However, further research is still necessary in this field.

TARGETED APPROACHES TO TNBC RESISTANT TO THERAPY: FOCUSING ON "WEAK POINTS" OF AGGRESSIVE CANCERS

Traditionally, the standard CHT used to treat patients with high-risk and locally advanced or metastatic TNBC has been composed of anthracyclines, alkylating agents, and taxanes [9]. However, recently, some other therapeutic classes, such as **immune checkpoint inhibitors (ICI), poly ADP-ribose polymerase (PARP) inhibitors**, and **antibody-drug conjugate (ADC)**, have been explored in phase III **randomized controlled trials (RCTs)**, and revealed certain beneficial outcomes [26 - 31]. As a result, many of these therapeutic options have been approved by the **US Food and Drug Administration (FDA)** as targeted therapies for selected subsets of patients with TNBC (Table **1**) [26 - 31].

It should be highlighted that the combinations of certain therapeutic agents from various pharmacologic classes and sequences, in which they are used, can be crucial to "awakening" the antitumor immune response of the host [32]. As a consequence, such a strong response may help in the transformation of immunologically "cold" into "hot" tumor areas in metastatic TNBC [32]. Due to rapid advances in this field, many women with metastatic, previously incurable TNBC may now have some reasonable hope that durable responses to ICI can be achieved [33]. Such progress may happen, especially when the ICI are used in combination with CHT, depending on the individual patient scenario, in which the immune system can be invigorated [33].

Immune Checkpoint Inhibitors (ICI) (Atezolizumab and Pembrolizumab)

According to recent RCTs data, ICI that target the **programmed death ligand-1 (PD-L1)** and **programmed death receptor-1 (PD-1)** have shown clinical benefits for patients with advanced and metastatic TNBC (*e.g.*, in combination with CHT) (Table **1**) [26, 27].

Table 1. Phase III RCTs investigating the effects of therapies with immune checkpoint inhibitors, PARP inhibitors, and antibody-drug conjugate for patients with advanced or metastatic TNBC.

RCT Name Identifier Ref.	Targeted Therapy (or Combination)	Usual adverse effects Monitoring tests	RCT's main outcomes or trends	Safety precautions Therapeutic actions
IMpassion130 NCT02425891 [26]	Anti-PD-L1 monoclonal antibody **Atezolizumab + nab-paclitaxel** (CHT)	Alopecia, fatigue, peripheral neuropathies, nausea, vomiting, < appetite, diarrhea, headache, anemia, neutropenia, pyrexia, arthralgia; ALT, AST, t. bilirubin, CBC	Atezolizumab + nab-paclitaxel *vs.* placebo + nab-paclitaxel for therapy of pts with previously untreated advanced or metastatic TNBC; adding atezolizumab to 1-st-line CHT (nab-paclitaxel) prolonged m PFS in the ITT group (7.2 *vs.* 5.5 ms) & in pts with PD-L--positive tumors (7.4 *vs.* 4.8 ms); ORR was higher in the ITT group (56.0% *vs.* 45.9%) & in PD-L1-positive subgroup (58.9% *vs.* 42.6%); a trend of improved m OS with atezolizumab in the ITT group (21.0 *vs.* 18.7 ms) & in the PD-L1-positive pts (25.0 *vs.* 18.0 ms); the PD-L1 expression in immune cells is a predictor of treatment response (PFS & OS improved in PD-L1–positive pts)	Immune-mediated pneumonitis or interstitial lung disease Use prednisone (taper it); > liver function tests, immune-mediated hepatitis Monitor for symptoms of hepatitis, use corticosteroids; Immune-mediated colitis or diarrhea; Observe, but if symptoms persist >5 days or recur, use steroids

(Table 1) cont.....

RCT Name Identifier Ref.	Targeted Therapy (or Combination)	Usual adverse effects Monitoring tests	RCT's main outcomes or trends	Safety precautions Therapeutic actions
KEYNOTE-522 NCT03036488 [27]	Anti-PD-1 monoclonal antibody **Pembrolizumab** + CHT	Alopecia, fatigue, peripheral neuropathies, nausea, vomiting, < appetite, diarrhea, headache, anemia, neutropenia,, pyrexia, arthralgia; ALT, AST, t. bilirubin, CBC	pCR rate was 64.8% in the pembrolizumab + CHT group *vs.* 51.2% in the placebo + CHT group; the disease progression rate was 7.4% in the pembrolizumab + CHT group *vs.* 11.8% in the placebo + CHT group	Immune-mediated pneumonitis or interstitial lung disease Use prednisone (taper it); > liver function tests, immune-mediated hepatitis Monitor for symptoms of hepatitis, use corticosteroids; Immune-mediated colitis or diarrhea; Observe, but if symptoms persist >5 days or recur, use steroids
KEYNOTE-355 NCT02819518 [28]	Anti-PD-1 monoclonal antibody **Pembrolizumab** + CHT preliminary findings	Alopecia, fatigue, peripheral neuropathies, nausea, vomiting, < appetite, diarrhea, headache, anemia, neutropenia,, pyrexia, arthralgia; ALT, AST, t. bilirubin, CBC	Comparison of pembrolizumab + CHT (nab-paclitaxel, paclitaxel, or emcitabine/carboplatin) to placebo + CHT in pts (previously untreated) with recurrent inoperable/metastatic TNBC; the addition of pembrolizumab to CHT improved PFS compared to CHT alone (9.7 *vs.* 5.6 ms).	Immune-mediated pneumonitis or interstitial lung disease Use prednisone (taper it); > liver function tests, immune-mediated hepatitis Monitor for symptoms of hepatitis, use corticosteroids; Immune-mediated colitis or diarrhea; Observe, but if symptoms persist >5 days or recur, use steroids

(Table 1) cont.....

RCT Name Identifier Ref.	Targeted Therapy (or Combination)	Usual adverse effects Monitoring tests	RCT's main outcomes or trends	Safety precautions Therapeutic actions
OlympiAD NCT02000622 [29]	PARP1 inhibitor **Olaparib**	Anemia, leukopenia, fatigue, nausea, vomiting, diarrhea, abdominal pain; CBC	Efficacy & safety of olaparib *vs.* CHT (capecitabine, vinorelbine, or eribulin) in pts with g*BRCA* mutation and HER2-negative metastatic BC (who had received no more than 2 previous lines of CHT or treatments of doctor's choice); m PFS was prolonged by 2.8 ms in olaparib arm; m OS was 19.3 ms in olaparib arm *vs.* 17.1 ms in CHT arm; OS benefit with olaparib, in pts who did not receive CHT for metastatic BC	Pneumonitis; Interrupt olaparib if pneumonitis is suspected, or stop olaparib, if it is confirmed; Rare MDS/AML; If MDS/AML is confirmed, stop olaparib;
EMBRACA NCT01945775 [30]	PARP inhibitor **Talazoparib**	Fatigue, nausea, headache, headache, alopecia, back pain, anemia, neutropenia, thrombocyte-penia, vomiting, diarrhea, < appetite; CBC	efficacy & safety of talazoparib *vs.* CHT (capecitabine, eribulin, gemcitabine or vinorelbine) in pts with g*BRCA* mutation, HER2-negative locally advanced/metastatic BC, who previously received CHT; m PFS was prolonged by 3 ms in the talazoparib arm; ORR was doubled in the talazoparib arm *vs.* CHT arm	Coadministration with amiodarone, carvedilol, verapamil, clarithromycin, or itraconazole should be avoided; if such agents are necessary, < the dose of talazoparib

(Table 1) cont.....

RCT Name Identifier Ref.	Targeted Therapy (or Combination)	Usual adverse effects Monitoring tests	RCT's main outcomes or trends	Safety precautions Therapeutic actions
ASCENT NCT02574455 [31]	Antibody-drug conjugate **Sacituzumab govitecan-hziy**	Neutropenia, anemia, nausea, vomiting, diarrhea, fatigue, increased AST, ALT, alkaline phosphatase, alopecia, < Mg, Ca CBC, liver panel, electrolytes, if diarrhea, evaluate for infectious causes	efficacy & safety of sacituzumab govitecan-hziy; pts treated with sacituzumab govitecan-hziy had PFS of 5.6 ms *vs.* 1.7 ms, in those, who were given CHT Improved PFS, OS, ORR, & durable objective responses in heavily pretreated pts with metastatic TNBC (without brain metastasis)	Premedicate for prevention of CHT-induced nausea/vomiting; In case of severe neutropenia, withhold if ANC<1,500/mm3 or neutropenic fever; can use G-CSF for secondary prophylaxis; give anti-infective agents in febrile neutropenia; If severe diarrhea - provide fluids/ electrolytes & atropine or loperamide (if no infection)

AKT, protein kinase B; ALT, Alanine transaminase; AML, Acute Myeloid Leukemia; ANC, Absolute Neutrophil Count; AST, Aspartate transaminase; BC, breast cancer; CBC, Complete Blood Count; CHT, chemotherapy, DOR, duration of response; FDA, Food and Drug Administration; g, germline; G-CSF, Granulocyte colony stimulating factor; ITT, intention-to-treat; m, median; MDS, Myelodysplastic Syndromes; ms, months; ORR, overall response rate; OS, overall survival; PARP, poly (ADP-ribose) polymerase; PD-1, programmed cell death protein-1; PD-L1, programmed death ligand 1; PFS, progression-free survival, pts, patients; RCT, randomised controlled trial; ref., reference; t., total; TNBC; triple negative breast cancer; *vs.*, versus.

In TNBC, **PD-L1** is usually expressed on the **tumor-infiltrating immune cells (TILs)**, and malignant tumor cells, while **PD-1** is commonly expressed on **T-cells** [26, 27]. When the PD-L1 binds to PD-1, an inhibitory signal is being sent that causes T-cell suppression [34]. To counteract the undesirable immune system suppression, **ICI,** such as the **PD-L1 inhibitor, atezolizumab**, or the **PD-1 inhibitor, pembrolizumab,** in combination with CHT, can be considered to treat women with locally advanced, recurrent, and metastatic TNBC (rather earlier than later in the disease course) [26, 27]. In fact, elevated TILs or expression of PD-L1/PD-1 immune checkpoint complexes is often related to a higher anti-tumor immunity, and a better patient prognosis [33]. This can be considered a biomarker, detecting potential candidates for treatment with ICI [33]. PD-L1, which is expressed in about 40% of TNBC, has become a novel therapeutic target, especially in metastatic TNBC [32, 33].

The **IMpassion130 trial** illustrates the favorable effects of adding **atezolizumab** (an **anti-PD-L1 monoclonal antibody**), to **nab-paclitaxel (CHT)** (compared to nab-paclitaxel alone, as first-line therapy) for women with metastatic TNBC (Table **1**) [26].

Similarly, the **KEYNOTE-522** trial has explored the addition of **pembrolizumab** (an **anti-PD-1 monoclonal antibody**) to CHT (neoadjuvant CHT, and continued adjuvant CHT) in untreated patients with stage II or III TNBC, showing some promising effects (Table **1**) [27]. It should be highlighted that in contrast to the **IMpassion130** trial, the addition of pembrolizumab to standard CHT in the **KEYNOTE-522** trial has revealed improvements in pCR [27]. Likewise, the ongoing **KEYNOTE-355** trial, investigating the addition of **pembrolizumab** to **CHT**, among patients with untreated, locally recurrent, inoperable or metastatic TNBC, has revealed some encouraging preliminary results (Table **1**) [28].

POLY-ADP-RIBOSE POLYMERASE (PARP) INHIBITORS (OLAPARIB AND TALAZOPARIB)

Based on recent RCTs, some PARP inhibitors, targeting specific genetic mutations or molecular signaling pathways (which govern malignant cell growth), have been applied in monotherapy, or in combination with CHT, in patients with metastatic TNBC [29, 30]. *BRCA1* and *BRCA2* are tumor suppressor genes that play a key role in the repair of DNA breaks [35]. The *BRCA1/2* mutations are related to increased familial inheritance, early onset, high tumor aggression, and poor TNBC prognosis [35]. As a result of this loss of function mutations, TNBC tumors that carry the mutated *BRCA1/2* genes, are unable to repair their damaged DNA [35]. In these circumstances, blocking off the PARP enzymes, *via* the PARP inhibitors causes the lethal accumulation of irreparable DNA breaks, and cytotoxic PARP-DNA complexes in the tumor [36]. Recently PARP inhibitors (olaparib and talazoparib) have been approved as targeted therapy that can be used in almost 20% of patients with TNBC (who have germline *BRCA1/2* mutations) [29, 30].

The **OlympiAD** trial has explored the efficacy of **olaparib**, in patients with metastatic, germline *BRCA* mutated, HER2-negative BC, who had received no more than two previous lines of CHT [29]. According to this study's results, olaparib monotherapy revealed beneficial effects, compared to standard CHT (*e.g.*, median PFS was almost three months longer and the risk of disease progression or death was over 40% lower in women, who received olaparib, compared to those who received standard **CHT** (Table **1**) [29].

Similarly, the **EMBRACA** trial examined the efficacy of **talazoparib**, in women with advanced BC and germline *BRCA1/2* mutations (who previously received CHT) [30]. The **EMBRACA** trial has shown that patients who were treated with talazoparib had improved PFS compared to those, who received CHT (Table **1**) [30]. Moreover, the most favorable responses were reported in a subset of patients with TNBC, who harbored germline *BRCA1/2* mutations. In addition, PARP inhibitors, used in combination with CHT, can be particularly helpful in the treatment of breast tumors with not only germline *BRCA1/2* mutations, but also with *PALB2, RAD51, p53,* and *CHEK2* gene mutations [37].

Anti-Trop-2 Antibody-drug Conjugate (ADC) (Sacituzumab Govitecan-hziy)

Trophoblast cell-surface antigen (Trop-2) is a glycoprotein overexpressed in several epithelial cancers, including TNBC, in which it plays the role of the growth-stimulating signal [31]. **Sacituzumab govitecan-hziy** is an **antibody-drug conjugate (ADC)** that combines a humanized monoclonal antibody that targets the Trop-2 with an active metabolite of **irinotecan**, which is a **topoisomerase I inhibitor (SN-38)**, *via* the cleavable linker [31]. Upon binding to Trop-2, the SN-38 is transported to the breast tumor cells. Subsequently, *via* the cleavable linker, the SN-38 is deployed into the tumor itself and the **tumor's microenvironment (TME)** [31].

According to the **ASCENT** trial, the efficacy and safety data of sacituzumab govitecan-hziy (*e.g.*, improved PFS, OS, and durable objective response (DOR)) in heavily pretreated patients with metastatic TNBC have been revealed (Table **1**) [31]. Sacituzumab govitecan has been the first ADC, approved for patients with relapsed or refractory metastatic TNBC (who have failed two prior CHTs) [31].

SELECTED ACTIONABLE PHARMACOLOGIC TARGETS AND EMERGING THERAPIES ON THE HORIZON

There are several emerging therapies, which target the tumor-driving signaling networks in TNBC. For instance, it has been reported that the **phosphoinositide-3 kinase (PI3K)** and **protein kinase B (PKB or AKT)** signaling pathways may represent novel actionable targets in TNBC. In fact, in approximately one-fourth of primary TNBCs, activating mutations (*e.g.*, *PIK3CA* and *AKT1)* occur in these pathways [38]. In an attempt to solve this challenge, PI3K inhibitors have been examined in RCTs and revealed some benefits in patients with advanced TNBC, in whom breast tumors harbored *PIK3CA* mutations [38]. In addition, **the PI3KCA inhibitor, alpelisib,** has improved PFS in patients with hormone receptor (HR)-positive, HER2-negative, *PIK3CA*-mutated advanced or metastatic BC [39].

Similarly, the **AKT inhibitors** (*e.g.*, **ipatasertib** and **capivasertib**) have shown favorable clinical effects with regard to patients with high-risk TNBC [40, 41]. In particular, in the **LOTUS** trial (a phase II RCT) patients with advanced or metastatic TNBC were treated with ipatasertib and paclitaxel *vs.* placebo and paclitaxel. The LOTUS study has reported that women with metastatic TNBC, in the ipatasertib arm had an improved median PFS, compared to the placebo arm (6.2 months *vs.* 4.9 months) [40]. Notably, in the subset of patients with metastatic TNBC and *PIK3CA/AK1/PTEN* mutations, women treated with ipatasertib (and paclitaxel) had a median PFS of 5.3 months *vs.* 3.7 months in those, who received the placebo (and paclitaxel) [40].

Likewise, the **PAKT** trial (a phase II RCT) has examined the efficacy of another **AKT inhibitor, capivasertib,** in combination with the same CHT agent (paclitaxel), compared to a placebo and paclitaxel, in a group of women with untreated metastatic TNBC [41]. Based on the PAKT study report, an addition of capivasertib to paclitaxel resulted in improving the median PFS (5.9 months *vs.* 4.2 months) and OS (19.1 months *vs.* 12.6 months) compared to the paclitaxel alone arm. It should be highlighted that the advantages of capivasertib (with paclitaxel) were even more evident in the subset of women with TNBC, whose tumors harbored *PIK3CA/AK1/PTEN* mutations (*e.g.*,. among these particular patients, a median PFS was 9.3 months *vs.* 3.7 months, in those, who were treated with paclitaxel only) [41].

Notably, the **mesenchymal (M)** subtype of **TNBC** has been related to **abnormal PI3K/ mammalian target of rapamycin (mTOR) pathway** activation and poor clinical outcomes. In this context, adding **the mTOR inhibitors** (*e.g.*, **temsirolimus** or **everolimus**) has been examined, in combination with **CHT** (*e.g.*, a liposomal formulation of doxorubicin) and an anti-**vascular endothelial growth factor (VEGF) antibody (bevacizumab)** [42]. However, these agents are still undergoing clinical investigations, and they have not been incorporated into the standard of care TNBC treatment.

CONCLUSION

In summary, the majority of TNBCs are characterized by a negative or very low AR expression. The AR-negative TNBC represents a highly aggressive QNBC phenotype. Presumably, placing QNBC into a distinct category from the TNBC subtype could be a reasonable step forward. Unfortunately, the absence of expression of ER, PR, AR, and HER2 has reduced, for many years, the TNBC and QNBC pharmacologic treatment options for cytotoxic CHT.

However, at present, in some novel therapies, which target the host immune tumor surveillance system (*e.g.*, *via* PD-L1 and PD-1 **ICI**, such as **atezolizumab** and

pembrolizumab), the damaged DNA repair machinery secondary to ***BRCA1/2*** **mutations** (*e.g.*, **by PARP** inhibitors, like **olaparib** and **talazoparib**), and the Trop-2 (*e.g.*, *via* an **ADC, sacituzumab govitecan-hziy**) represent desirable breakthrough strategies. However, further large-scale clinical studies are necessary to explore these therapies, in various clinical contexts.

- To take advantage of the novel **targeted immune therapies**, women with advanced or **metastatic TNBC** should be tested for the expression of **PD-L1**;
- Patients with advanced or **metastatic TNBC** need to be tested for the presence of germline ***BRCA1/2* mutations** to determine whether or not they would qualify for **PARP inhibitors**, as one of the therapeutic options, which could maximize their chances for improved outcomes;
- It is critically important to **share knowledge** about promising research advances and **clinical applications in the TNBC and QNBC** in the medical communities (*e.g.*, among the physicians, nurses, and other members of treatment teams) and the patients at risk, or afflicted by TNBC or QNBC, as well as their families and caregivers;
- A strong **proactive approach** can help more adequately represent various ethnic groups of women with TNBC or QNBC in future clinical trials, to bridge the gap in the field of research, **diagnosis**, and **therapy** for this devastating female malignancy.

REFERENCES

[1]   Garrido-Castro AC, Lin NU, Polyak K. Insights into molecular classifications of triple-negative breast cancer: Improving patient selection for treatment. Cancer Discov 2019; 9(2): 176-98.
        [http://dx.doi.org/10.1158/2159-8290.CD-18-1177] [PMID: 30679171]

[2]   Kohler BA, Sherman RL, Howlader N, *et al*. Annual report to the nation on the status of cancer, 1975–2011, featuring incidence of breast cancer subtypes by race/ethnicity, poverty, and state. J Natl Cancer Inst 2015; 107(6): djv048.
        [http://dx.doi.org/10.1093/jnci/djv048] [PMID: 25825511]

[3]   Gupta GK, Collier AL, Lee D, *et al*. Perspectives on triple-negative breast cancer: Current treatment strategies, unmet needs, and potential targets for future therapies. Cancers 2020; 12(9): 2392.
        [http://dx.doi.org/10.3390/cancers12092392] [PMID: 32846967]

[4]   Siddharth S, Sharma D. Racial disparity and triple-negative breast cancer in African-American women: A multifaceted affair between obesity, biology, and socioeconomic determinants. Cancers 2018; 10(12): 514.
        [http://dx.doi.org/10.3390/cancers10120514] [PMID: 30558195]

[5]   Bhattarai S, Saini G, Gogineni K, Aneja R. Quadruple-negative breast cancer: Novel implications for a new disease. Breast Cancer Res 2020; 22(1): 127.
        [http://dx.doi.org/10.1186/s13058-020-01369-5] [PMID: 33213491]

[6]   Lehmann BD, Jovanović B, Chen X, *et al*. Refinement of triple-negative breast cancer molecular subtypes: Implications for neoadjuvant chemotherapy selection. PLoS One 2016; 11(6): e0157368.
        [http://dx.doi.org/10.1371/journal.pone.0157368] [PMID: 27310713]

[7]   Burstein MD, Tsimelzon A, Poage GM, *et al*. Comprehensive genomic analysis identifies novel

subtypes and targets of triple-negative breast cancer. Clin Cancer Res 2015; 21(7): 1688-98.
[http://dx.doi.org/10.1158/1078-0432.CCR-14-0432] [PMID: 25208879]

[8]   Echavarria I, López-Tarruella S, Picornell A, *et al.* Pathological response in a triple-negative breast cancer cohort treated with neoadjuvant carboplatin and docetaxel according to Lehmann's refined classification. Clin Cancer Res 2018; 24(8): 1845-52.
[http://dx.doi.org/10.1158/1078-0432.CCR-17-1912] [PMID: 29378733]

[9]   Sharma P. Biology and management of patients with triple-negative breast cancer. Oncologist 2016; 21(9): 1050-62.
[http://dx.doi.org/10.1634/theoncologist.2016-0067] [PMID: 27401886]

[10] Bhattarai S, Klimov S, Mittal K, *et al.* Prognostic role of androgen receptor in triple negative breast cancer: A multi-institutional study. Cancers 2019; 11(7): 995.
[http://dx.doi.org/10.3390/cancers11070995] [PMID: 31319547]

[11] Elebro K, Bendahl PO, Jernström H, Borgquist S. Androgen receptor expression and breast cancer mortality in a population-based prospective cohort. Breast Cancer Res Treat 2017; 165(3): 645-57.
[http://dx.doi.org/10.1007/s10549-017-4343-0] [PMID: 28643022]

[12] Peters AA, Buchanan G, Ricciardelli C, *et al.* Androgen receptor inhibits estrogen receptor-alpha activity and is prognostic in breast cancer. Cancer Res 2009; 69(15): 6131-40.
[http://dx.doi.org/10.1158/0008-5472.CAN-09-0452] [PMID: 19638585]

[13] Hon JD, Singh B, Sahin A, *et al.* Breast cancer molecular subtypes: From TNBC to QNBC. Am J Cancer Res 2016; 6(9): 1864-72.
[PMID: 27725895]

[14] Gucalp A, Tolaney S, Isakoff SJ, *et al.* Phase II trial of bicalutamide in patients with androgen receptor-positive, estrogen receptor-negative metastatic breast cancer. Clin Cancer Res 2013; 19(19): 5505-12.
[http://dx.doi.org/10.1158/1078-0432.CCR-12-3327] [PMID: 23965901]

[15] Traina TA, Miller K, Yardley DA, *et al.* Enzalutamide for the treatment of androgen receptor-expressing triple-negative breast cancer. J Clin Oncol 2018; 36(9): 884-90.
[http://dx.doi.org/10.1200/JCO.2016.71.3495] [PMID: 29373071]

[16] Yu Q, Niu Y, Liu N, *et al.* Expression of androgen receptor in breast cancer and its significance as a prognostic factor. Ann Oncol 2011; 22(6): 1288-94.
[http://dx.doi.org/10.1093/annonc/mdq586] [PMID: 21109569]

[17] Bonnefoi H, Grellety T, Tredan O, *et al.* A phase II trial of abiraterone acetate plus prednisone in patients with triple-negative androgen receptor positive locally advanced or metastatic breast cancer (UCBG 12-1). Ann Oncol 2016; 27(5): 812-8.
[http://dx.doi.org/10.1093/annonc/mdw067] [PMID: 27052658]

[18] Lim B, Seth S, Huo L, *et al.* Comprehensive profiling of androgen receptor-positive (AR+) triple-negative breast cancer (TNBC) patients (pts) treated with standard neoadjuvant therapy (NAT) +/- enzalutamide. J Clin Oncol 2020; 38(15_suppl): 517.
[http://dx.doi.org/10.1200/JCO.2020.38.15_suppl.517]

[19] Dehm SM, Tindall DJ. Alternatively spliced androgen receptor variants. Endocr Relat Cancer 2011; 18(5): R183-96.
[http://dx.doi.org/10.1530/ERC-11-0141] [PMID: 21778211]

[20] Antonarakis ES, Lu C, Wang H, *et al.* AR-V7 and resistance to enzalutamide and abiraterone in prostate cancer. N Engl J Med 2014; 371(11): 1028-38.
[http://dx.doi.org/10.1056/NEJMoa1315815] [PMID: 25184630]

[21] Hickey TE, Robinson JLL, Carroll JS, Tilley WD. Minireview: The androgen receptor in breast tissues: Growth inhibitor, tumor suppressor, oncogene? Mol Endocrinol 2012; 26(8): 1252-67.
[http://dx.doi.org/10.1210/me.2012-1107] [PMID: 22745190]

[22] Barton VN, Christenson JL, Gordon MA, *et al.* Androgen receptor supports an anchorage-independent, cancer stem cell-like population in triple-negative breast cancer. Cancer Res 2017; 77(13): 3455-66.
[http://dx.doi.org/10.1158/0008-5472.CAN-16-3240] [PMID: 28512248]

[23] Gass P, Lux MP, Rauh C, *et al.* Prediction of pathological complete response and prognosis in patients with neoadjuvant treatment for triple-negative breast cancer. BMC Cancer 2018; 18(1): 1051.
[http://dx.doi.org/10.1186/s12885-018-4925-1] [PMID: 30373556]

[24] Pelizzari G, Gerratana L, Basile D, *et al.* Post-neoadjuvant strategies in breast cancer: From risk assessment to treatment escalation. Cancer Treat Rev 2019; 72: 7-14.
[http://dx.doi.org/10.1016/j.ctrv.2018.10.014] [PMID: 30414986]

[25] Angajala A, Mothershed E, Davis MB, *et al.* Quadruple negative breast cancers (qnbc) demonstrate subtype consistency among primary and recurrent or metastatic breast cancer. Transl Oncol 2019; 12(3): 493-501.
[http://dx.doi.org/10.1016/j.tranon.2018.11.008] [PMID: 30594038]

[26] Schmid P, Rugo HS, Adams S, *et al.* Atezolizumab plus nab-paclitaxel as first-line treatment for unresectable, locally advanced or metastatic triple-negative breast cancer (IMpassion130): Updated efficacy results from a randomised, double-blind, placebo-controlled, phase 3 trial. Lancet Oncol 2020; 21(1): 44-59.
[http://dx.doi.org/10.1016/S1470-2045(19)30689-8] [PMID: 31786121]

[27] Schmid P, Cortes J, Pusztai L, *et al.* Pembrolizumab for early triple-negative breast cancer. N Engl J Med 2020; 382(9): 810-21.
[http://dx.doi.org/10.1056/NEJMoa1910549] [PMID: 32101663]

[28] Cortes J, Cescon DW, Rugo HS, *et al.* Pembrolizumab plus chemotherapy versus placebo plus chemotherapy for previously untreated locally recurrent inoperable or metastatic triple-negative breast cancer (KEYNOTE-355): A randomised, placebo-controlled, double-blind, phase 3 clinical trial. Lancet 2020; 396(10265): 1817-28.
[http://dx.doi.org/10.1016/S0140-6736(20)32531-9] [PMID: 33278935]

[29] Robson ME, Tung N, Conte P, *et al.* OlympiAD final overall survival and tolerability results: Olaparib versus chemotherapy treatment of physician's choice in patients with a germline BRCA mutation and HER2-negative metastatic breast cancer. Ann Oncol 2019; 30(4): 558-66.
[http://dx.doi.org/10.1093/annonc/mdz012] [PMID: 30689707]

[30] Litton JK, Rugo HS, Ettl J, *et al.* Talazoparib in patients with advanced breast cancer and a germline BRCA mutation. N Engl J Med 2018; 379(8): 753-63.
[http://dx.doi.org/10.1056/NEJMoa1802905] [PMID: 30110579]

[31] Bardia A, Mayer IA, Vahdat LT. Sacituzumab govitecan-hziy in refractory metastatic triple-negative breast cancer. N Engl J Med 2019; 380(8): 741-51.
[http://dx.doi.org/10.1056/NEJMoa1814213] [PMID: 30786188]

[32] Killock D. Chemotherapy as a TONIC to invigorate PD-1 inhibition in TNBC. Nat Rev Clin Oncol 2019; 16(8): 464.
[http://dx.doi.org/10.1038/s41571-019-0232-2] [PMID: 31114036]

[33] Thomas R, Al-Khadairi G, Decock J. Immune checkpoint inhibitors in triple negative breast cancer treatment: Promising future prospects. Front Oncol 2021; 10: 600573.
[http://dx.doi.org/10.3389/fonc.2020.600573] [PMID: 33718107]

[34] Marra A, Viale G, Curigliano G. Recent advances in triple negative breast cancer: The immunotherapy era. BMC Med 2019; 17(1): 90.
[http://dx.doi.org/10.1186/s12916-019-1326-5] [PMID: 31068190]

[35] Hatano Y, Tamada M, Matsuo M, Hara A. Molecular trajectory of BRCA1 and BRCA2 mutations. Front Oncol 2020; 10: 361.

[http://dx.doi.org/10.3389/fonc.2020.00361] [PMID: 32269964]

[36]   McCann KE, Hurvitz SA. Advances in the use of PARP inhibitor therapy for breast cancer. Drugs Context 2018; 7: 1-30.
[http://dx.doi.org/10.7573/dic.212540] [PMID: 30116283]

[37]   Shi Y, Jin J, Ji W, Guan X. Therapeutic landscape in mutational triple negative breast cancer. Mol Cancer 2018; 17(1): 99.
[http://dx.doi.org/10.1186/s12943-018-0850-9] [PMID: 30007403]

[38]   Pascual J, Turner NC. Targeting the PI3-kinase pathway in triple-negative breast cancer. Ann Oncol 2019; 30(7): 1051-60.
[http://dx.doi.org/10.1093/annonc/mdz133] [PMID: 31050709]

[39]   André F, Ciruelos E, Rubovszky G, *et al.* Alpelisib for PIK3CA-mutated, hormone receptor-positive advanced breast cancer. N Engl J Med 2019; 380(20): 1929-40.
[http://dx.doi.org/10.1056/NEJMoa1813904] [PMID: 31091374]

[40]   Kim SB, Dent R, Im SA, *et al.* Ipatasertib plus paclitaxel versus placebo plus paclitaxel as first-line therapy for metastatic triple-negative breast cancer (LOTUS): A multicentre, randomised, double-blind, placebo-controlled, phase 2 trial. Lancet Oncol 2017; 18(10): 1360-72.
[http://dx.doi.org/10.1016/S1470-2045(17)30450-3] [PMID: 28800861]

[41]   Schmid P, Abraham J, Chan S, *et al.* Capivasertib plus paclitaxel versus placebo plus paclitaxel as first-line therapy for metastatic triple-negative breast cancer: The PAKT trial. J Clin Oncol 2020; 38(5): 423-33.
[http://dx.doi.org/10.1200/JCO.19.00368] [PMID: 31841354]

[42]   Basho RK, Gilcrease M, Murthy RK, *et al.* Targeting the PI3K/AKT/mTOR pathway for the treatment of mesenchymal triple-negative breast cancer. JAMA Oncol 2017; 3(4): 509-15.
[http://dx.doi.org/10.1001/jamaoncol.2016.5281] [PMID: 27893038]

CHAPTER 3

Liquid Biopsy: Insights Into Monitoring Tumor Dynamics and Response to Therapy in Patients with Breast Cancer

Abstract: The ability to identify the molecular features of metastatic breast cancer (BC) provides a unique insight into a patient's therapeutic options and the opportunity to follow the BC progress over time. A classical **tissue biopsy** remains the standard procedure to describe tumor biology and guide treatment choices.

However, a **liquid biopsy**, which can provide medical practitioners with the opportunity to **detect genomic mutations** and **monitor therapeutic effect**s, can play a prominent role in the diagnosis, therapy, and prognosis of patients with different malignancies, including metastatic BC. In fact, the liquid-biopsy-based therapeutic interventions led to the approval of **alpelisib (a PI3K inhibitor)** in patients with **hormone receptor (HR)-positive, human epidermal growth factor receptor2 (HER2)-negative,** advanced or **metastatic BC**, in whom BC had progressed on or after therapy with an **aromatase inhibitor (AI)**.

This chapter describes a **liquid biopsy in BC**. It explores its potential for clinical applications in early **diagnosis, monitoring treatment response, detecting minimal residual lesions, predicting risk of progression** or **recurrence,** and **estimating prognosis**. It compares a **liquid biopsy** with a **tissue biopsy**, and outlines the **benefits** and **limitations** of each of these procedures, focusing on patients with metastatic BC. Moreover, this chapter analyses the results from recent studies relevant to liquid biopsies in BC (*e.g.,* **circulating tumor cells (CTCs)** and **circulating tumor DNA (ctDNA))**.

Keywords: Alpelisib (A PI3K Inhibitor), Breast cancer (BC), Circulating tumor cells (CTCs), Circulating tumor DNA (ctDNA), Liquid biopsy, Targeted therapy.

INTRODUCTION

A classical **tissue biopsy** still remains the standard procedure to assess **tumor biology** and **guide treatment choices** in patients with cancer [1]. Recently, it has been suggested that **liquid biopsy** provides some valuable **insights into malignant tumor dynamics,** and thus, it can play a **beneficial role in personalized oncology management**.

At present, many research efforts are being made to understand how to use **liquid biopsy** as a surveillance instrument for women with **breast cancer (BC)**. However, a lot of work still needs to be done before applying **liquid biopsy** as a standard tool to clinical practice. According to a recent systematic review, **liquid biopsy** has been particularly useful for the early **detection of genomic mutations** and **timely monitoring of the treatment effects** [1]. Such information may be skillfully combined with the **traditional tumor tissue biopsy** to allow physicians to make the most accurate **decisions** regarding possible **targeted therapy** options, in given clinical contexts. However, the liquid biopsy has some **limitations** for its common use in clinical practice (*e.g.*, a liquid biopsy may not be sensitive enough to detect some relevant mutations), and thus, it **has not yet been incorporated into routine clinical diagnostics** for patients with malignancies [1]. Nevertheless, the liquid biopsy, as a potential **diagnostic** and **prognostic aid**, has a great chance to become a valuable tool for the management of women with metastatic **BC** [1].

In brief, a **liquid biopsy** is a process of **obtaining tumor-derived materials,** including DNA, RNA, intact tumor cells, or extracellular vesicles from body fluids such as blood, urine, saliva, stool, or cerebrospinal fluid [2]. Currently, the progress in highly sensitive assays, which can identify a very small amount of tumor-derived materials, in the body fluids, has augmented the significance of liquid biopsy as a reasonable modality that can be added to traditional tumor biopsy (*e.g.*, in women with metastatic BC) [2]. In particular, a liquid biopsy allows for the detection of **circulating tumor cells (CTCs)** and **circulating tumor DNA (ctDNA)** in the circulating blood (plasma fraction) [2]. It is a noninvasive or only mini-invasive procedure since such materials are obtained *via* a blood draw or body fluid collection. Moreover, it represents a convenient and attractive methodology, for both the patients and the medical staff [2]. Some other remarkable benefits include its ability to "decipher" the puzzle **of tumor heterogeneity**, *via* sampling the entire genome of the tumor [2]. In addition, it can be repeated over time, enabling long-term monitoring of the malignant tumor, together with its reactions to the applied antineoplastic therapies (Fig. **1**) [2].

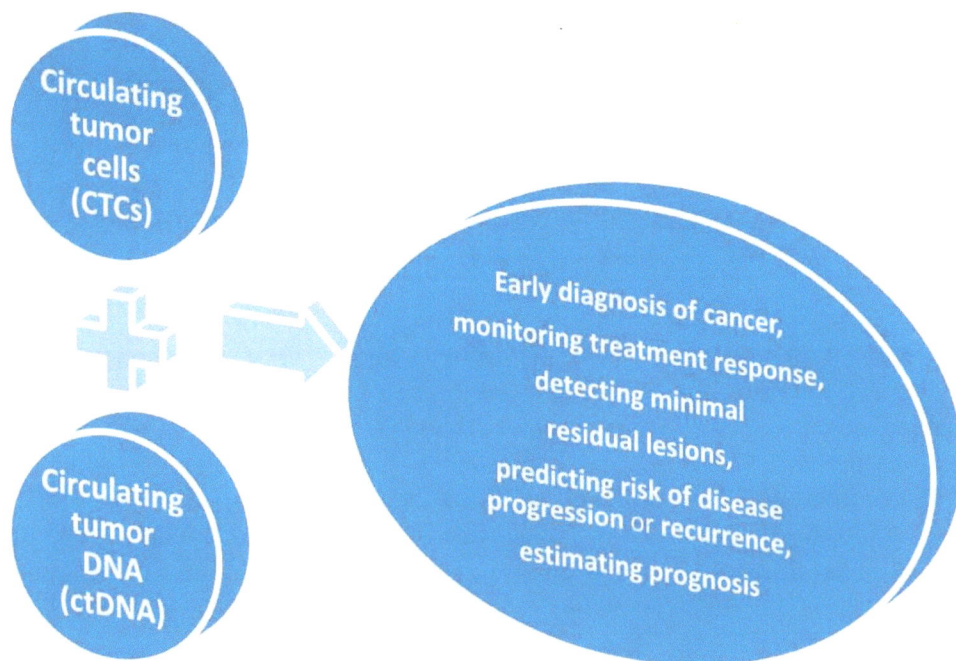

Fig. (1). Exemplary applications of liquid biopsy in the management of patients with cancer.

The aim of this chapter is to present the potential of **liquid biopsy** in patients with metastatic **BC** and explore its clinical applications (*e.g.*, for early **diagnosis, monitoring treatment response, detecting minimal residual lesions, predicting risk of disease progression** or **recurrence,** and **estimating prognosis**). In addition, this chapter compares a **liquid biopsy** with a **tissue biopsy**, and outlines **the benefits** and **limitations** of each of these procedures, for patients with metastatic BC. Moreover, it analyses the results from recent studies relevant to liquid biopsies in BC, focusing on **circulating tumor cells (CTCs)** and **circulating tumor DNA (ctDNA)**.

HOW LIQUID BIOPSY CAN BE USED IN MONITORING METASTATIC BC PROGRESSION AND TREATMENT?

Recently, the US **Food and Drug Administration (FDA)** approved the first companion diagnostic test, **Therascreen PIK3CA RGQ polymerase chain reaction assay,** for tissue and liquid biopsies [3, 4]. In short, the **therascreen PIK3CA RGQ PCR** is a laboratory test used to detect 11 mutations in the *PIK3CA* gene in tumor tissue or in the blood, obtained from patients with advanced or metastatic BC. In BC tissue, mutations in the *PIK3CA* gene create an altered form of the PIK3CA protein, leading to its abnormal functioning [3, 4]. Since the **therascreen** can detect *PIK3CA* gene mutations in patients' **ctDNA, it can help** determine whether or not these patients should receive a targeted therapy for these genetic alterations, such as the **PI3K inhibitor, alpelisib,** along with **the endocrine therapy (ET)** agent, **fulvestrant** [3, 4]. If *PIK3CA* mutations are not detected in the plasma specimens of patients with advanced or **metastatic BC,** then the patient's eligibility for treatment with **alpelisib** needs to be determined *via* testing the tumor tissue sample [3, 4].

In addition, the US FDA approved two other liquid biopsy tests, known as **Guardant360 CDx** [4], and **FoundationOne Liquid CDx** [5]. It should be noted that in the **Guardant360 CDx** the concordance between this new test and the traditional tissue testing was greater than 90% (for the four biomarkers corresponding with FDA-approved therapies) [4]. In addition, the turnaround time was approximately one week faster with the use of Guardant360 CDx compared to the standard-of-care (SOC) tissue test [4]. Another FDA-approved test, **FoundationOne Liquid CDx**, is a companion diagnostic that analyzes over 300 genes and can help guide treatment strategies and predict patients' responses [5].

TRANSLATING A LEARNING EXPERIENCE FROM THE SOLAR-1 TRIAL INTO CLINICAL PRACTICE: THE APPROVAL OF ALPELISIB AND THERASCREEN

SOLAR-1 (NCT02437318) is a **randomized, controlled trial (RCT)** (a phase 3), of **alpelisib** plus **fulvestrant** *vs.* **placebo** plus **fulvestrant** conducted in 572 patients (*e.g.*, mostly postmenopausal women, with HR-positive, HER2-negative, advanced or metastatic BC, in whom BC had progressed on or after therapy with an **aromatase inhibitor (AI))** [6]. In **SOLAR-1,** the **therascreen**, as a **companion diagnostic test** was applied to mark the early stages of using liquid biopsy to match the target treatment to genetic abnormalities in metastatic BC. Based on the **SOLAR-1** data, it was found that the **PI3K inhibitor, alpelisib,** plus the **endocrine therapy (ET) agent, fulvestrant** almost doubled the **progression-free survival (PFS)** (11 *vs.* 5.7 months in the placebo-fulvestrant group) in women with *PIK3CA*-mutated, hormone receptor (HR)-positive, human epidermal growth factor receptor2 (HER2)-negative, advanced or metastatic BC, and thus, the **alpelisib** and **therascreen** were then approved by the **FDA**, for patients with *PIK3CA*-mutated, HR-positive, HER2-negative advanced or metastatic BC (Fig. **2**) [6].

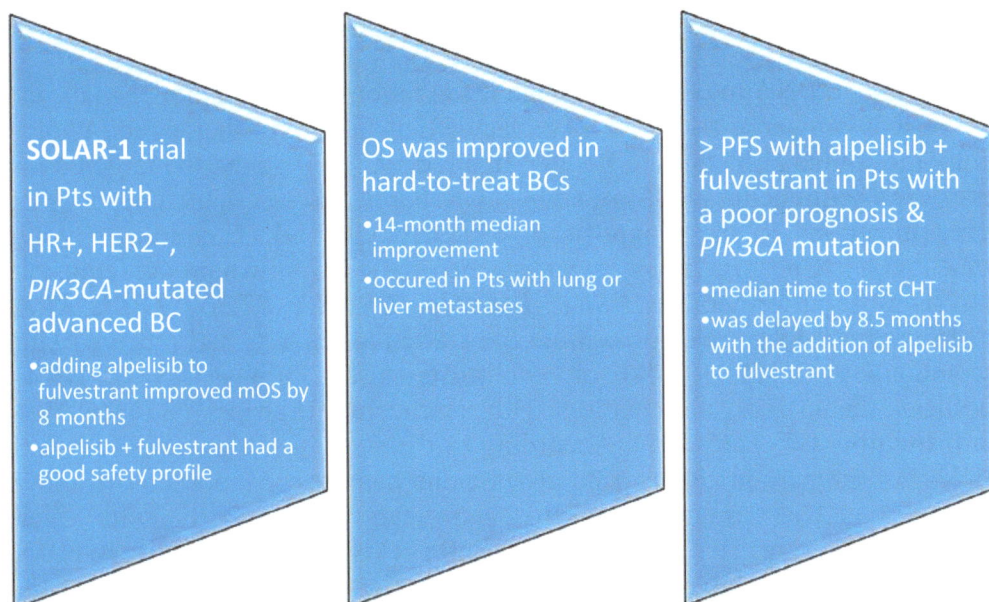

Fig. (2).   The main practical messages from the SOLAR-1 trial. mOS, median overall survival; PFS, progression-free survival; Pts, patients; BC, breast cancer; CHT, chemotherapy; HR+, hormone receptor-positive; HER2−, human epidermal growth factor receptor-2-negative.

A key message conveyed from this trial to a "real life" clinical practice is that detecting a patient's targetable mutations (*e.g.*, *PIK3CA*) represents now the main application of liquid biopsy. As a consequence, eligible patients could be offered both the tissue and liquid biopsy at the time of their metastatic BC diagnosis. Such a complementary use of the tissue and liquid biopsy tests may allow a more comprehensive insight into a patient's personalized case management [6]. An invasive tissue biopsy enables targeting of a spectrum of BC biomarkers, while a less invasive liquid biopsy permits to follow the BC evolution and to monitor patients' treatment response over time. As a result, this approach can allow for the detection of signs of BC recurrence prior to the development of metastatic lesions [6, 7]. Therefore, depending on a given patient's context, a possible blending of these two tests appears beneficial, and merits exploration in further clinical trials [6, 7].

AN IMPORTANCE OF CTDNA MUTATIONAL ANALYSIS IN THE MANAGEMENT OF PATIENTS WITH METASTATIC BC

Some studies focused on fluctuations of **ctDNA** levels, during the course of BC, have shown their correlations with the response to treatment. For instance, an early increase in **ctDNA,** which represents an independent biomarker of BC progression, prior to detectable radiologic or clinical signs of malignant progression, may be a "warning signal" for some women with metastatic BC [8].

Furthermore, ctDNA may offer valuable information about mutational analysis of ctDNA that can serve as a predictive factor that facilitates therapeutic choices, during the course of metastatic BC [9]. In a recent, small study, the targeted **next generation sequencing (NGS)** of ctDNA was applied to assess the impact of BC-driven mutations on the prognosis of metastatic BC [9]. This study involved women with ER-positive, HER2-negative metastatic BC, in whom the sequencing analysis was performed for *ESR1, PIK3CA, ERBB2, PTEN, TP53, KRAS, HRAS,* and *NRAS* [9]. As a baseline, the study participants had received either chemotherapy (**CHT**) (34%) or **cyclin-dependent kinase 4/6 (CDK4/6) inhibitor** therapy in combination with **endocrine therapy (ET) (CDK4/6 inhibitor plus ET)** (66%) [9]. According to the study findings, over two-thirds (64.4%) of the participants carried at least one pathogenic mutation. Moreover, numerous **ctDNA** mutations were significantly associated with worse **progression-free survival (PFS)** and **overall survival (OS)**. In addition, **ctDNA** load (meaning the number of mutant ctDNA molecules per one mL of plasma), was significantly correlated with PFS and OS. Also, the mutational status of *ESR1* and *TP53* predicted PFS and OS, in a statistically significant manner. These findings indicate an important clinical value of **ctDNA** mutational analysis in the management of patients with metastatic BC [9].

CIRCULATING TUMOR DNA ANALYSIS TO HELP DIRECT THERAPY IN ADVANCED BC (PLASMAMATCH): THE UNIQUE TOOL TO IDENTIFY SENSITIVITY

The recent Plasma Based Molecular Profiling of Advanced Breast Cancer to Inform Therapeutic Choices (plasmaMATCH) (a phase 2) platform trial (NCT03182634), focused on ctDNA testing, is in line with a potential future "adoption" into a diagnostic work-up in the clinical practice [10]. It offers rapid genotyping that allows the selection of mutation-directed therapies (*e.g.*, targeted therapies against rare *HER2* and *AKT1* mutations). The results of the plasmaMATCH study have confirmed that these mutations could be targetable for BC treatment [10]. With regard to predicting responses to treatment, the **plasmaMATCH trial** [10] evaluated ctDNA in over a thousand women with advanced BC for mutations in ESR1, HER2, and AKT1 (*via* **polymerase chain reaction (PCR)** and Guardant360 CDx).

The results have shown that over one-third of the study patients had potentially targetable aberrations. An agreement between the PCR and Guardant360 CDx testing was 96%-99%, and the liquid biopsy showed 93% sensitivity (compared with tumor biopsy). In addition, the liquid biopsy findings were used to match the participants' mutations to targeted therapies (*e.g.*, **fulvestrant** - for the ones with ESR1 mutations, **neratinib** - for those with HER2 mutations, and the selective AKT inhibitor, **capivasertib**,- for those with ER–positive tumors with *AKT1* mutations). The results of the **plasmaMATCH trial** indicate that ctDNA testing can provide an accurate tumor genotyping, which is compatible with the tissue biopsy.

This suggests that ctDNA testing is suitable for a "real-life" clinical practice. In essence, ctDNA testing allows for the detection of relatively common (*e.g.*, *ESR1*) and rare (*e.g.*, *HER2* and *AKT1*) genetic mutations. Therefore, it can precisely guide therapeutic choices, especially in some difficult clinical cases, which involve about 5% of women with advanced BC [10].

AN IMPACT OF THE LIQUID BIOPSY ON THE PERSONALIZED TREATMENT OF WOMEN WITH METASTATIC BC

Another recent study has shown that liquid biopsy can identify clinically relevant *ESR1* mutations, which are prevalent in women with newly diagnosed metastatic BC and local recurrence of BC that was treated with ET [11]. The *ESR1* mutations may subsequently guide the treatment selection [11]. Furthermore, it should be emphasized that according to a recent study, the **NGS** of ctDNA, in patients with HR-positive metastatic BC, HER2-positive metastatic BC, or triple-negative breast cancer (TNBC) the *ESR1* mutations were detected in 14% of the study participants [12].

Notably, the *ESR1* mutations were found only in women with **HR-positive** BC, who had already obtained ET. In addition, this study investigated *PIK3CA* mutations, which occurred in about 30% of the participants. It was also shown that the *ESR1* mutations were correlated with hepatic and bone metastases [12]. Importantly, this trial has revealed some differences in tumor biology across *ESR1* and *PIK3CA* genetic variants [12].

Useful Ways of Predicting the Patients' Survival and BC Recurrence

It should be highlighted that a liquid biopsy can be helpful for predicting patient outcomes and monitoring for early signs of BC recurrence (prior to the occurrence of overt metastatic lesions) [13]. Following tumor mutations *via* plasma circulating **cell-free DNA** variants **(cfDNA)** can augment the detection of **minimal residual disease (MRD)** (Fig. **3**) [13]. In the clinical setting, optimal systemic therapy for women with an early-stage BC still represents an unmet need. In an attempt to overcome this challenging issue, a study exploring an ultrasensitive blood test for **MRD** was conducted, aimed at identifying patients, who could take advantage of the use of additional systemic therapy (**escalation** group) *vs.* no additional systemic therapy (**de-escalation** group). According to the study findings, it has been revealed that this blood test for **MRD** was 100-fold more sensitive than the **droplet digital PCR** test. However, its sensitivity depends on the number of mutations available to assess in cfDNA. Notably, the MRD detection in the study participants (treated for an early-stage BC in the postoperative period, and one-year post-surgery) was related to distant BC recurrence. Importantly, clinical sensitivity was highest among patients, who had most mutations identified from their tissue biopsies, which had assessed **cfDNA**. This approach might guide future, personalized therapeutic interventions, in patients, who would otherwise develop metastatic BC recurrence [13]. However, further studies on this topic are necessary.

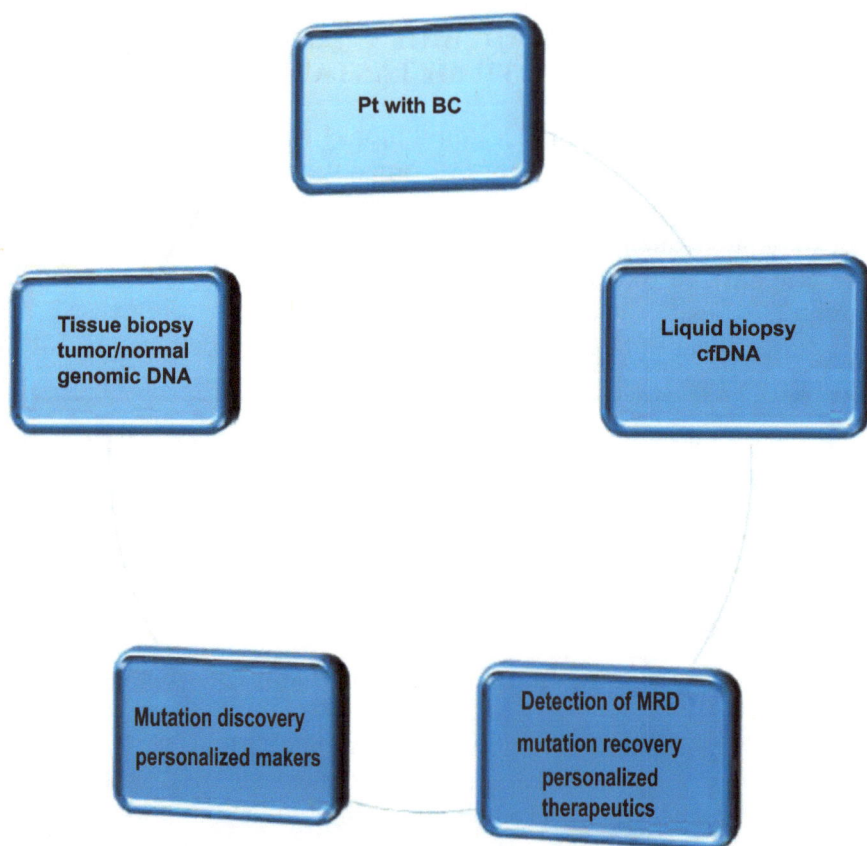

Fig. (3). Detection of Minimal Residual Disease in Patients Treated for Early-Stage Breast Cancer. BC, Breast Cancer; cfDNA cfDNA, cell-free DNA; MRD, Minimal Residual Disease; Pt, Patient.

Can the Circulating Tumor Cell (CTC) Count be Used for a Selection of the First-line Therapy (CHT or ET) in Women with HR–positive, HER2-negative Metastatic BC?

Traditionally, the choice between CHT and ET as first-line treatment for HR–positive, HER2-negative metastatic BC depends on the presence of clinical factors related to a poor BC prognosis. However, based on an earlier study in this area, it was reported that patients with metastatic BC who had ≥5 CTCs/7.5 mL of whole blood, prior to receiving the first-line therapy had a much shorter median OS (10 *vs.* > 18 months) and PFS (2.7 *vs.* 7.0 months) than those with <5 CTCs/7.5 mL [14]. Therefore, it was suggested that the number of CTCs before treatment can serve as an independent predictor of OS and PFS, in patients with metastatic BC [14].

Similarly, based on the results of a recent **STIC CTC** RCT (NCT01710605), the CTC count can be considered to be a valuable biomarker for making a therapeutic decision with regard to the CHT and single-agent ET, as the first-line treatment in patients with HR–positive, HER2-negative metastatic BC [15]. This RCT (phase 3) was aimed to compare the efficacy of a clinician-driven treatment choice (the control arm) *vs.* the CTC-driven choice (in which, patients received CHT or ET, based on the CTC count, as follows: CHT if ≥5 CTCs/7.5 mL or ET if <5 CTCs/7.5 mL, for the first-line treatment). Findings from this RCT have revealed that the CTC count can be a reliable biomarker for guiding the therapeutic choice between CHT and ET (as the first-line treatment in HR–positive, HER2-negative metastatic BC). In this scenario, an elevated CTC count (≥5 CTCs/7.5 mL) was a strong negative prognostic factor for OS and PFS [15].

Can ctDNA Monitoring During the Neoadjuvant Chemotherapy (CHT) Course Reveal a Patient's Risk for Distant BC Metastases?

Similarly, in a retrospective study, patients who remained **ctDNA**-positive after three weeks of neoadjuvant CHT were more prone to have residual BC, after completion of this therapy than those, who cleared ctDNA at the early stage of their therapeutic course. It should be underscored that the presence of ctDNA in the period between the start and completion of treatment was correlated with a higher risk for BC metastatic recurrence. In contrast, the clearance of **ctDNA** during or after neoadjuvant CHT use was related to better patient survival [16].

Can Lack of ctDNA Clearance in Early Period of Neoadjuvant Chemotherapy (NAC) be a Predictor of Poor Response to Treatment?

It should be underscored that detectable ctDNA levels during **Neoadjuvant Chemotherapy (NAC)** have been associated with poor patient outcomes. In practical terms, a failure to clear ctDNA after NAC has been correlated with worse **disease-free survival (DFS)**. In contrast, the clearance of ctDNA has been associated with improved survival, even in patients who did not achieve **pathological complete response (pCR)** [16]. Therefore, personalized monitoring of ctDNA during NAC, among high-risk patients with early BC, may help in the ongoing evaluation of therapeutic response and enable to the refinement of pCR as a surrogate measure of survival [16]. In patients with **post-NAC residual TNBC**, more than a quarter exhibited a detectable amount of ctDNA after curative surgery and ctDNA kinetics can serve as a biomarker for optimizing adjuvant treatment [17].

Similarly, it has been indicated that monitoring patients' ctDNA levels after NAC and surgery may help predict their risk for relapse and progression to metastatic BC stages [18]. A study that monitored a small group of women with BC after surgery, revealed that the ongoing ctDNA testing contributed to an accurate differentiation between the women, who ultimately developed metastatic BC *vs.* those, who might have a long-term **DFS** (with 93% sensitivity and 100% specificity) [18]. For instance, no ctDNA was detectable at any time-point after surgery, among patients with long-term DFS. In addition, **ctDNA** test detected metastatic BC almost one year earlier than the imaging studies, for over 80% of the study patients [18]. Moreover, serial measurements of ctDNA have been shown to be quite accurate biomarkers for the occult metastatic BC lesions, in women with **primary (non-metastatic)** BC. This indicates that the sequential ctDNA levels represent valuable quantitative risk factors for adverse patient outcomes [18]. However, further trials to address these issues are needed.

How to Predict the BC Metastatic Relapse Before the Clinical Recurrence?

Predicting whether or not a patient with **BC** will have a relapse still remains very challenging. At present, ctDNA circulating in the blood may provide some hints about possible residual BC. In particular, malignant cells, which have survived anticancer treatments, can initiate the development of new BC tumors. In an attempt to help solve this clinical problem, a personalized ctDNA assay was developed [19]. This ctDNA test was based on **digital PCR** to follow genetic mutations over time, in women with early-stage BC, who had obtained curative treatments (*e.g.*, surgery or CHT). The study findings have revealed that the serial mutation tracking was able to accurately predict BC metastatic relapse, on average by eight months before the clinical relapse. This early prediction may help introduce some specific treatment interventions, prior to the reappearance of malignancy, especially in high-risk patients with BC [19].

CONCLUSION

A **liquid biopsy** can serve as a **tool to monitor patients with cancer** and **predict, who will have a desirable response to treatment *vs.* resistance to therapy** (that should be immediately addressed by a treatment team).

Fortunately, the landscape of BC today differs significantly from the one in the past years. At present, **ctDNA, CTCs,** and **NGS** play a promising role in "fine-tuning" the diagnosis, monitoring, and treatment of cancer, as well as in gaining new knowledge about **tumor biology,** and **its multifactorial causes,** and **possible preventive strategies**.

Due to recent advances in technologies, which can isolate a minute amount of tumor-derived materials, liquid biopsies can play an increasing **role in personalized care for many women with metastatic BC**.

It should be underscored that a great advantage of liquid biopsy is its **ability to detect molecular alterations before imaging studies can show any suspicious lesions or overt clinical symptoms** that may appear. In this way, a liquid biopsy can identify those women, who have an increased risk of BC recurrence. Moreover, a chance to prevent metastatic BC, *via* finding **minimal residual disease (MRD)** at its early stages, is one of the most remarkable features of liquid biopsy. This approach may favorably change the course of BC for many afflicted women.

Although an increasing number of studies show that **ctDNA** and **CTCs are prognostic for BC recurrence**, a big dilemma still exists, in relation to the patients with elevated levels of ctDNA or CTCs, but without the evidence of overt BC, based on imaging studies or clinical evaluation. Whether or not the therapy, based on the results of liquid biopsy, will prevent or delay the development of metastatic BC, or will positively affect the survival and quality of life would require future, large-scale prospective studies, in various populations of women with metastatic BC.

It is encouraging that the **SOLAR-1** trial, which led to the approval of **alpelisib** (the **PI3K inhibitor**) and **therascreen** (the companion diagnostic test), found that the PI3K inhibitor plus fulvestrant almost doubled progression-free survival (PFS) (11 *vs.* 5.7 months in the placebo-fulvestrant group) in patients with *PIK3CA*-mutated, HR-positive, HER2-negative advanced BC.

In addition, **lack of ctDNA clearance** was a significant predictor of poor response to treatment and BC metastatic recurrence, while **clearance of ctDNA** was associated with improved survival even in patients who did not achieve pCR.

Therefore, personalized monitoring of ctDNA during NAC of high-risk patients with early BC may help in the ongoing evaluation of therapeutic response and can refine pCR as a surrogate measure of survival.

Hopefully, in the future, the **liquid biopsy** will shed more light on the genetic events driving BC metastases and will enable researchers and physicians to timely analyze the clinically important data, which can precisely guide the diagnosis and therapy, as well as predict the prognosis of numerous patients with a **metastatic BC**.

Liquid biopsies have revealed some promising results in the management of patients with **metastatic BC**.

- The modern diagnostic methods, including new molecular testing and **liquid biopsy, facilitate a choice of personalized anticancer treatments**, which are available today.
- Liquid biopsies in BC are promising, particularly in **monitoring treatment response** and **predicting disease progression or relapse** in numerous patients with BC.
- With continued advancements in isolation tumor-derived materials, liquid biopsies may play a key role in BC clinical management.
- Many large analyses confirmed that the **elevated CTC counts are independent prognostic factors** in several patients with BC.
- **High CTC** numbers during systemic treatment are associated with an **early BC progression**.
- The **ctDNA-driven therapy** selection has been approved in clinical practice, and **alpelisib** was the first targeted treatment indicated on the basis of a ctDNA test.
- CTCs and ctDNA can predict clinical outcomes and have the potential to improve personalized therapy choices in metastatic BC.
- It has been shown that the presence of **ctDNA in plasma after NAC and surgery** was able to **predict a metastatic BC relapse** by almost eight months prior to the BC clinical manifestations.
- The latest developments in this area offer new **hope to many women afflicted by the most aggressive types of BC.**

REFERENCES

[1]   Arneth B. Update on the types and usage of liquid biopsies in the clinical setting: A systematic review. BMC Cancer 2018; 18(1): 527.
        [http://dx.doi.org/10.1186/s12885-018-4433-3] [PMID: 29728089]

[2]   Tay TKY, Tan PH. Liquid biopsy in breast cancer: A focused review. Arch Pathol Lab Med 2021; 145(6): 678-86.
        [http://dx.doi.org/10.5858/arpa.2019-0559-RA] [PMID: 32045277]

[3]   Banys-Paluchowski M, Fehm TN, Grimm-Glang D, Rody A, Krawczyk N. Liquid Biopsy in metastatic breast cancer: current role of circulating tumor cells and circulating tumor DNA. Oncol Res Treat 2022; 45(1-2): 4-11.
[http://dx.doi.org/10.1159/000520561] [PMID: 34718243]

[4]   Guardant 360 CDx. Available at: https://www.fda.gov/news-events/press-announcements/fda-approves-first-liquid-biopsy-next-generation-sequencing-companion-diagnostic-test (Accessed on: 2022).

[5]   FoundationOne Liquid CDx. Available at: https://www.foundationmedicine.com/test/foundationone-liquid-cdx (Accessed on: 2022).

[6]   André F, Ciruelos EM, Juric D, *et al.* Alpelisib plus fulvestrant for PIK3CA-mutated, hormone receptor-positive, human epidermal growth factor receptor-2–negative advanced breast cancer: Final overall survival results from SOLAR-1. Ann Oncol 2021; 32(2): 208-17.
[http://dx.doi.org/10.1016/j.annonc.2020.11.011] [PMID: 33246021]

[7]   Banys-Paluchowski M, Krawczyk N, Fehm T. Liquid biopsy in breast cancer. Geburtshilfe Frauenheilkd 2020; 80(11): 1093-104.
[http://dx.doi.org/10.1055/a-1124-7225] [PMID: 33173237]

[8]   Velimirovic M, Juric D, Niemierko A, *et al.* Rising circulating tumor dna as a molecular biomarker of early disease progression in metastatic breast cancer. JCO Precis Oncol 2020; 4(4): 1246-62.
[http://dx.doi.org/10.1200/PO.20.00117] [PMID: 35050782]

[9]   Muendlein A, Geiger K, Gaenger S, *et al.* Significant impact of circulating tumour DNA mutations on survival in metastatic breast cancer patients. Sci Rep 2021; 11(1): 6761.
[http://dx.doi.org/10.1038/s41598-021-86238-7] [PMID: 33762647]

[10]   Turner NC, Kingston B, Kilburn LS, *et al.* Circulating tumour DNA analysis to direct therapy in advanced breast cancer (plasmaMATCH): A multicentre, multicohort, phase 2a, platform trial. Lancet Oncol 2020; 21(10): 1296-308.
[http://dx.doi.org/10.1016/S1470-2045(20)30444-7] [PMID: 32919527]

[11]   Zundelevich A, Dadiani M, Kahana-Edwin S, *et al.* ESR1 mutations are frequent in newly diagnosed metastatic and loco-regional recurrence of endocrine-treated breast cancer and carry worse prognosis. Breast Cancer Res 2020; 22(1): 16.
[http://dx.doi.org/10.1186/s13058-020-1246-5] [PMID: 32014063]

[12]   Gerratana L, Davis AA, Velimirovic M, *et al.* Uncovering the differential impact of *ESR1* and *PIK3CA* codon variants on the clinical phenotype of metastatic breast cancer (MBC) through circulating tumor DNA (ctDNA) next-generation sequencing (NGS). J Clin Oncol 2021; 39(15_suppl): 1033-3.
[http://dx.doi.org/10.1200/JCO.2021.39.15_suppl.1033]

[13]   Parsons HA, Rhoades J, Reed SC, *et al.* Sensitive detection of minimal residual disease in patients treated for early-stage breast cancer. Clin Cancer Res 2020; 26(11): 2556-64.
[http://dx.doi.org/10.1158/1078-0432.CCR-19-3005] [PMID: 32170028]

[14]   Cristofanilli M, Budd GT, Ellis MJ, *et al.* Circulating tumor cells, disease progression, and survival in metastatic breast cancer. N Engl J Med 2004; 351(8): 781-91.
[http://dx.doi.org/10.1056/NEJMoa040766] [PMID: 15317891]

[15]   Bidard FC, Jacot W, Kiavue N, *et al.* Efficacy of circulating tumor cell count–driven *vs.* clinician-driven first-line therapy choice in hormone receptor–positive, erbb2-negative metastatic breast cancer. JAMA Oncol 2021; 7(1): 34-41.
[http://dx.doi.org/10.1001/jamaoncol.2020.5660] [PMID: 33151266]

[16]   Magbanua MJM, Swigart LB, Wu HT, *et al.* Circulating tumor DNA in neoadjuvant-treated breast cancer reflects response and survival. Ann Oncol 2021; 32(2): 229-39.
[http://dx.doi.org/10.1016/j.annonc.2020.11.007] [PMID: 33232761]

[17] Kim H, Kim YJ, Park D, *et al.* Dynamics of circulating tumor DNA during postoperative radiotherapy in patients with residual triple-negative breast cancer following neoadjuvant chemotherapy: A prospective observational study. Breast Cancer Res Treat 2021; 189(1): 167-75.
[http://dx.doi.org/10.1007/s10549-021-06296-3] [PMID: 34152505]

[18] Olsson E, Winter C, George A, *et al.* Serial monitoring of circulating tumor DNA in patients with primary breast cancer for detection of occult metastatic disease. EMBO Mol Med 2015; 7(8): 1034-47.
[http://dx.doi.org/10.15252/emmm.201404913] [PMID: 25987569]

[19] Garcia-Murillas I, Schiavon G, Weigelt B. Mutation tracking in circulating tumor DNA predicts relapse in early breast cancer. Sci Transl Med 2015; 7(133): 302.
[http://dx.doi.org/10.1126/scitranslmed.aab0021] [PMID: 26311728]

CHAPTER 4

Importance of Biomarker Conversions as "Road Signs" to Manage Women with Metastatic Breast Cancer: How To Use Them for Personalized Care of These Patients?

Abstract: During a metastatic progression of **breast cancer (BC)**, and upon application of various antineoplastic therapies, the initial status of biomarkers can be altered. Awareness of changes in **hormone receptors (HR)** and **human epidermal growth factor receptor 2 (HER2)** is very important, because they may have an impact on patient management. However, the procedures for monitoring these changes in women with metastatic BC still remain unclear.

According to the guidelines for clinical practice from the **American Society of Clinical Oncology (ASCO),** the reevaluation of metastatic BC lesions, is of great importance, and it has been recommended that the biopsies of multiple metastatic lesions need to be performed.

The **aim** of this chapter is to highlight the role of **retesting receptor status in BC metastases** and the impact that this approach may have on the **selection of therapeutic strategies**, in the individualized **management plans for patients with metastatic BC**. In addition, this chapter concisely presents some novel biomarkers linked with targeted therapies for metastatic BC.

Keywords: Biomarkers, Breast cancer (BC), Estrogen receptor (ER), Hormone receptors (HR), Human epidermal growth factor receptor 2 (HER2), Progesterone receptor (PR), Triple-negative breast cancer (TNBC), Targeted therapies, Tumor heterogeneity.

INTRODUCTION

Systemic therapy is the basis of treatment for a majority of women with metastatic **breast cancer (BC)**. It is not considered to be curative, but some recent diagnostic and therapeutic efforts have ameliorated the patient survival (*e.g.*, a median **overall survival (OS)** has increased from about a year in 1985 to almost three years in 2016) [1].

In general, an effective systemic treatment of metastatic BC should be focused on improving patient's symptoms, **quality of life (QoL)**, and survival, as well as minimizing toxic effects. Depending on the BC subtype, it includes traditional **chemotherapy (CHT), poly(ADP-ribose) polymerase (PARP) inhibitors, immune checkpoint inhibitors (ICIs), endocrine therapy (ET), small molecule signal transduction inhibitors, targeted monoclonal antibodies**, and **antibody-drug conjugates (ADCs)** [1]. It has been reported that during a **metastatic progression** of BC, and upon using different **anticancer therapies**, the initial status of BC **biomarkers** can undergo some specific **changes** [1].

It has been noted that changes in biomarker status in BC are not uncommon, and typically occur in an **undesirable** direction (*e.g.*, as a **negative conversion**) in the BC metastatic lesions [1, 2]. It should be highlighted that the awareness of such changes is clinically important, since it can influence many critical decisions relevant to the patient management. According to the guidelines for clinical practice from the **American Society of Clinical Oncology (ASCO)**, the **reevaluation of metastatic BC lesions (including biomarkers)** is of great importance, and it has been recommended that the **biopsies of multiple metastatic lesions** should be performed [2].

The aim of this chapter is to explain the prognostic value of **biomarker's status re-evaluation** and the influence that this approach can have on the **selection of therapeutic strategies**, in the management of patients with BC. Moreover, this chapter highlights some features of **tumor heterogeneity**, with special emphasis on its pathologic findings. In addition, it provides insights into the clinical significance of molecular and cellular mechanisms of tumor heterogeneity. Furthermore, it concisely presents some novel **biomarkers** for the most adequate treatment tailoring in individual patients.

COMMON CONVERSIONS OF BIOMARKER'S STATUS IN METASTATIC BREAST CANCER

According to a recent article, approximately 15% changes in clinically meaningful receptors, such as **hormone receptors (HR)** (*e.g.*, **estrogen receptor [ER]** and **progesterone receptor [PR]**), as well as **human epidermal growth factor receptor 2 (HER2)** occur between primary and metastatic BC lesions [3]. In particular, **the negative conversion, from ER/PR-positive to ER/PR-negative** status (more frequent) usually signalizes that the present treatment is no longer effective, and requires an adjustment [1 - 3]. Also, a negative conversion of the **ER** status can indicate a worse patient's outcome. On the other hand, a **positive conversion** (less common) can indicate some new, **specific treatment directions**, which should be followed [1 - 3]. For this with reason, it is **beneficial to timely re-assess changes in biomarker status** in women BC, for both prognostic and therapeutic purposes [1 - 3].

Since such alterations require new decisions about treatment strategies, a **tumor tissue biopsy** and **systemic biomarkers should be re-evaluated**, in the course of a patient's metastatic BC. This is particularly important in cases of ER-positive to ER-negative BC conversion, and in HER2-positive to HER2-negative, borderline or low HER2 expression [3]. However, there is no "predetermined" schedule, according to which, a follow-up test should be done. In fact, a **repeated biopsy** needs to be considered before making any new decision about the selection of therapeutic options [3].

ALTERATIONS OF THE BIOMARKER'S STATUS IN METASTATIC BREAST CANCER AND THEIR POTENTIAL ROLE IN THE PROGNOSIS AND THERAPY

It has been noted that some biomarkers, such as *PI3K*, usually do not change over time. In practical terms, *PI3K* can predict therapeutic benefits of a *PI3K*-**inhibitor, alpelisib** [4]. At present, only *PIK3CA* **mutations** have shown a **predictive value for treatment with α-selective and β-sparing PI3K inhibitors**, in females with the advanced BC [4]. Moreover, biomarkers, such as *ESR1* **mutations**, may serve as **predictors for lack of benefits from treatment with aromatase inhibitors (AI)** (*e.g.*, a single-agent tamoxifen) [5].

It should be highlighted that clonal selection for hotspot *ESR1* mutations can occur at the early stages of both metastatic and locally recurrent BC. Such mutations may occur during or after an **adjuvant ET** or during **neoadjuvant ET** of primary BC lesions, possibly indicating a worse prognosis [5]. These findings carry some clinical implications for the future monitoring strategies to improve patients' outcomes [5]. Hopefully, further studies in the early recurrent BC phases will guide both researchers and clinicians how to provide the most suitable therapies in such patients.

Similarly, germline mutations of *BRCA1* and *BRCA2* genes are reliable **predictors for benefits with PARP inhibitors** [6]. In short, **PARP inhibitors** are the first FDA-approved **DNA damage response (DDR)-targeted** agents that have revolutionized treatment landscape for many patients with BC and ovarian cancer. **DDR deficiencies** represent a common factor that plays a key role in tumorigenesis. However, the **DDR deficiencies** are also a "weak spot" that can be "strategically " used as a therapeutic target [6]. Furthermore, there are some recent findings that **somatic *BRCA* mutations** may also predict some benefits from PARP inhibitors (Table **1**) [7]. In fact, the effectiveness of PARP inhibitors extends beyond the therapy of **germline *BRCA1/2* mutations**, involving **homologous recombination deficiency (HRD)** [7].

Table 1. Examples of common biomarkers (or their combinations) and matching targeted treatments in patients with metastatic breast cancer.

Biomarkers/combinations of biomarkers matched with targeted therapies		
Targetable mutations or therapeutic targets for patients with mBC	**Targeted therapeutic class Remarks**	**Examples of targeted therapeutics**
HER2-positive mBC	TKIs disrupt the signal transduction pathways of protein kinases	TKI – tucatinib, neratinib effective against activating mutations in *HER2*
ER-positive, HER2-negative mBC, & mutations in *PIK3CA*	PI3KCA inhibitors block PI3K enzymes (part of the PI3K/AKT/mTOR signal pathway, regulating cellular growth & survival) SERDs for the treatment of endocrine-resistant BC	PI3K inhibitor - alpelisib + SERD - fulvestrant
ER-positive HER2-negative BC	mTOR inhibitors block PI3K enzymes, which regulate cellular metabolism, growth, proliferation + AI (steroidal)	mTOR inhibitor - everolimus + AI - exemestane
Activating mutations in *ESR1*	SERDs as above	SERD - fulvestrant for pts with activating mutations in *ESR1*
mHR-positive BC or TNBC with germline *BRCA1/2* mutations	PARP inhibitors block PARP enzymes; cancer cells are more dependent on PARP than regular cells, making PARP a target for anticancer therapy	PARP inhibitor - olaparib & talazoparib
mTNBC the cell surface protein TROP2	ADC a monoclonal antibody attached to a topoisomerase I inhibitor payload - exatecan derivative (SN-38) with a cleavable linker	ADC - Sacituzumab govitecan
mTNBC with PD-L1	ICIs antibodies that unleash an immune system attack on cancer cells + CHT anticancer treatment that uses various chemotherapeutics	ICI - atazolizumab + CHT – nab-paclitaxel

m, metastatic; ADC, antibody-drug conjugates; CHT, chemotherapy; ICI, immune checkpoint inhibitors; SERD, selective estrogen receptor degrader; TKIs, tyrosine kinase inhibitors; ER, estrogen receptor; PR, progesterone receptor, HER2, human epidermal growth factor receptor 2; PARP, poly(ADP-ribose) polymerase; TNBC, Triple-Negative Breast Cancer; Trop-2, transmembrane glycoprotein 2; AI, aromatase inactivator.

COMMON BIOMARKERS OR THEIR COMBINATIONS MATCHED WITH TARGETED TREATMENTS FOR BREAST CANCER

Biomarkers can be obtained from the **tumor biopsy** or **liquid biopsy (circulating tumor DNA (ctDNA)** from the blood), depending on the clinical situation [8]. In addition, in the field of precision medicine, the **next generation sequencing (NGS)** along with **protein expression analysis** represent fundaments of targeted therapy in women with metastatic BC [8]. According to a recent retrospective study report, a comprehensive genomic profiling combined with protein expression analysis in patients with metastatic BC, permitted the use of personalized therapy for 50% of the study patients.

These findings may link the individual genetic alterations combined with protein expression, to detect the potential **targets** for **personalized therapy,** such as HER2-directed therapy with **trastuzumab emtansine** and **lapatinib**, or a *PI3K*-**inhibitor, alpelisib**, in combination with a selective estrogen receptor degrader (**SERD**), **fulvestrant** [8]. However, in the future, some novel, accurate tools, which will enable clinicians to correctly interpret the genomic alterations (*e.g.*, identified by NGS, in concert with protein expression or other factors), need to be investigated [8].

At this point, knowing that for many women, the motivation to undergo genetic testing is often related to the new diagnosis of BC, physicians should use this opportunity, especially for patients at particularly high risk of aggressive BC to beneficially change the BC trajectory for them and their family members.

BIOMARKERS' SHIFTS IN METASTATIC BREAST CANCER AND THEIR REASSESSMENT: A POTENTIAL ROLE IN THE PROGNOSIS AND TREATMENT

As previously mentioned, in many patients with **metastatic BC, alterations in the ER, PR, and HER2 biomarkers** usually display a direction **from a positive to a negative status**, while the changes of **Ki-67**, mainly occur **from a low to high index** [1]. Apparently, there are no differences in the frequencies of biomarker alterations, based on the metastatic sites. Furthermore, a **negative conversion of ER** represents an independent **poor prognostic factor among women with primary ER-positive BC** [9]. Based on a small study (conducted by the **Dutch Distant Breast Cancer Metastases Consortium**) that analyzed distant metastases in patients with metastatic BC, over one third of them revealed a **discordance in ER alpha and PR status** [10]. These findings indicate that **multiple metastases may require a biopsy to re-evaluate receptors** in the most accurate manner [10].

According to another clinical study of women with metastatic BC, a conversion from the HR–positive status in the primary tumor to the HR–negative in the metastasis occurred in over 20% of patients [11]. In contrast, the HR–negative to HR–positive conversion occurred only in less than 4% of patients [11]. In addition, the **HER2 status** was **discordant between primary and metastatic BC lesions** in 12.5% of patients [11]. Also, a recent meta-analysis of almost forty studies evaluating receptor conversion from primary tumors to distant metastases, in women with BC, has shown some differences in the incidence of HR conversion between studies (*e.g.*, for ER alpha, PR, and *HER2*, the positive to negative conversions were equal to 22.5%, 49.4%, and 21.3%, while the negative to positive conversions were 21.5%, 15.9%, and 9.5%, respectively) [12].

Nevertheless, it should be underscored that **ER alpha discordance** was higher in the **central nervous system (CNS)** and **bone** than in hepatic metastases (*e.g.*, 20.8% and 29.3% vs. 14.3%, respectively). In contrast, **PR discordance** was higher in **bone** (*e.g.*, 42.7%) and **liver metastases** (*e.g.*, 47.0%) than in the CNS metastases (*e.g.*, 23.3%) [12]. Since the receptor conversions for ER alpha, PR, and HER2 often occur during the BC metastatic progression, further prospective studies, exploring the reasons for these **receptor conversions and** impact of such conversions on therapeutic efficacy of different agents and clinical outcomes are merited [12].

Traditionally, a **systemic treatment of metastatic BC** has been mainly based on ER, PR, and HER2 receptor status. However, recently, in addition to this classical approach, some therapies for metastatic BC have been targeted certain biomarker-driven signaling pathways (*e.g.*, **cyclin-dependent kinase (CDK) 4/6**, and **phosphoinositide 3-kinase (PI3K)/protein kinase B (AKT)/mammalian target of rapamycin (mTOR)**). Also, targeted therapies focused on synthetic lethality, with **PARP inhibitors**, in patients with BC, who carry *BRCA1/2* mutations, and the novel **antibody-drug conjugates (ADCs)** have been added to the treatment strategies (Fig. **1**) [13].

Modern tools (*e.g.*, genomic sequencing like **NGS**) can help with individualized treatment selection and with evaluating potential **resistance to therapy**. Constant progress in the area of **biomarker-** and **genomic-driven therapeutic approaches** may override the historical **subtype-** and **line-based strategies**. Moreover, **surgical treatment** of the metastatic BC also undergoes transition (*e.g.*, an aggressive approach to locoregional BC or ablation procedures for oligometastatic BC, based on individual evaluation of medical context of a given patient), and thus, more studies are necessary to explore clinical outcomes related to these methodologies [13].

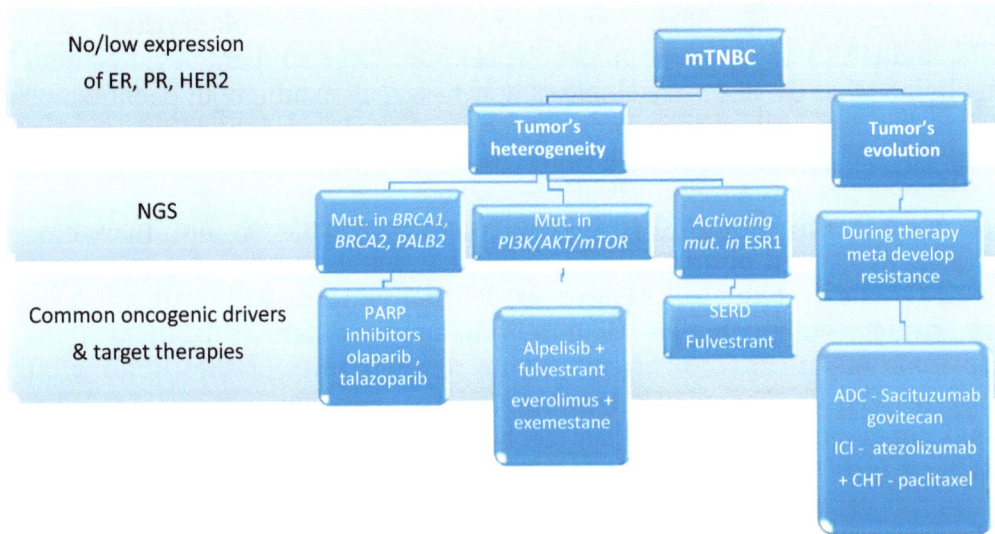

Fig. (1). Matching the TNBC with target therapies at the time of metastatic diagnosis; ER, estrogen receptor; PR, progesterone receptor, HER2, human epidermal growth factor receptor 2; ADC, antibody-drug conjugates; ICI, immune checkpoint inhibitors; mut, mutations; m, metastatic; NGS, next-generation sequencing; PI3K/AKT/ mTOR, phosphoinositide 3-kinase/protein kinase B/mammalian target of rapamycin; PARP, poly(ADP-ribose) polymerase; SERD, selective estrogen receptor degrader; CHT, chemotherapy; TNBC, Triple-Negative Breast Cancer.

CONSIDERATIONS OF INTERTUMOR AND INTRATUMOR HETEROGENEITY: CHALLENGES AND OPPORTUNITIES

Tumor heterogeneity including both **intertumor** and **intratumor** components is one of the hallmarks of malignancy [14, 15]. It should be highlighted that BC displays its heterogeneous nature and varies among different women (that reflects the **intertumor heterogeneity**) and additionally, within each individual tumor (the **intratumor heterogeneity**) [14, 15]. **Intertumor heterogeneity** is frequently noted in women with BC from different female populations. It should be underscored that the **intertumor heterogeneity of BC** is illustrated by **clinical staging** of BC, based on physical examination and imaging studies (*e.g.*, the TNM [Tumor size, regional lymph Node status, and distant Metastases] staging system) [15]. These established **clinicopathologic parameters** influence the patient **survival** and affect variability in clinical **outcomes** of women with BC. Current standards of BC treatment are based on the tumor characteristics, such as clinical stage, histopathologic features, and biomarker profile.

In addition, the patient's age, menopausal status, and general health (*e.g.*, comorbidities, genetic predispositions, and environmental or behavioral factors) affect treatment choices and results. A clinical and morphologic intertumor heterogeneity is reflected *via* staging systems and histopathologic classification of BC. As a consequence, **heterogeneity in the expression of biomarkers**, such as HRs, and HER2 oncoprotein guides the relevant targeted therapies. It should be highlighted that BC cells in a single tumor mass may exhibit both phenotypic and genetic heterogeneity, while only a limited number of such cells gains a metastatic potential and creates metastatic lesions [14, 15].

In contrast, **intratumor heterogeneity** is secondary to the **presence of heterogeneous cell populations within a particular tumor** of a given patient with BC. The detection of **intratumor cell populations** with different features (*e.g.*, **tumorigenicity, metastatic potential,** and **treatment resistance**) allows to find some important factors, contributing to **variability in the tumor clinical behavior** and its **therapeutic response**, in the individual patient [14]. Further exploring of molecular and cellular mechanisms of the **intratumor heterogeneity** and their **interrelations with the diagnosis, prognosis, and therapy of BC** is critical for designing a well-balanced, personalized approach for each patient with BC [14].

Intratumor heterogeneity is usually manifested at the **genomic, transcriptomic, proteomic, and morphologic levels**, causing both diagnostic and therapeutic difficulties. In fact, **molecular classifications** indicate the **genetic tumor heterogeneity**, which can be tested *via* **multigene assays**, and can contribute to a more accurate **stratification** into low- and high-risk populations, in which **personalized therapies** can be used. Moreover, it is critical to identify the **molecular** and **cellular mechanisms of tumor heterogeneity**, which are related to the development of **therapeutic resistance** [14, 15]. It should be underscored that the reporting biomarkers allows to maximize patient eligibility for targeted therapies. However, a failure to consider the **intratumor heterogeneity** (*e.g.*, not adding the molecular classification of BC to the routine procedures of clinical practice) may result in incomplete clinical picture of a given patient [14, 15].

Tumor Evolution and Its Connections with Changing of the Biomarker's Status in Metastatic Breast Cancer

Numerous patients with metastatic BC may have several active areas of malignancy, which could undergo different processes of evolution. For instance, tumors can change over time, as they become more biologically aggressive or resistant to therapies. It should be underscored that during each line of BC treatment, only some metastatic lesions might develop therapeutic resistance. In particular, when a patient's **hepatic metastases** begin to grow, the therapeutic changes should be implemented rapidly. However, when a patient's single **bone metastasis** starts to grow and the hepatic metastases have shown a good response to therapy, then only a local therapy (*e.g.*, radiation therapy (RT) for the bone metastatic lesion) should be applied. It should be underscored that the resistance mutations can often occur when the ER becomes hormonally independent. This happens due to a chronic estrogen deprivation (*e.g.*, due to ET), during which, the ER evolves to become independent of estrogen stimulation. Under these circumstances, the BC tumor develops **resistance to ET** (*e.g.*, in cases of **activating mutations** in *ESR1*) [5, 10].

If biomarker status is heterogeneous in the primary tumor and is associated with different metastatic potential, then it can also change during metastatic progression. Selection pressure from treatment is another possible reason for receptor conversion [16].

Many patients diagnosed with metastatic BC receive endocrine or HER2-targeted therapy and approximately 50% of HER2-positive BCs are also ER-positive [17]. A role of cross-communication between the ER and HER2 signaling pathways may represent a missing "piece of the puzzle" to the development of resistance to endocrine therapies (ET). The approach that simultaneously inhibits both signaling pathways would be the best strategy to prevent or overcome the ET or anti-HER2 therapy resistance [18]. For instance, PI3K and CDK4/6 are suitable targets, which act downstream of the ER and HER2 signaling pathways [18]. Moreover, the evaluation of efficacy and safety findings from studies with anti-HER2 agents combined with ET, as well as studies investigating small molecules targeting these signaling pathways appear promising.

CONCLUSION

As new therapeutic options continue to emerge, bringing some hope for women with metastatic BC, it is essential to find biomarkers for the most adequate treatment tailoring. Recent research findings focused on **changing biomarker status have critical influence on the decision-making about personalized therapies for women with metastatic BC**. The exact causes or **receptor conversion** during BC metastatic progression are still poorly understood, and thus, prospective large-scale studies, evaluating the influence of receptor conversion on therapeutic efficacy and clinical outcomes are merited.

Since the **receptor status in BC** is often related to the patient's therapy, it is crucial to timely detect any new alterations in **HR** and **HER receptors** among patients with metastatic BC, during their BC therapeutic journey. It should be highlighted that the **negative conversions** (more frequent) usually inform that the **present treatment is no longer effective**, and requires an individualized adjustment. On the other hand, **positive conversions** (less common) can indicate some new, **specific treatment** directions which should be followed. In spite of remarkable advances in the understanding of the malignant breast tumor heterogeneity and its evolution over time, there has been only moderate progress in diagnostic and prognostic approaches for patients with metastatic BC. Therefore, it is necessary to refine effective targeted therapies, as novel oncogenic drivers, tumor-specific proteins, and DNA repair deficits are being identified.

At present, one of the most significant advances has been the development of efficient and affordable genome sequencing, which has led to the **selection of gene panels** and identification of new **therapeutic targets**. Furthermore, determining some **genetic predispositions** for patients with BC, beyond *BRCA1/2*, would allow to advise patients and their relatives about BC risks and provide more accurate recommendations for BC screening. This, in turn, should lead to making well-balanced, personalized choices for the therapy (*e.g.*, that will target some DNA repair deficits, detected in a given patients with BC).

However, to accomplish such progress, the patients, their families, and treatment teams need to be engaged in continuous educational efforts. Moreover, it is critical to disseminate knowledge to "bridge the gap" between the recent research developments in diagnostic and therapeutic fields and the medical and personal needs of women with metastatic BC, as well as their oncology teams, in the "real-life" oncology practice setting. Hopefully, **re-evaluation of biomarkers in the management of metastatic BC** will be an important step to enable a more personalized treatment for many women with metastatic BC, in the near future.

An assessment of different biomarkers and their changes in women with metastatic BC is very important. To take advantage from recent research studies, the patients with BC and their medical teams need to:

Go forward with knowledge about a positive *BRCA1* or *BRCA2* mutation & find out what to do about it – here are some examples:

• If a woman has the new diagnosis of BC, learning about her **genetic profile** may positively influence her choice of targeted treatment of the BC subtype and possible prevention of some other cancers (*e.g.*, ovarian cancer);

• **A test for *BRCA* gene mutation** can be done from a blood sample; *BRCA* mutations are found in **5% -10%** of **BCs** and up to **20%** in **TNBC** subtype;

• Counseling about the practical meaning of *BRCA* positive genetic test is critical because **PARP inhibitors**, such as **olaparib** and **talazoparib** (that are administered **orally** and usually **well tolerated**), are **improving outcomes for *BRCA* mutation carriers with BC** in the **metastatic** setting and also in the **early-stages of BC;**

- For patients with ***BRCA*** mutations and **early-stages BCs** (potentially curable), a systemic treatment with **PARP inhibitors** and should be given and **bilateral mastectomy** can be considered.

Discover benefits of immune checkpoint inhibitors (ICIs) or antibody-drug conjugates (ADCs) & possibly apply them – here are some example:

- **PD-L1 status is a predictor of benefit from ICI (atezolizumab)** in **metastatic TNBC.**
- For treatment planning in case of **metastatic TNBC,** it is important to know **PD-L1 status** since it plays the role of **predictive biomarker** (*e.g.*, **CPS ≥ 10** is the companion diagnostic test for **pembrolizumab**).
- **PD-L1 status** is not necessary to determine eligibility for neoadjuvant **pembrolizumab**, which should be considered for the use in **early-stage of TNBC.**
- **Sacituzumab govitecan (SG)** is a therapeutic **antibody** that can attach to a specific Trop-2 target on the surface of BC cells. The antibody carries a medication (SN-38), which is released within and around the cancer cells, causing their destruction.
- Patients with **advanced TNBC**, who took **SG** may **live longer** than those who took a different CHT regimen.
- Patients with an **ER-positive metastatic BC** may have some **benefits** from **SG.**

REFERENCES

[1]   Woo JW, Chung YR, Ahn S, *et al.* Changes in biomarker status in metastatic breast cancer and their prognostic value. J Breast Cancer 2019; 22(3): 439-52.
[http://dx.doi.org/10.4048/jbc.2019.22.e38] [PMID: 31598343]

[2]   Andre F, Ismaila N, Henry NL, *et al.* Use of biomarkers to guide decisions on adjuvant systemic therapy for women with early-stage invasive breast cancer: Asco clinical practice guideline update—integration of results from tailoRx. J Clin Oncol 2019; 37(22): 1956-64.
[http://dx.doi.org/10.1200/JCO.19.00945] [PMID: 31150316]

[3]   Walter V, Fischer C, Deutsch TM, *et al.* Estrogen, progesterone, and human epidermal growth factor receptor 2 discordance between primary and metastatic breast cancer. Breast Cancer Res Treat 2020; 183(1): 137-44.
[http://dx.doi.org/10.1007/s10549-020-05746-8] [PMID: 32613540]

[4]   Brandão M, Caparica R, Eiger D, de Azambuja E. Biomarkers of response and resistance to PI3K inhibitors in estrogen receptor-positive breast cancer patients and combination therapies involving PI3K inhibitors. Ann Oncol 2019; 30 (10): x27-42.
[http://dx.doi.org/10.1093/annonc/mdz280] [PMID: 31859350]

[5]   Zundelevich A, Dadiani M, Kahana-Edwin S, *et al.* ESR1 mutations are frequent in newly diagnosed metastatic and loco-regional recurrence of endocrine-treated breast cancer and carry worse prognosis. Breast Cancer Res 2020; 22(1): 16.
[http://dx.doi.org/10.1186/s13058-020-1246-5] [PMID: 32014063]

[6]   Pilié PG, Gay CM, Byers LA, O'Connor MJ, Yap TA. PARP Inhibitors: Extending benefit beyond *BRCA* -mutant cancers. Clin Cancer Res 2019; 25(13): 3759-71.

[http://dx.doi.org/10.1158/1078-0432.CCR-18-0968] [PMID: 30760478]

[7]   Eoh KJ, Kim HM, Lee JY, *et al.* Mutation landscape of germline and somatic BRCA1/2 in patients with high-grade serous ovarian cancer. BMC Cancer 2020; 20(1): 204.
        [http://dx.doi.org/10.1186/s12885-020-6693-y] [PMID: 32164585]

[8]   Hempel D, Ebner F, Garg A, *et al.* Real world data analysis of next generation sequencing and protein expression in metastatic breast cancer patients. Sci Rep 2020; 10(1): 10459.
        [http://dx.doi.org/10.1038/s41598-020-67393-9] [PMID: 32591580]

[9]   Fujii K, Watanabe R, Ando T, *et al.* Alterations in three biomarkers (estrogen receptor, progesterone receptor and human epidermal growth factor 2) and the Ki67 index between primary and metastatic breast cancer lesions. Biomed Rep 2017; 7(6): 535-42.
        [http://dx.doi.org/10.3892/br.2017.1003] [PMID: 29188058]

[10]   Hoefnagel LDC, van der Groep P, van de Vijver MJ, *et al.* Discordance in ERα, PR and HER2 receptor status across different distant breast cancer metastases within the same patient. Ann Oncol 2013; 24(12): 3017-23.
        [http://dx.doi.org/10.1093/annonc/mdt390] [PMID: 24114857]

[11]   Chang HJ, Han SW, Oh DY, *et al.* Discordant human epidermal growth factor receptor 2 and hormone receptor status in primary and metastatic breast cancer and response to trastuzumab. Jpn J Clin Oncol 2011; 41(5): 593-9.
        [http://dx.doi.org/10.1093/jjco/hyr020] [PMID: 21406492]

[12]   Schrijver WAME, Suijkerbuijk KPM, van Gils CH, van der Wall E, Moelans CB, van Diest PJ. Receptor conversion in distant breast cancer metastases: A systematic review and meta-analysis. J Natl Cancer Inst 2018; 110(6): 568-80.
        [http://dx.doi.org/10.1093/jnci/djx273] [PMID: 29315431]

[13]   Savard MF, Khan O, Hunt KK, Verma S. Redrawing the lines: The next generation of treatment in metastatic breast cancer. Am Soc Clin Oncol Educ Book 2019; 39(39): e8-e21.
        [http://dx.doi.org/10.1200/EDBK_237419] [PMID: 31099662]

[14]   Ramón y Cajal S, Sesé M, Capdevila C, *et al.* Clinical implications of intratumor heterogeneity: Challenges and opportunities. J Mol Med 2020; 98(2): 161-77.
        [http://dx.doi.org/10.1007/s00109-020-01874-2] [PMID: 31970428]

[15]   Turashvili G, Brogi E. Tumor heterogeneity in breast cancer. Front Med 2017; 4: 227.
        [http://dx.doi.org/10.3389/fmed.2017.00227] [PMID: 29276709]

[16]   Schrijver WAME, Schuurman K, van Rossum A, *et al.* Loss of steroid hormone receptors is common in malignant pleural and peritoneal effusions of breast cancer patients treated with endocrine therapy. Oncotarget 2017; 8(33): 55550-61.
        [http://dx.doi.org/10.18632/oncotarget.15548] [PMID: 28903441]

[17]   El Sayed R, El Jamal L, El Iskandarani S, Kort J, Abdel Salam M, Assi H. Endocrine and targeted therapy for hormone-receptor-positive, HER2-negative advanced breast cancer: Insights to sequencing treatment and overcoming resistance based on clinical trials. Front Oncol 2019; 9: 510.
        [http://dx.doi.org/10.3389/fonc.2019.00510] [PMID: 31281796]

[18]   Montagna E, Colleoni M. Hormonal treatment combined with targeted therapies in endocrine-responsive and HER2-positive metastatic breast cancer. Ther Adv Med Oncol 2019; 11.
        [http://dx.doi.org/10.1177/1758835919894105] [PMID: 31897091]

CHAPTER 5

Putting It All Together: Clinical Pearls of Recently Approved Therapies for Triple-Negative Breast Cancer

Abstract: Three recently approved therapies for the treatment of **triple-negative breast cancer (TNBC)**, including **poly(ADP-ribose) polymerase (PARP) inhibitors, immunotherapy**, and **antibody-drug conjugates (ADC)** have changed the management of several patients with advanced, metastatic, and even early-stage TNBC.

PARP inhibitors, such as **olaparib** and **talazoparib**, have been approved as therapies for *BRCA*-**mutated human epidermal growth factor receptor 2 (HER2)-negative metastatic breast cancer (BC)**.

Immunotherapy has been approved for patients with **programmed death ligand 1 (PD-L1)-positive, metastatic TNBC. Immune checkpoint inhibitors (ICIs)**, such as **atezolizumab** and **pembrolizumab** demonstrated a significant improvement in **progression-free survival (PFS)** (in combination with chemotherapy).

An **antibody-drug conjugate (ADC), sacituzumab govitecan (SG)** (that **targets trophoblast cell surface antigen 2 (Trop-2)**), has shown efficacy and prolonged **PFS** and **overall survival (OS)** in patients with **metastatic TNBC.**

The goal of this chapter is to briefly review some of the most promising therapies available for the treatment of TNBC, including PARP inhibitors, ICIs, and ADCs. Considerations of choosing these therapeutic options and their sequence, in the context of the *BRCA* mutation and the **PD-L1 positivity**, in patients with TNBC have been discussed.

Keywords: Atezolizumab, Antibody drug conjugates (ADCs), Human epidermal growth factor receptor 2 (HER2), Immune checkpoint inhibitors (ICIs), Olaparib, Poly (ADP-ribose) polymerase (PARP) inhibitors, Pembrolizumab, Programmed death ligand 1 (PD-L1), Sacituzumab govitecan, Talazoparib, Triple-negative breast cancer (TNBC).

Katarzyna Rygiel

INTRODUCTION

Triple-negative breast cancer (TNBC) is more common in young women (*e.g.*, under 40 years of age), premenopausal, those who are of African or Hispanic ancestry, and the ones, who harbor a germline mutation in the *BRCA1* gene [1]. **TNBC** is characterized by rapid growth, spread, and negative patient outcomes [1]. Also, **TNBC** has a higher risk of recurrence after therapy (*e.g.*, especially for early-stage **TNBC)** and poor survival (*e.g.*, for patients diagnosed with advanced and metastatic TNBC) [1].

Traditionally, **TNBC** has been defined by what it does **not express** (*e.g.*, the **estrogen receptor (ER), progesterone receptor (PR)**, and **human epidermal growth factor receptor (HER2)**) [1]. At present, this characteristic has been "enriched" by specifying what TNBC does express, such as *BRCA1* or *BRCA2* **gene mutations**, and **PD-L1** marker. Unfortunately, treatment options in TNBC have been limited, compared to some other forms of BC (*e.g.*, hormone receptor (HR)-positive BC, and HER2-positive BC) [1].

However, it should be underscored that three recently approved therapies for the treatment of **TNBC**, including **PARP inhibitors, immunotherapy**, and **antibody-drug conjugates (ADCs)** have changed the management strategy for several patients with advanced, metastatic, and even early-stage TNBC [1].

For instance, inhibitors of **poly(ADP-ribose) polymerase (PARP)**, such as **olaparib** and **talazoparib**, have been approved as therapies for patients with *BRCA*-mutated **HER2-negative metastatic breast cancer (BC)** [2].

In addition, **immune checkpoint inhibitors (ICIs)** were initially explored in **TNBC** rather than in HR-positive BC. This is because, in contrast to the other BC subtypes, **TNBC** is more **immunogenic** (*e.g.*, it has **a higher tumor mutational burden**, more abundant **tumor-infiltrating lymphocytes**, and higher **programmed death ligand 1 (PD-L1) expression**) [3]. In consequence, adding **immunotherapy** to chemotherapy **(CHT)** in patients with **TNBC**, who have tumors that are **PD-L1-positive** has shown beneficial effects [3].

Moreover, **antibody-drug conjugates (ADCs)** that **target trophoblast cell surface antigen 2 (Trop-2)** have shown efficacy for patients with **metastatic TNBC**. In particular, an **ADC, sacituzumab govitecan (SG)**, has revealed improved **progression-free survival (PFS)** and **overall survival (OS)** for women with **metastatic TNBC** [4].

The goal of this chapter is to briefly review some of the most promising therapies available for the treatment of TNBC, including PARP inhibitors, immune checkpoint inhibitors (ICIs), and antibody-drug conjugates (ADCs). Considerations of choosing these therapeutic options and their sequence, in the context of the *BRCA* mutation and the PD-L1 positivity, in patients with TNBC are discussed.

A SPECIAL TASK OF PARP INHIBITORS: TARGETING ENZYMES THAT REPAIR DNA DAMAGE

To understand what are the **PARP inhibitors**, one has to first understand what the **poly (ADP-ribose) polymerase (PARPs)** is [2]. Simply put, **PARP** is a class of nuclear enzymes involved in the pathogenesis of various malignant tumors. In particular, **PARP1** and **PARP2** are the two most recognized members of this enzymatic family [2]. **PARP1** and **PARP2** are activated by DNA damage and can repair it (*e.g.*, single-strand DNA breaks). However, if **PARP1** and **PARP2** are suppressed, then the unrepaired single DNA base pairs degrade into double-stranded DNA breaks [2]. As a consequence, in patients who carry a *BRCA* gene mutation, the **PARP inhibitors** prevent the damaged cancer cells from the ability to repair their DNA breaks, leading to the *BRCA*-mutated cell death, and subsequently, to cancer's destruction [2].

WHO CAN BENEFIT THE MOST FROM PARP INHIBITORS? - GOOD NEWS FROM THE OLYMPIAD AND THE EMBRACA TRIALS FOR WOMEN WITH METASTATIC *BRCA*-POSITIVE TNBC

The **OlympiAD** trial has led to the approval of **olaparib** in **metastatic *BRCA*-positive BC** [5]. Patients included in this study had deleterious, **germline *BRCA* mutations** and **advanced HER2-negative BC (hormone receptor (HR)-positive** or **TNBC**). Previously, they received up to two lines of CHT for metastatic BC [5]. The participants of the **OlympiAD** trial were randomized to receive **olaparib (300 mg twice a day) or CHT of the physician's choice (capecitabine, vinorelbine, or eribulin)** [5]. The **PFS** was improved significantly in the olaparib group compared to the CHT. In addition, women with TNBC had the most beneficial effects from the olaparib therapy [5].

Concurrently, the **EMBRACA** trial examined **talazoparib** *vs.* CHT in women with deleterious, germline, *BRCA* mutation, with HER2-negative BC, who had received the previous CHT for metastatic BC [6]. They were randomized to receive **talazoparib** (1 mg a day) *vs.* **CHT of the physician's choice (capecitabine, vinorelbine, eribulin,** or **gemcitabine)**. The women who received **talazoparib** had a better **PFS** [6].

The **TBCRC 048** examined the patients who had **somatic *BRCA* mutations** or **other germline mutations** (*e.g.*, *PALB2, ATM,* and *CHEK2)*, to see whether or not these patients could also benefit from **olaparib** [7]. The **TBCRC 048** study has revealed that the **somatic *BRCA* mutations** may benefit from **olaparib,** similar to the **germline *BRCA* mutation carriers** [7]. In addition, women with ***PALB2* mutations in the germline setting** had significant benefits from **olaparib** therapy. However, based on the **TBCRC 048** study findings, the *ATM* and *CHEK2* **mutation carriers** had no benefits from **olaparib** [7].

It should be underscored that **PARP inhibitors** are helping women not only live longer but also live better (*e.g.*, the **quality of life (QoL)** was better with the **PARP inhibitors** compared to CHT) [8, 9]. The advantages of therapy with **olaparib** or **talazoparib** over CHT also include improved **PFS** and more **manageable adverse effects (AEs)** [8, 9]. The main AEs of **olaparib** or **talazoparib** are cytopenia, fatigue, nausea, and indigestion. These AEs need to be clearly explained to patients upfront, to give the patients a chance to manage them proactively. PARP inhibitors are easier to take due to the oral form of administration [8, 9]. In addition, the majority of women taking **PARP inhibitors** do not suffer from hair loss which may be particularly important for many younger patients [8, 9].

Shifting Gears to Immunotherapy: Who Can Be A Winner?

Immunotherapy has been approved for patients with **PD-L1-positive, metastatic TNBC** [10]. **Immune checkpoint inhibitors (ICIs)** such as **atezolizumab** and **pembrolizumab** have demonstrated a significant improvement in **PFS** when immunotherapy was combined with standard of care chemotherapy (CHT) in the first-line metastatic setting (*e.g.*, atezolizumab and nab-paclitaxel improved **PFS** and **overall survival (OS)** for those patients, who were treated with **atezolizumab + nab-paclitaxel**) [10].

IMpassion130 study took patients, who were receiving treatment (the first-line therapy) for their **metastatic TNBC** and randomized them to *nab*-**paclitaxel** with or without **atezolizumab**. This trial required that patients would be at least 12 months out from their adjuvant therapy or would have de novo metastatic disease. Patients were stratified based on their **PD-L1** status. The endpoints of the study were **PFS** and **OS** [10]. In short, adding **atezolizumab to *nab*-paclitaxel improved PFS**, and this improvement was mostly seen in the PD-L1-positive subgroup, while there was no improvement in PFS in the PD-L1-negative subgroup (Fig. **1**) [10].

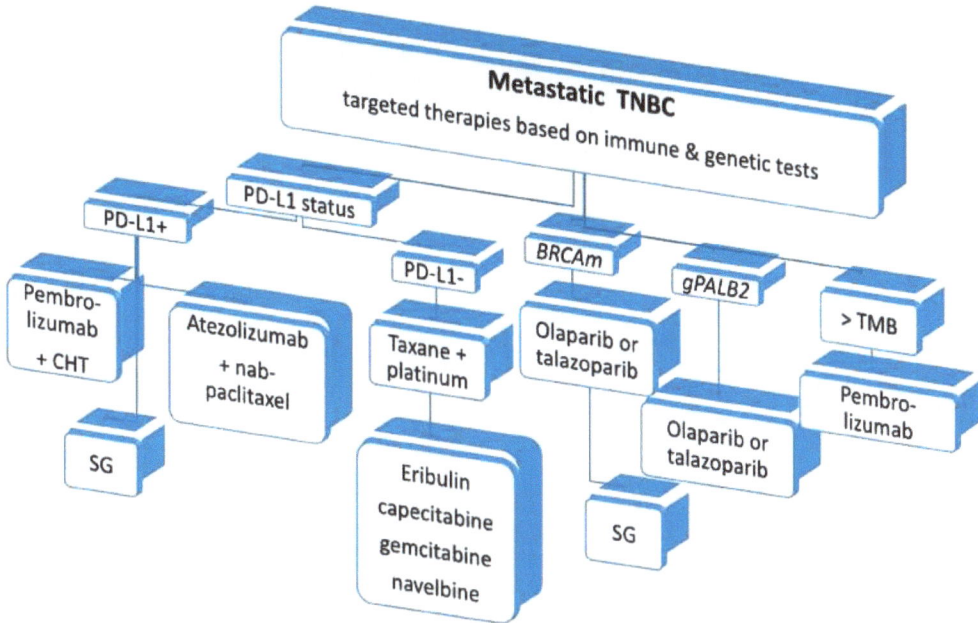

Fig. (1). Current targeted/personalized treatment strategies for patients with metastatic TNBC, based on immune and genetic tests; CHT, chemotherapy; g, germline; m, mutation, PD-L1, programmed death ligand 1; SG, sacituzumab govitecan; TMB, tumor mutation burden; TNBC, triple-negative breast cancer.

In the **KEYNOTE-355** trial, **pembrolizumab** was added to different CHT agents, including **nab-paclitaxel, paclitaxel,** or **carboplatin + gemcitabine** doublet therapy. In the **KEYNOTE-355** trial, patients with **PD-L1-positive metastatic TNBC** had a significantly improved **PFS** and **duration of response** of 12 months (for those patients, who were treated with **pembrolizumab + CHT**). As a consequence, pembrolizumab was approved for **PD-L1-positive metastatic TNBC** (Fig. **1**) [11].

Similar to the experience with PARP inhibitors, once ICIs demonstrate effectiveness in the advanced or **metastatic BC** setting, they will be moved into the **early-stage BC** setting [12]. As noted in the **KEYNOTE-355** and the **Impassion-031** trials, adding **pembrolizumab** or **atezolizumab** to a standard of care neoadjuvant CHT improves **the pathologic complete response (pCR)** rates [11, 13]. It should be underscored that some other trials have shown that the **addition of immunotherapy to a standard of care neoadjuvant CHT for patients with early-stage TNBC** improved **pCR** rates and **long-term outcomes** [12]. In particular, **KEYNOTE-522** was a practice-changing study, in which patients with **early-stage, high-risk TNBC** received **paclitaxel** and **carboplatin** followed by **anthracycline/cyclophosphamide** with or without **pembrolizumab** in the **neoadjuvant** setting. Subsequently, the study patients had surgery (**pCR** was an endpoint). Patients, who were randomized to the **pembrolizumab,** also received **adjuvant pembrolizumab,** for one year [12]. **KEYNOTE-522** findings revealed that (based on pCR reports) whether patients had a CPS < 1, ≥ 1, or ≥ 10, the addition of **pembrolizumab** contributed to higher pCR rates, compared to CHT alone [12]. In addition, the **KEYNOTE-522 study** has shown that there was a clinically meaningful **improvement** (almost 40%) in **event-free survival (EFS), irrespective of PD-L1** status, in **early-stage TNBC.** This **EFS benefit** included **fewer local** and **distant recurrences** (practically meaning that fewer patients had BC progression on **ICI** therapy), whether the tumor was PD-L1 positive or PD-L1 negative [12]. Moreover, **immunotherapy**, similarly to **PARP inhibitors**, can be a part of the treatment armamentarium that may help cure women with **early-stage TNBC** [12, 14].

The Role of Ventana and Dako Assay in PD-L1 Testing

In a patient who has metastatic TNBC, the **PD-L1** status needs to be tested, since such a patient can benefit from the use of **immunotherapy** (in the case of a PD-L1-positive tumor) [10, 11]. In addition, performing **genetic testing** to find out if she can be a candidate for the use of **PARP inhibitors** (in case of germline *BRCA* **mutations**) [6, 7]. Also, a biopsy (to make sure that this is metastatic TNBC and not a new malignancy), and a confirmation of the receptor status (to find out whether or not the receptor status has been changed) are needed in cases of TNBC recurrence. This extended diagnostic approach is critical since it can impact future patient management by applying ICIs or PARP inhibitors.

Since there are two approved immunotherapy agents, **atezolizumab** and **pembrolizumab,** in combination with CHT, two different **PD-L1 assays** can be used, such as **the Ventana** and **the Dako** assay [10, 11]. Importantly, **atezolizumab** has been approved for patients who have an **SP142 test with an immune cell (IC) score that's greater than or equal to 1,** while **pembrolizumab** has been **approved with a companion diagnostic, the 22C3 antibody, with a combined positive score (CPS) greater than or equal to 10** [10, 11]. In practical terms, for a precise choice of targeted therapy, doing a **PD-L1** assay and testing for *BRCA1/2* is helpful (Fig. 1) [6, 10, 11]. In addition, for motivated women, with good performance status, genetic testing for *PALB2* is useful, especially if they intend to find a suitable clinical study [7]. Also, **next-generation sequencing (NGS)** can be helpful, especially if a woman may consider a potential participation in the relevant clinical trial exploring new, more personalized therapeutic options [7, 14].

Sacituzumab Govitecan - An Antibody Drug Conjugate (ADC) Starting the "Optimistic Wave" of Therapy for Patients with Metastatic TNBC

Antibody-drug conjugates (ADCs) represent new promising therapeutic options on the **TNBC** horizon. Their first "family member", **sacituzumab govitecan (SG)**, which has recently been approved, is targeting **trophoblast cell surface antigen 2 (Trop-2)** and delivers an **SN38 payload (**using a **topoisomerase**) [15]. An advantage of **SG** is a high **drug-to-antibody ratio (7:1**) and the ability to work by the **bystander effect,** meaning the partial release of the payload in the **tumor microenvironment (TME)** (Fig. **1**) [15]. The **ASCENT** trial that compared **SG** to CHT (of physician's choice) was designed for patients with metastatic TNBC, who were pretreated with two prior lines of CHT [15]. However, if a patient had relapsed at any time of her adjuvant CHT, then such a patient only needed to have one line of CHT, in the metastatic setting, to be eligible to participate in the **ASCENT** trial (in which, the patients who received the second-line or third-line therapy and beyond, were mostly included) [15].

Importantly, in the **ASCENT** trial, a significant difference was seen with regard to **PFS** in the **SG arm** compared to the **physician's choice CHT arm (**5.6 months *vs.* only 1.7 months) [15]. Moreover, the **OS** was extended from 6.7 to 12 months in the **SG arm,** reflecting a desirable result. Since **SG is targeting Trop-2**, it appears "natural" that the level of Trop-2 expression could predict the SG's treatment effects. However, the benefits in favor of SG, compared to the CHT of the physician's choice arm, were seen regardless of the degree of Trop-2 expression [15]. In essence, the good news for women with metastatic TNBC is that they do not need to be tested for Trop-2 expression, since the therapy with SG has been beneficial for all of the patients, who received such treatment. Overall, the **ASCENT** trial's results revealed an **improvement in PFS** and **OS** among patients, who received therapy with SG [15].

A Spotlight on HER2-low BC: Diagnostic Challenges to HER2 Status Interpretation

About 20% of invasive BC cases are characterized by **HER2 protein overexpression** or *HER2* **gene amplification** [16]. HER2 is a predictive biomarker for the use of HER2-directed treatments in women with BC [17]. Unfortunately, an accurate interpretation of the HER2 status can be problematic in many patients with BC, and these difficulties can be due to various factors, such as HER2 **intratumoral heterogeneity (ITH)** and changes in HER2 status in the process of BC metastatic progression or post neoadjuvant chemotherapy (CHT [17].

At present, HER2 **immunohistochemistry (IHC)** is applied for **screening** purposes, and *in situ* **hybridization (ISH)** serves as a **confirmation**, if the HER2 IHC test results are equivocal (this has usually been determined *via* HER2 **fluorescence** *in situ* **hybridization (FISH) or silver** *in situ* **hybridization (SISH)** probes) [18]. Furthermore, when there is a discrepancy between the results of HER2 status between primary and metastatic BC lesions, FISH or SISH tests should be conducted [18]. To address these issues, the American Society of Clinical Oncology/College of American Pathologists (ASCO/CAP) guidelines have incorporated some modified recommendations for a precise interpretation of the HER2 status (Table **1**) [18, 19].

Table 1. Interpretation of HER2 status by using immunohistochemistry and dual-probe *in situ* hybridization tests (based on the ASCO/CAP 2018 guidelines) [18, 19].

HER2 by Immunohistochemistry (IHC) [18]		
Tips for Assessment of HER2 Heterogeneity in BC		Recommended actions [19]
NEGATIVE [-]	No staining observed, incomplete membrane staining (faint) & within ≤10% of the invasive tumor cells.	Review the entire HER2 IHC slide.
NEGATIVE [1+]	Incomplete membrane staining (faint) & within >10% of the invasive tumor cells.	Find areas with potential HER2 amplification.
EQUIVOCAL [2+]	Weak to moderate complete membrane staining in >10% of tumor cells.	Scan the entire HER2 ISH slide prior to counting.
POSITIVE [3+]	Circumferential membrane staining (complete, intense) & in >10% of tumor cells.	The ISH report documents a proportion of amplified cells within a tumor.
HER2 by *in situ* Hybridization (ISH) [18]		
Test Result		Recommended actions [19]
Negative [-]	-	-
No Equivocal	-	-
Positive	SISH or CISH are beneficial for the assessment of HER2 heterogeneity (since such tests can be conveniently matched with HER2 IHC slide under the optical microscope).	In case of finding a subpopulation of tumor cells with HER2 amplification (including > 10% of tumor cells on the slide), perform a separate counting in this subpopulation; Provide separate calculations for the HER2/CEP17 ratios and HER2 gene copy number for the amplified & non-amplified areas.

ASCO, American Society of Clinical Oncology; BC, Breast Cancer; CAP, College of American Pathologists; HER2, Human Epidermal Growth Factor Receptor 2; IHC, Immunohistochemistry; ISH, *In Situ* Hybridization; CEP17, Chromosome Enumeration Probe 17; CISH, Chromogenic *In Situ* Hybridization; SISH, Silver *In Situ* Hybridization.

The Remarkable Place of ADCs for Patients with Metastatic TNBC and HER2-low BC

In addition to SG, there are other novel **ADCs** under investigation for patients with advanced or metastatic **TNBC** and **HER2-low-expression BC**, such as **trastuzumab deruxtecan** [20]. It should be underscored that **trastuzumab deruxtecan** has been evaluated in women with **HER2-low positive BC cases** (meaning 1+ or 2+ expression for HER2 and no FISH- amplification) and has shown favorable effects (*e.g.*, the response rates to **trastuzumab deruxtecan** therapy were close to 40% in women with **HER2-low BC**) [20].

It should be highlighted that for the most difficult cases of symptomatic women with advanced or metastatic TNBC, who previously received CHT, immunotherapy or PARP inhibitors, the next option to consider would be SG (since SG demonstrated significant benefits, including prolonged OS, compared to standard CHT) [15].

Likewise, another ADC, **DS-1062** also targets **Trop-2** and has a **topoisomerase** payload that may offer a promising treatment option, but more studies are needed to further explore this issue [21]. Furthermore, some other **ADCs targeting HER3-positive BC** (*e.g.*, **U3-1402**) have been intensely explored in research studies [22].

How to Put Immune Checkpoint Inhibitors and PARP Inhibitors Into Perspective? Considerations of Targeted Therapeutic Options and Their Sequence in Patients with TNBC Associated With the *BRCA* Mutation and PD-L1 Positivity

If a woman with TNBC has the *BRCA* **gene mutation** and **PD-L1 positivity**, this means that many therapeutic options are available for her. However, there is often a dilemma about what to do first, if a patient has PD-L1-positive BC and a germline alteration in *BRCA* genes. It appears that **ICIs** should be used in the **first-line setting** (due to the survival benefit ICIs), and **PARP inhibitors** should be used **second** [23]. It seems that even if the PARP inhibitor is not applied first, this can be done later. In general, considering the use of CHT and ICIs first, and then PARP inhibitors looks reasonable (with the exception of some frail patients, who might not tolerate the CHT and ICI) [23].

CONCLUSION

A recent explosion of new **targeted** therapies for patients with advanced or **metastatic TNBC** poses a **challenging task to** properly diagnose patients and sequence these therapies in the face of individual clinical contexts and the personal needs of each patient.

In this situation, detecting groups of patients (using relevant tests), who have **germline *BRCA* or *PALB2* alterations, or somatic *BRCA* mutations** can indicate the potential candidates for therapies with PARP inhibitors. **PARP inhibitors** (*e.g.*, **olaparib**) should be incorporated into therapy for patients with germline *BRCA1* and *BRCA2* mutations (about 10%).

TNBC is more **immunogenic** (*e.g.*, it has a **higher tumor mutational burden,** more abundant **tumor-infiltrating lymphocytes,** and **higher PD-L1 expression**). Performing the **PD-L1** assay can indicate the candidates for possible immunotherapy (*e.g.*, **ICI** in combination with **CHT,** such as **atezolizumab + nab-paclitaxel)** in the first-, second-, and beyond-line settings (regardless of patients having germline alterations in *BRCA1/2* and possible ongoing therapy with **PARP inhibitors**).

Also, **antibody-drug conjugates (ADCs)** have shown efficacy and survival benefits for patients with **metastatic TNBC.** The first member of this class, **sacituzumab govitecan (SG)** (that is targeting **TROP2)** has been approved in the second-line and beyond setting, for treatment of all patients with metastatic **TNBC.** In the future, the use of ADCs in monotherapy *vs.* combination therapy requires further investigation.

• New **targeted therapies** for women with advanced or **metastatic TNBC** need to be individually considered, depending on their clinical status, personal preferences, **immune markers,** and **genetic mutations**;

• **PARP inhibitors** were the **first targeted therapies** approved for the management of women with **metastatic TNBC** associated with a **germline *BRCA1/2* mutation;**

• **Immunotherapy** has been approved for patients with **PD-L1-positive TNBC** (*e.g.*, **advanced or metastatic);**

• If a woman has **PD-L1-positive** BC and a germline alteration in *BRCA* genes, **immunotherapy** (which improves survival) should usually be used first, and **PARP inhibitors** could be incorporated second into her treatment;

• **Antibody-drug conjugates (ADCs)** revealed benefits for patients with **TNBC;**·

• An **ADC, sacituzumab govitecan,** has been approved in the second-line and beyond setting, for treatment of all patients with metastatic **TNBC;**

• Some **targeted therapies,** such as **PARP inhibitors** (*e.g.*, oral forms of **olaparib** and **talazoparib)** allow women to live longer, experience fewer side effects, and enjoy a better **quality of life (QoL).**

REFERENCES

[1]   American Cancer Society (ACS) Triple-Negative Breast Cancer. Available at: https://www.cancer. org/cancer/breast-cancer/about/types-of-breast-cancer/triple-negative.html (Accessed on: 2022).

[2]   Morales J, Li L, Fattah FJ, *et al.* Review of poly (ADP-ribose) polymerase (PARP) mechanisms of action and rationale for targeting in cancer and other diseases. Crit Rev Eukaryot Gene Expr 2014; 24(1): 15-28.
[http://dx.doi.org/10.1615/CritRevEukaryotGeneExpr.2013006875] [PMID: 24579667]

[3]   Cimino-Mathews A, Thompson E, Taube JM, *et al.* PD-L1 (B7-H1) expression and the immune tumor microenvironment in primary and metastatic breast carcinomas. Hum Pathol 2016; 47(1): 52-63.
[http://dx.doi.org/10.1016/j.humpath.2015.09.003] [PMID: 26527522]

[4]   Nagayama A, Vidula N, Ellisen L, Bardia A. Novel antibody–drug conjugates for triple negative breast cancer. Ther Adv Med Oncol 2020; 12.
[http://dx.doi.org/10.1177/1758835920915980] [PMID: 32426047]

[5]   Robson M, Im SA, Senkus E, *et al.* Olaparib for metastatic breast cancer in patients with a germline BRCA mutation. N Engl J Med 2017; 377(6): 523-33.
[http://dx.doi.org/10.1056/NEJMoa1706450] [PMID: 28578601]

[6]   Litton JK, Hurvitz SA, Mina LA, *et al.* Talazoparib versus chemotherapy in patients with germline BRCA1/2-mutated HER2-negative advanced breast cancer: final overall survival results from the EMBRACA trial. Ann Oncol 2020; 31(11): 1526-35.
[http://dx.doi.org/10.1016/j.annonc.2020.08.2098] [PMID: 32828825]

[7]   Tung NM, Robson ME, Ventz S, *et al.* TBCRC 048: phase II study of olaparib for metastatic breast cancer and mutations in homologous recombination-related genes. J Clin Oncol 2020; 38(36): 4274-82.
[http://dx.doi.org/10.1200/JCO.20.02151] [PMID: 33119476]

[8]   Robson M, Ruddy KJ, Im SA, *et al.* Patient-reported outcomes in patients with a germline BRCA mutation and HER2-negative metastatic breast cancer receiving olaparib versus chemotherapy in the OlympiAD trial. Eur J Cancer 2019; 120: 20-30.
[http://dx.doi.org/10.1016/j.ejca.2019.06.023] [PMID: 31446213]

[9]   Ettl J, Quek RGW, Lee KH, *et al.* Quality of life with talazoparib versus physician's choice of chemotherapy in patients with advanced breast cancer and germline BRCA1/2 mutation: patient-reported outcomes from the EMBRACA phase III trial. Ann Oncol 2018; 29(9): 1939-47.
[http://dx.doi.org/10.1093/annonc/mdy257] [PMID: 30124753]

[10]   Emens LA, Adams S, Barrios CH, *et al.* LBA16 IMpassion130: Final OS analysis from the pivotal phase III study of atezolizumab + nab-paclitaxel *vs.* placebo + nab-paclitaxel in previously untreated locally advanced or metastatic triple-negative breast cancer. Ann Oncol 2020; 31 (4): S1148.
[http://dx.doi.org/10.1016/j.annonc.2020.08.2244]

[11]   Cortes J, Cescon DW, Rugo HS, *et al.* Pembrolizumab plus chemotherapy versus placebo plus chemotherapy for previously untreated locally recurrent inoperable or metastatic triple-negative breast cancer (KEYNOTE-355): A randomised, placebo-controlled, double-blind, phase 3 clinical trial. Lancet 2020; 396(10265): 1817-28.
[http://dx.doi.org/10.1016/S0140-6736(20)32531-9] [PMID: 33278935]

[12]   Schmid P, Cortes J, Dent R, *et al.* Event-free survival with pembrolizumab in early triple-negative breast cancer. N Engl J Med 2022; 386(6): 556-67.
[http://dx.doi.org/10.1056/NEJMoa2112651] [PMID: 35139274]

[13]   Miles D, Gligorov J, André F, *et al.* Primary results from IMpassion131, a double-blind, placebo-controlled, randomised phase III trial of first-line paclitaxel with or without atezolizumab for unresectable locally advanced/metastatic triple-negative breast cancer. Ann Oncol 2021; 32(8): 994-1004.
[http://dx.doi.org/10.1016/j.annonc.2021.05.801] [PMID: 34219000]

[14]   Bergin ART, Loi S. Triple-negative breast cancer: Recent treatment advances. F1000Res 2019; 8: 1342.
[http://dx.doi.org/10.12688/f1000research.18888.1] [PMID: 31448088]

[15]   Bardia A, Tolaney SM, Loirat D. ASCENT: A randomized phase 3 study of sacituzumab govitecan *vs.* treatment of physician's choice in patients with previously treated triple-negative breast cancer. Ann Oncol 2020; 31 (4): S1142-215.
[http://dx.doi.org/10.1016/j.annonc.2020.08.2245]

[16]   National Comprehensive Cancer Network (NCCN). Available at: https://www.nccn.org/professionals/physician_gls/pdf/breast.pdf (Accessed on: 2022).

[17]   Van Poznak C, Somerfield MR, Bast RC, *et al.* Use of biomarkers to guide decisions on systemic therapy for women with metastatic breast cancer: American society of clinical oncology clinical practice guideline. J Clin Oncol 2015; 33(24): 2695-704.
[http://dx.doi.org/10.1200/JCO.2015.61.1459] [PMID: 26195705]

[18]   Wolff AC, Hammond MEH, Allison KH, *et al.* Human epidermal growth factor receptor 2 testing in breast cancer: American society of clinical oncology/college of american pathologists clinical practice guideline focused update. J Clin Oncol 2018; 36(20): 2105-22.
[http://dx.doi.org/10.1200/JCO.2018.77.8738] [PMID: 29846122]

[19]   Starczynski J, Atkey N, Connelly Y, *et al.* HER2 gene amplification in breast cancer: A rogues' gallery of challenging diagnostic cases: UKNEQAS interpretation guidelines and research recommendations. Am J Clin Pathol 2012; 137(4): 595-605.
[http://dx.doi.org/10.1309/AJCPATBZ2JFN1QQC] [PMID: 22431536]

[20]   Modi S, Park H, Murthy RK, *et al.* Antitumor activity and safety of trastuzumab deruxtecan in patients with HER2-low-expressing advanced breast cancer: Results from a phase Ib study. J Clin Oncol 2020; 38(17): 1887-96.
[http://dx.doi.org/10.1200/JCO.19.02318] [PMID: 32058843]

[21]   First-in-human Study of DS-1062a for Advanced Solid Tumors (TROPION-PanTumor01). Available at: https://clinicaltrials.gov/ct2/show/NCT03401385 (Accessed on: 2022).

[22]   Phase I/II Study of U3-1402 in Subjects With Human Epidermal Growth Factor Receptor 3 (HER3) Positive Metastatic Breast Cancer. Available at: https://clinicaltrials.gov/ct2/show/NCT02980341 (Accessed on: 2022).

[23]   Shen M, Pan H, Chen Y, Xu YH, Yang W, Wu Z. A review of current progress in triple-negative breast cancer therapy. Open Med 2020; 15(1): 1143-9.
[http://dx.doi.org/10.1515/med-2020-0138] [PMID: 33336070]

CHAPTER 6

The Way Out From the Labyrinth of Anticancer Therapies for Patients with Breast Cancer: How Can We Improve Their Cardiac Safety and Quality of Life?

Abstract: Patients with **Breast cancer (BC)** often experience a spectrum of **adverse, anticancer therapy-related symptoms**, which deteriorate their **quality of life (QoL)**. Therefore, effective strategies for BC are needed. Personalized medicine offers many therapeutic options (*e.g.*, targeted therapies) that can be tailored to the individual needs of a given patient.

This chapter aims to briefly present typical **side effects of current anticancer treatments**, which often reduce the QoL of patients with BC and survivors. In particular, it addresses pain (including chemotherapy (CHT)-induced peripheral neuropathy (PN) and lymphedema), depression, cognitive dysfunction, premature menopause, and CHT-induced menopause. It focuses on the adverse effects of the BC therapies, such as **chemotherapy (CHT), immunotherapy (IT)**, and some **targeted therapies.** In addition, several issues related to **cardiovascular toxicity** induced by anticancer treatments and **cardioprotective measures** for women with BC are addressed. This chapter also touches on the recent advances in precision medicine and provides some future directions, aimed at fulfilling unmet needs of patients with BC. The described approaches may be helpful in planning personalized treatment, facilitating the patient's tolerability of many available anticancer therapies, optimizing the medication selection, and improving the patient's QoL.

Keywords: Breast Cancer (BC), Chemotherapy (CHT), Cardiovascular toxicity, Cardioprotection, Cardio-oncology, Depression, Immunotherapy (IT), Pain, Peripheral neuropathy (PN), Personalized medicine approach, Precision medicine, Precision oncology, Quality of life (QoL), Targeted therapies.

INTRODUCTION

Over the last decade, **breast cancer (BC)** has been the most common type of malignancy in women worldwide [1]. According to the presence of certain BC-associated biomarkers (*e.g.*, estrogen receptor (ER), progesterone receptor (PR), and human epidermal receptor 2 (HER2)) detected in breast tumors, BC can be classified into different sub-types [2]. Due to the growing prevalence of BC, the development of safe and effective therapeutic strategies for BC is of utmost importance.

In addition to well-established treatment options (*e.g.*, surgery, radiation therapy (RT), endocrine therapy (ET) chemotherapy (CHT), some modern strategies, which influence the pathways of tumor signaling (*e.g.*, immunotherapy (IT) and targeted therapies), have been applied, contributing to the improved outcomes and longer survival rates of many patients with BC [3].

However, many challenges still remain with regard to targeted therapies and IT. In addition to the development of resistance to treatment, leading to patient relapses, the occurrence and severity of adverse effects of the standard and emerging anti-BC therapies often represent barriers to their application [4]. Risks for developing **long-term side effects post-BC treatments** are multifactorial, including the woman's age at the time of diagnosis, comorbid conditions with their therapies, and type, dose, and duration of the antineoplastic treatment [4]. In contrast to the "one size fits all" approach to patients with BC, individualized approaches should play the main role. In line with this concept, **precision medicine** presents strategies for the treatment and prevention of serious, chronic diseases (such as malignancies) that include the patient's genetics, cancer biological features, tumor microenvironment characteristics, patient's comorbidities, lifestyle, and quality of life (QoL) [5]. Furthermore, in **precision oncology**, the purpose is to **individualize each patient's management** (according to a detailed assessment of the risk of progression or recurrence of that patient's malignancy), during every step of diagnostic work-up, treatment process, and survivorship journey [5]. At present, several commonly used anticancer therapies (*e.g.*, CHT) cause various, undesirable symptoms, which negatively influence the QoL of BC patients or survivors (Fig. **1**) [4, 6].

This chapter aims to briefly present typical side effects of current anticancer treatments, which often reduce the QoL of patients with BC and survivors. In particular, it addresses pain (including chemotherapy (CHT)-induced **peripheral neuropathy (PN)** and **lymphedema**), **depression, cognitive dysfunction, premature menopause,** and **CHT-induced menopause**. It focuses on adverse effects of BC therapies, such as chemotherapy (CHT), immunotherapy (IT), and some targeted therapies. Also, several issues related to **cardiovascular toxicity induced by anticancer treatments and cardioprotective measures** for women with BC are addressed. In addition, it touches on the recent advances in precision medicine and provides some future directions to novel therapies, aimed at fulfilling unmet needs of patients with BC. The described approaches may be helpful in **planning personalized treatment**, facilitating the patient's tolerability of many available anticancer therapies, optimizing the medication selection, and improving the patient's QoL.

FREQUENT SIDE EFFECTS OF ANTICANCER TREATMENTS AND THEIR PERCEPTION IN PATIENTS WITH BREAST CANCER

Several patients with BC often experience treatment-related, unpleasant symptoms (Fig. **1**) [4, 6]. The effects of CHT on the QoL, among patients with BC and BC survivors, were assessed using the QoL evaluation forms (*e.g.*, physical and psychological parameters) at certain time points (*e.g.*, before CHT, after the 3-rd cycle of CHT, within two-three weeks of completing adjuvant CHT, and at least 8 years post CHT). Based on this study's results, **pain, fatigue**, and **depressive symptoms**, were increased in the participating pre-and peri-menopausal women with BC at all stages of their therapeutic process [7]. In addition, many disturbing symptoms, as well as their adverse impact on the patient's functional status, corresponding with BC worse outcomes, were noted in these patients [8].

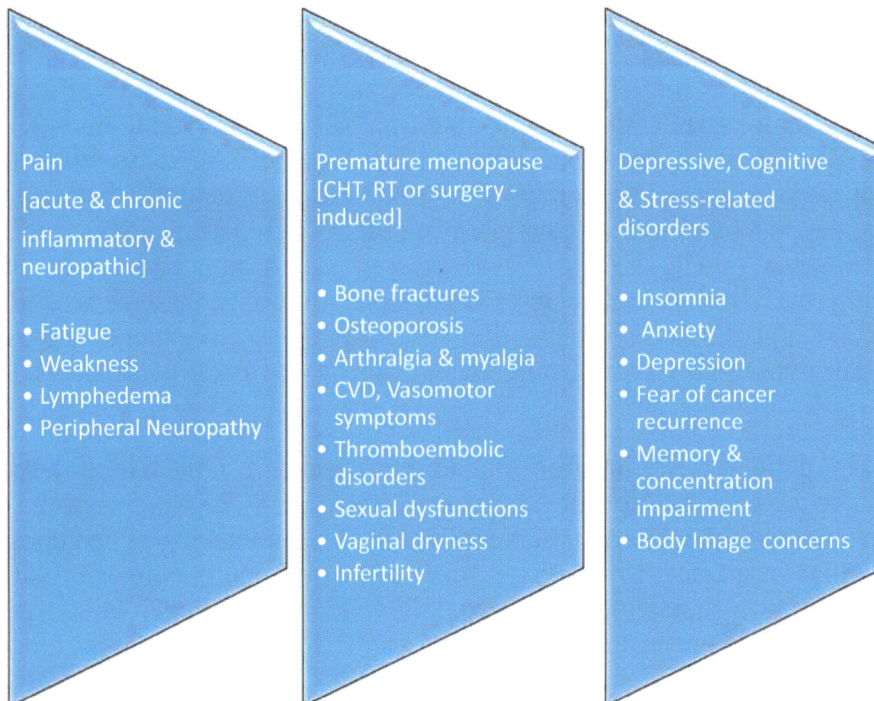

Fig. (1). Frequent adverse effects of breast cancer treatments that decrease the patients quality of life; CVD, cardiovascular diseases; CHT, chemotherapy; RT, radiotherapy.

It should be noted that the patients with BC, who have been diagnosed with different BC stages, revealed **various perceptions of the BC treatment-associated side effects**. For instance, certain negative effects may seem more acceptable to patients at the **early stage of BC**, mostly due to the anticipated positive treatment results and hope of curing the BC. In contrast, the similar side effects, in patients with a metastatic stage of BC, need to be promptly addressed and effectively managed. This is because **metastatic BC** has usually poor outcome, and thus, focusing on satisfactory QoL is one of the main priorities for such patients and their medical teams and family caretakers. Under these circumstances, it is critically important to understand the context of the BC treatment-related adverse effects. Physicians and other treatment team members need to pay special attention to timely provide helpful solutions to minimize the toxicity of BC therapies for patients with metastatic BC stages.

A SPOTLIGHT ON TWO "FACES" OF PAIN SECONDARY TO ANTICANCER THERAPIES IN PATIENTS WITH BREAST CANCER: PERIPHERAL NEUROPATHY AND LYMPHEDEMA

Pain that is often induced by the anticancer therapies is one of the most typical symptoms experienced by numerous patients with BC. This is often because of the chemotherapy (CHT)-induced **peripheral neuropathy (PN)**. It has been noted that in PN, the changes in neurotransmission and pro-inflammatory cytokine's actions reflect the main abnormalities in peripheral nerves, which adversely influence motor and sensory functions of the extremities [9]. In addition, according to a recent meta-analysis, it has been reported that some other risk factors, such as axillary lymph node dissection, lymphedema, receiving different kinds of CHT, RT, or ET, as well as obesity, and lower level of education, may lead to a more intense pain perception, in patients with BC and BC survivors [10]. Even six years after finishing of such treatments, almost 50% of BC survivors had reported numbness in the distal parts of their extremities [11].

Moreover, patients suffering from PN are more prone to falls and bone fractures [12]. Since the neuropathic pain caused by CHT, such as PN, represents an unmet need in women with BC, some therapies using antioxidants have been considered as potential strategies to alleviate this refractory neuropathy. Similarly, an oxidative-stress-associated mitochondrial dysfunction was shown to be a possible contributor to the neuropathic pain, induced by CHT [13]. In addition, it has been found that the hormone melatonin (secreted by the pineal gland) works as a powerful antioxidant, and can possibly reduce mitochondrial damage as well as neuropathic pain caused by paclitaxel (based on animal study findings) [13]. However, further studies are necessary to explore this area.

Lymphedema that is a swelling of the extremities, induced by BC treatments, presents a common problem among patients with BC and survivors [14]. Based on a recent study, the BC survivors with lymphedema are characterized by certain biochemical parameters (*e.g.*, an increased level of total polyunsaturated fatty acids (PUFA), elevated activity of fatty acid desaturase, and a higher ratio between arachidonic acid and eicosapentaenoic acid) [15]. These findings may indicate a possible association between the risk of lymphedema and fatty acid metabolism. Also, it is possible that the PUFA status of women with BC may play the role of a biomarker for targeting pain levels experienced by these patients. That may indicate a potential modification of the PUFA nutritional intake, which may be helpful in decreasing lymphedema-associated pain in women with BC. However, further studies in patients with BC are necessary to determine these results.

HOW CAN WE APPROACH DEPRESSION AND COGNITIVE IMPAIRMENT IN PATIENTS WITH BREAST CANCER FROM DIFFERENT PERSPECTIVES?

Depression is a serious psychological problem, which is frequently associated with other symptoms, such as pain, fatigue, insomnia, anxiety, and cognitive deterioration in patients with BC undergoing anticancer therapies (*e.g.*, CHT) [16]. Mild to moderate levels of depression were also reported in about 50% of BC survivors, often in combination with cognitive dysfunctions [16]. In addition, these mental or emotional symptoms, and impairment of the QoL were noted in women with BC, during the anticancer therapy, and after its completion [17].

From the personalized perspective, a gene coding for **brain-derived neurotrophic factor (BDNF)** was suggested to play a role of potential biomarker for depression [18]. Moreover, a genetic polymorphism in the BDNF gene is related to the blood level of **C-reactive protein (CRP)**. This may help predict the severity level of depression [18]. Also, a polymorphism in the BDNF gene may be used as an early indicator for the introduction of anti-depressive treatments (*e.g.*, before the occurrence of full-blown depressive symptoms) [18]. In a practical setting, these patients should undergo screening for depression, and then, treatment strategies should be matched with the needs of individual patients (*e.g.*, pharmacotherapy or psychotherapy) [18].

Cognitive impairment is a complex problem associated with CHT, ET, and anesthesia during surgery, in which the patient's age, comorbid conditions and medications, and genetic factors are strongly related to the risk for mental decline in patients with BC [19]. Deterioration of cognition, including difficulties with memory, concentration, and executive functions, has also been reported in approximately 30% of BC survivors (*e.g.*, after CHT completion) [19]. According to a recent study, a **polymorphism** in the ***IL1R1* gene (*IL1R1*** gene product participates in promoting inflammation) is related to a higher level of cognitive functions in BC survivors [20]. This finding suggests a possible biomarker, which can detect patients receiving CHT, who may have a low risk of cognitive dysfunction, and thus, would not require additional interventions for this reason.

HOW CAN WE ADDRESS THE MANAGEMENT OF MENOPAUSAL SYMPTOMS IN YOUNGER WOMEN UNDERGOING CHEMOTHERAPY FOR BREAST CANCER?

Many younger women with BC, who underwent CHT, have a higher risk of developing premature menopause (**chemotherapy-induced menopause (CIM)**), which leads to various gynecologic symptoms, increased risk of osteoporosis, bone fractures, and cardiovascular conditions, which often decrease their QoL [21]. Premature menopause is caused by the decline of ovarian functions (a deficiency in estrogen and progesterone production) in young patients (*e.g.*, below 40 years of age) with BC, who were treated with CHT [21]. It appears that the identification of genetic polymorphisms, which are related to production and metabolism of estrogen may provide some novel genetic biomarkers. These biomarkers can be helpful to address symptoms of premature menopause or CIM, among women with BC. For instance, a recent study has shown that single nucleotide polymorphisms (SNPs) in the **genes coding for estrogen receptors (*ESR1*** and ***ESR2*)** were related to premature ovarian failure (which is a component of premature menopause) [22]. These findings may indicate potential biomarkers, which can be targeted for the treatment of patients with BC, who suffer from premature menopause. In the future, this approach may yield useful information for the development of personalized therapies, which can improve the management of menopausal symptoms among such women [22].

HOW TO ASSESS CARDIOTOXICITY RELATED TO TREATMENTS FOR BREAST CANCER?

Anticancer-treatment-related cardiotoxicity is a serious concern for numerous patients with BC, receiving various types of therapy. This cardiotoxicity is often superimposed on the pre-existing **cardiovascular diseases (CVD)** or **cardiovascular (CV) risk factors** [23]. CHT, RT, ET, and certain targeted BC treatments (*e.g.*, anti-HER-2 therapies, CDK4/6 inhibitors), are related to an increased risk of developing cardiotoxicity [24]. Similarly, RT has also been related to different CV complications, such as **pericardial, myocardial,** and **valvular diseases**, as well as **CHD, HF,** and **cardiac arrhythmias** [25].

Also, BC survivors are at higher risk for thromboembolic disorders, due to increased platelet adherence and thrombus formation in arteries, after RT [24]. Moreover, adjuvant ET (*e.g.*, tamoxifen) can augment the risk of **venous thromboembolism** and its adverse consequences [25]. The most prevalent CV complications of anticancer therapies are **arterial hypertension, cardiac arrhythmias, coronary heart disease (CHD), heart failure (HF), valvular diseases, peripheral vascular disease (PVD), stroke, pulmonary hypertension,** and **pericardial diseases** [26]. In addition, premature menopause (*e.g.*, CHT-induced) predisposes women to higher risk of CVD [25].

Moreover, women with BC and their treatment teams should be aware of the **cardiotoxicity profiles of the anticancer treatments for BC**. Identification of high-risk patients, modification of their CV risk factors, detection of early signs of CV abnormalities (*e.g., via* regular cardiac exams, imaging tests, such as echocardiography and cardiac magnetic resonance imaging for monitoring left ventricular function and circulating cardiac biomarkers) and rapid introduction of effective CV treatment strategies (*e.g., via* pharmacologic agents, nutrition, and exercise programs) are necessary to improve the CV and BC outcomes in the afflicted patients [25].

It should be emphasized that an early, comprehensive evaluation of patients with BC, who are scheduled to receive cardiotoxic anticancer therapies (*e.g.*, anthracycline-based CHT) needs to be conducted, and then, such patients require a regular, long-term treatment-and monitoring (Tables **1-3**) [26 - 30].

Table 1. Exemplary imaging techniques of the heart for initial evaluation and follow-up of patients scheduled to receive cardiotoxic treatments for breast cancer.

Imaging Test	Practical Remarks	Advantages	Limitations
2D Echocardiography	Measures cardiac structure & function, • chamber size, • wall thickness, • heart valves, • pericardium, • LVEF, • diastolic function	Safe (no radiation) Available Cost-effective	Intra- & inter-observer variability (*e.g.*, in the LVEF evaluation) • variability in the estimation of cardiac parameters, • suboptimal image quality • (*e.g.*, in pts with BC, post mastectomy) • changes in hemodynamic status, myocardial contractility, loading conditions can affect the results • unable to detect early stages of cardiac dysfunction, or subclinical cardiotoxicity

(Table 1) cont.....

Imaging Test	Practical Remarks	Advantages	Limitations
3D Echocardiography	More precise than the 2D ECHO for measurements of LVEF & LV volumes, the preferred method for serial monitoring of cardiotoxicity.	• Accurate & reproducible • Low variability of intra-, inter-observer, • High correlation with CMR	Expensive Training of medical staff is needed.
Strain Speckle-Tracking Echocardiography	Strain and strain rate can be measured in 3 dimensions. Reveals early abnormalities in cardiac mechanics, secondary to anticancer therapies.	Reproducible Able to detect subclinical LV dysfunction	Hemodynamic status and preload/afterload conditions can affect the results, expensive Advanced technical training is needed.
MUGA scan	Not accurate for HF prediction, cannot be used for the accurate evaluation of RV function due to the the overlap between RV and RA.	High reproducibility	Exposure to radiation that will cumulate when performing serial scans during the course of CHT.
CMR	The reference standard in the evaluation of LV volumes and LVEF • epicardial & endocardial contours can be traced in end-diastole and end-systole, • calculations of LVEF %, ventricular volumes, and LV mass can be performed concurrently, • should be considered if the assessment *via* ECHO is inadequate	• Safety (absence of radiation), • superior spatial resolution of cardiac structures, • ability to identify myocardial fibrosis and edema, • reproducible assessment of cardiac chamber size	High cost, time-consuming test, specialized training of medical personnel is needed, difficult access

BC, breast cancer; HF, heart failure; 2D, Two-dimensional echocardiography; ECHO, echocardiography; 3D, Three-dimensional echocardiography; GLS, global longitudinal strain; LV, left ventricle; LVEF, left ventricular ejection fraction; pts, patients; RA, right atrium; RV, right ventricle; SSTE, strain speckle-tracking echocardiography; MUGA, Multiple Gated Acquisition; CMR, cardiac magnetic resonance (imaging test).

According to the **2021 European Society of Cardiology (ESC) Guidelines for the Diagnosis and Treatment of Heart Failure (HF), the updated recommendations**, relevant to **patients with cancer, who receive chemotherapeutic agents** (and thus, are at risk for cardiotoxicity), need to be **evaluated by a cardio-oncologist** (or a **cardio-oncology team**) before the initiation of cardiotoxic anticancer therapies, and then, carefully monitored, depending on the individual patient's status (Table **3**) [26 - 30].

Table 2. Clinical role of selected cardiac biomarker testing.

Cardiac Biomarker	Biologic Action	Diagnostic Value	Practical Remarks
Brain natriuretic peptide (BNP)	a peptide hormone released by cardiomyocytes in response to heart muscle stretch or injury; BNP signals to the kidneys to release sodium and water to the urine to lower the blood volume & BP;	diagnosing HF predicting clinical outcomes; BNP rising is proportional to the CV risk level;	serum levels of BNP & its precursor NT-pro BNP can be quantified;
N-terminal pro-B-type natriuretic peptide (NT-pro BNP)	a marker of HF severity, NT-proBNP is released from over-worked heart muscle cells	an absence of a reduction in the BNP or NT-proBNP levels from hospital admission to discharge may detect high-risk patients, in whom a vigilant post-discharge monitoring is mandatory	a precursor of BNP; NT-proBNP is not a substrate for an enzyme neprilysin; endogenous BNP levels are increased due to effects of the sacubitril (inhibitor of neprilysin; however, the NT-proBNP levels are not affected by sacubitril
Cardiac troponins (cTnI & cTnT)	regulatory proteins related to cardiac muscle fibers; can be released to circulation upon cardiomyocyte injury or death;	the gold standard for detecting acute damage to the heart muscle (*e.g.*, MI); measurement of serum cTnT using a high-sensitivity assay (hs-cTnT) can be used in HF diagnosis & risk assessment;	may "leak" from myocytes during chronic diseases (*e.g.*, HF);
C-reactive protein (CRP)	CRP is secreted in response to inflammatory cytokines; its levels increase rapidly (in case of trauma, inflammation, & infection) & decrease upon the resolution of the condition	a pro-inflammatory marker, patients at risk of CHD might benefit from the measurement of CRP	more relevant in prognostic rather than diagnostic aspects, not specific for HF

BNP, Brain natriuretic peptide; BP, blood pressure; CV, cardiovascular; CVD, cardiovascular disease; HF, heart failure; MI, myocardial infarction; CHD, coronary heart disease.

MAY STANDARD PHARMACOTHERAPY FOR HEART FAILURE PROVIDE CARDIOPROTECTIVE EFFECTS FOR WOMEN WITH BREAST CANCER?

Reducing cardiotoxic effects, without compromising anticancer effects is an important treatment goal for women with BC (in particular those with preexisting CVD and elderly ones). Importantly, **angiotensin-converting enzyme inhibitors (ACEIs)**, **angiotensin receptor blockers (ARBs)** and **beta-blockers (BBs)** are recommended first-line agents for **heart failure (HF)** [26].

Table 3. The updated recommendations from 2021 ESC Guidelines for the Diagnosis and Treatment of Heart Failure, relevant to patients with cancer, receiving cardiotoxic therapies.

ESC Guidelines for the Diagnosis and Treatment of Heart Failure		
Focus on patients with cancer, who are exposed To cardiotoxicity		
-	**Clinical Remarks**	**Updated Recommendations**
1	HF with left ventricular ejection fraction (LVEF) of 41-49% is now revised to HF with mildly reduced EF (HFmEF)	HF with LVEF of 41-49% is HF with mildly reduced EF (HFmEF) HF with LVEF ≤40% is HF with reduced EF (HFrEF) HF with LVEF ≥50% is HF with preserved EF (HFpEF)
2	Cardiac magnetic resonance (CMR) test is recommended in Pts with poor acoustic windows (ECHO) or in Pts with suspected infiltrative cardiomyopathy, hemochromatosis, or myocarditis	Pts with suspected HF should have • ECG, ECHO, CXR, • blood tests: CBC, urea, electrolytes, iron studies, • metabolic tests: HbA1c, lipid, panel, thyroid panel, • biomarkers: BNP/NT-proBNP
3	Guideline-directed medical therapy (GDMT) is now modified & includes ARNI	For Pts with HFrEF & NYHA class II or worse, therapy includes • angiotensin receptor neprilysin inhibitor (ARNI) as a replacement for angiotensin-converting enzyme (ACE) inhibitors • addition of SGLT-2 inhibitors (dapagliflozin or empagliflozin)
4	Implantable cardioverter-defibrillators (ICDs) recommendations	ICDs are recommended for • primary prevention of sudden cardiac death for symptomatic ischemic or nonischemic cardiomyopathy with LVEF ≤35% (despite 3 ms of therapy) if expected survival is >1 year. ICD is NOT recommended • within 40 ds of a MI. • for Pts with NYHA class IV (who are not candidates for advanced therapies).
5	Cardiac resynchronization therapy (CRT) recommendations	CRT is recommended for • symptomatic HFrEF with EF <35% in sinus rhythm with an LBBB (> 150 msec). • in HFrEF with EF <35% irrespective of symptoms or QRS duration if there is a high-grade AV block with need for a pacemaker.

(Table 3) cont.....

ESC Guidelines for the Diagnosis and Treatment of Heart Failure		
Focus on patients with cancer, who are exposed To cardiotoxicity		
-	**Clinical Remarks**	**Updated Recommendations**
6	Therapies recommended for HFmEF & HFpEF	Recommended for HFmEF • diuretics - to relieve vascular congestion • ACE inhibitors/angiotensin-receptor blockers • ARNIs • beta-blockers • mineralocorticoid receptor antagonists (considered as additional therapy to < mortality & hospitalization). for HFpEF, diagnosis & treatment of contributing factors • hypertension, kidney disease, *etc.* • use of diuretics. No specific therapies have been proven to < mortality in HFpEF
7	For all Pts with HF, exercise & HF programs, home - or clinic-based, self-management are recommended; counseling against smoking, alcohol, drug use, & obesity	For prevention of HF - treatment of hypertension, • use of statins when indicated, • SGLT2 inhibitors in diabetics at high risk for or with CVD For acute decompensated HF, routine use of • inotropes is NOT recommended in the absence of cardiogenic shock. • opioids is NOT recommended. • intra-aortic balloon pump in post-MI cardiogenic shock is NOT recommended. For hospitalized Pts with acute HF, < volume overload prior to discharge (with follow-up within 1-2 weeks of discharge) is needed For Pts with AF • routine use of anticoagulation (for CHA2DS2-VASc ≥3 in women), with DOACs (except in the presence of a prosthetic mechanical valve or moderate or severe mitral stenosis) is recommended. • urgent cardioversion for Pts in AF with HF and hemodynamic compromise is recommended. All Pts with HF should be periodically screened for iron deficiency anemia.
8	Heart team approach	including catheter ablation to be considered for Pts with AF & symptoms of HF. For Pts with HF & severe aortic stenosis, transcatheter/surgical aortic valve replacement is recommended.

(Table 3) cont.....

ESC Guidelines for the Diagnosis and Treatment of Heart Failure		
Focus on patients with cancer, who are exposed To cardiotoxicity		
-	**Clinical Remarks**	**Updated Recommendations**
9	Heart team approach	For Pts with HF & secondary mitral regurgitation - percutaneous edge-to-edge mitral valve repair – is to be considered if severe symptoms persist despite therapy. For Pts with secondary mitral regurgitation & CAD who need revascularization - CABG & mitral valve surgery - to be considered
10	Cardio-oncology team evaluation	Pts with cancer, who need to receive CHT agents & are at risk for cardiotoxicity, should be evaluated by a cardio-oncologist prior to initiation of such therapies.

ESC, European Society of Cardiology; HF, Heart Failure; Pts, patients; ECG, electrocardiogm; ECHO, transthoracic echocardiogram; CXR, chest X-ray; CBC, complete blood cell count; HbA1c, glycated hemoglobin; BNP/NT-proBNP, B-type natriuretic peptide; LVEF, left ventricular ejection fraction; CMR, cardiac magnetic resonance; GDMT, guideline-directed medical therapy; NYHA, New York Heart Association; ICDs, Implantable cardioverter-defibrillators; ms, months; ds, days; MI, myocardial infarction; CRT, cardiac resynchronization therapy; LBBB, left bundle branch block; SR, sinus rhythm; AV, atrioventricular; CVD, cardiovascular disease; AF, atrial fibrillation; DOACs, direct-acting oral anticoagulants; CAD, coronary artery disease; CABG, coronary artery bypass grafting; CHT, chemotherapy; CHA2DS2-VASc, clinical prediction score for estimating the risk of ischemic stroke and systemic thromboembolism (IS/SE) in patients with atrial fibrillation (AF).

According to the results from **MANTICORE 101-Breast** trial for the prevention of **trastuzumab-associated cardiotoxicity**, an ACEI, **perindopril**, and BB, **bisoprolol**, were well tolerated in patients with **HER2-positive early BC**, who received **targeted therapy** with trastuzumab (Table **4**) [31]. In addition, perindopril and bisoprolol were protective against anticancer therapy-related declines in LVEF (Table **4**) [31].

Also, based on the results from the **PRADA** study, treatment with **anthracycline CHT** for **early BC** is associated with an increase in circulating cardiovascular biomarkers, but this increase is not associated with an early decline in ventricular function. Moreover, **BBs** (*e.g.*, **metoprolol)** may reduce early myocardial injury. However, it is unknown whether or not this reduction translates into decreased risk of developing ventricular dysfunction, in the long term. In addition, concomitant treatment with an **ARB**, **candesartan**, provides protection against an early decline in left ventricular function (Table **4**) [32]. It appears that the use of standard pharmacotherapy for HF, including **ACEIs (perindopril), ARBs (candesartan)** in combination with **BBs (carvedilol** or **metoprolol)** can decrease the risk of CHT-mediated cardiac dysfunction, but long-term clinical trials are needed to confirm these benefits [31, 32].

Table 4. Exemplary clinical trials investigating the protective role of certain classes of cardiac medications in patients with HER2-positive breast cancer.

Trial Name Reference	Anticancer Treatment Agent	Breast Cancer Type	Cardio-Protective Medications	Trial Purpose Outcomes	Clinical Implications
MANTICORE NCT01016886 [31]	**Trastuzumab**	HER2-positive early invasive	**ACEI - perindopril, BB - bisoprolol**	Testing cardiac meds in the prevention of trastuzumab-induced cardiotoxicity; The 12-month change in LV - end-diastolic volume (assessed by ECHO, CMR)	**Developing guidelines for the use of ACEIs & BBs in HER2-positive BC, treated with trastuzumab.**
PRADA NCT01434134 [32]	**Anthracycline-containing CHT** with or without **trastuzumab, & RT**	HER2-positive early stage	**ARB - candesartan, BB - metoprolol**	Change in LVEF (assessed by ECHO, MUGA scans, or CMR) from start to completion of adjuvant anti-cancer therapy	**Treatment with ARB - candesartan (but not with BB – metoprolol) provides protection against LVEF decline in patients with BC; further RCTs are needed to investigate the protective role of ARB, long-term.**

ACEI, angiotensin-converting enzyme inhibitor; ARB, angiotensin receptor blocker; BB, beta-blocker; BC, breast cancer; CHT, chemotherapy; CMR, cardiac magnetic resonance; ECHO, echocardiography; MUGA, multiple-gated acquisition scan; HER-2, human epidermal growth factor receptor-2; LVEF, left ventricular ejection fraction; meds, medications; RT, radiotherapy; RCT, Randomized Controlled Trial.

HOW TO REDUCE CARDIOTOXICITY RELATED TO TREATMENTS FOR BREAST CANCER? FOCUS ON CARDIO-ONCOLOGY, REHABILITATION, AND INTEGRATIVE INTERVENTIONS

The main components of integrative **Cardio-Oncology** care include an initial **evaluation of patient-related cardiovascular (CV) concerns and oncology therapy-specific risks,** followed by careful monitoring and management of the CV condition [33].

Cardiotoxicity is a big concern among possible **CV complications of anticancer therapies**. In particular, harmful mechanisms of CHT agents usually include

DNA damage, endothelial dysfunction, and oxidative stress. As a consequence, patients with BC often suffer from fatigue, weakness, and reduced fitness level, due to these toxic effects, tumor burden, and physical deconditioning [33]. Therefore, a prompt introduction of **cardioprotective approaches**, around BC therapies is needed to decrease cardiotoxicities associated with treatments for BC [33]. For instance, aerobic exercises might play a protective role, and thus, a supervised, group or individual, **physical activity** program appears to be the most feasible solution to apply. Such an optimal physical activity program needs to consider each patient's **personal motivations** and obstacles to regular physical exercises during and after treatment for BC [33]. To enhance the expected benefits, it is necessary to constantly reinforce **adherence** and maintain motivation. Further studies are needed to determine practical recommendations, which should be given to patients with BC by their treatment team members [33].

In addition, many patients with BC or survivors of BC require certain interventions to prevent them from weight gain, as well as help with weight loss and maintenance of the recommended body mass. Adding such interventions (*e.g.*, **lifestyle modifications to reduce obesity)** would decrease their risk of BC recurrence. These interventions (*e.g.*, combined nutritional and exercise programs) appear acceptable to patients with BC undergoing anticancer treatments as well as to BC survivors [34]. Moreover, in several patients with cancer, exercise training is usually safe and well-tolerated. It may counteract various side effects of anticancer therapies, and this is particularly important since protective pharmacologic treatments for combating cardiotoxicity induced by anticancer therapies are limited. Furthermore, exercise-induced modifications of gene expression contribute to better CV parameters and higher levels of cardiopulmonary fitness [34].

Also, numerous patients with cancer require specially tailored exercise programs, created by cardiologists and oncologists. Depending on the circumstances, in addition to the group programs, home-based **cardio-oncology rehabilitation programs** may be considered to fulfill the needs of individual patients [34].

FURTHER DIRECTIONS: EFFORTS TO DEVELOP THE "KNOWLEDGE NETWORK" FOR PERSONALIZED MEDICINE GOALS

To accomplish the personalized medicine goals, the development of the **"Knowledge Network"**, meaning a precise **disease classification system** (*e.g.*, based on molecular biology), will be created [35]. This network system will incorporate genomic information from several fields (*e.g.*, DNA sequencing, molecular biotechnologies, basic and clinical research data, reports from observational studies, and patients' medical records), which are crucial to analyze relations between the different data sets. As a consequence, a more accurate **classification of malignancies, such as BC, will enable a precise selection of possible targeted treatments** [35].

Also, to provide the best available treatment for every individual patient, the treatment teams will need to apply several resources, such as **sets of medical data** and link them with the given **patient's clinical and personalized context** [35].

Moreover, the genetic biomarkers need to be identified, to predict the individual risk of developing common adverse symptoms, associated with particular anticancer treatments [36]. Also, the detection of novel biomarkers, which can influence the treatment efficacy and severity of adverse symptoms is needed. For this reason, further studies in this field are merited to enable the development of novel approaches, which may refine anticancer therapies for many patients with BC, by increasing the treatment effectiveness and improving the QoL of women with BC, who suffer from discomfort due to complex diagnostic and therapeutic procedures, during their BC journey.

CONCLUSION

Precision medicine (the term that is preferable to "personalized medicine") means the creation of therapies, which are unique for a given patient (*e.g.*, a woman with certain BC subtype). This approach relates to the tailoring of medical treatment to the individual clinical and personal characteristics of each patient. In addition, precision medicine classifies patients with BC into subpopulations that vary in their response to particular therapeutic agents. In a result, **therapeutic** or potentially **preventive interventions** are focused on the individuals, who will benefit from such approaches and also, will experience relatively **minimal side effects**, leading to **improved QoL**.

Due to the numerous adverse effects of the currently used anticancer treatment regimens, many patients with BC suffer from different therapy-related symptoms. Since this situation may even cause the treatment termination, molecular-targeted therapy or immunotherapy, in addition to CHT or hormone therapy, merits special attention. Currently, various genomic changes, which may influence the adverse symptoms, among many individual patients with BC, have been detected. Since pain (*e.g.,*) is one of the most prevalent symptoms in patients with BC, the detection of novel biomarkers, which are associated with pain (caused by the BC treatment) will be helpful for the design of innovative personalized strategies for pain management among such patients. For instance, some possible avenues for **alleviation of pain** caused by lymphedema and chemotherapy-induced peripheral neuropathy (PN) have recently been considered. It appears that certain genes may represent innovative targets, relevant to the CHT-induced neurotoxicity, which may be helpful for the development of new interventions to reduce neuropathic pain due to CHT.

In addition, some cardiac biomarkers have been identified, which may serve as possible tools for guiding the best treatment selection and **reducing cardiotoxic side effects of anticancer therapies** for many patients with BC. Simultaneously, the updated recommendations from ESC Guidelines for the Diagnosis and Treatment of Heart Failure provide some helpful strategies for prevention, surveillance, and treatment of anticancer therapy-induced cardiotoxicity, and indicate approaches for cardioprotection, for patients with BC. Moreover, it should be encouraging for many women with BC that staying physically active can prevent, to some degree, BC treatment-induced cardiotoxicity.

Cardioprotective strategies, based on cardiac risk stratification, tailored to both the individual patient genetic predispositions, and the anticancer therapy-related risk factors need to be incorporated in **patient-centered,** comprehensive therapeutic plans. **Cardio-oncology team members** (*e.g.*, oncologists, cardiologists, primary care physicians, nurses, rehabilitation therapists, and pharmacists) and their patients with BC should be engaged in long-term, close cooperation.

• **Precision medicine** offers an individualized treatment for every woman with BC, as well as the development of helpful strategies, necessary to **combat many side effects** of therapies for BC.

• Individualized strategies for **the relief of pain, depression,** and **symptoms of premature menopause** (induced by anticancer therapies) need to be applied for patients with BC to reduce their discomfort and improve QoL.

• **Cardio-oncology care** involves an evaluation and management of patient-related cardiac concerns and oncology therapy-specific cardiac risks.

• The **benefit-risk ratio for any anticancer medication** has to be **analyzed for the individual patient's BC &cardiac condition**, together with regular monitoring of the patient's clinical symptoms and parameters (*e.g.*, arterial blood pressure, heart rate, left ventricular ejection fraction (LVEF), renal function parameters, and cardiac biomarkers).

• Introduction to **cardioprotective approaches** (*e.g.*, pharmacotherapy, weight control, and cardiac rehabilitation) around the BC therapies is necessary to decrease cardiotoxicities associated with many treatments for BC.

REFERENCES

[1]   Lei S, Zheng R, Zhang S, *et al.* Global patterns of breast cancer incidence and mortality: A population-based cancer registry data analysis from 2000 to 2020. Cancer Commun 2021; 41(11): 1183-94.
[http://dx.doi.org/10.1002/cac2.12207] [PMID: 34399040]

[2]   Cardoso F, Senkus E, Costa A, *et al.* 4th ESO–ESMO international consensus guidelines for advanced breast cancer (ABC 4). Ann Oncol 2018; 29(8): 1634-57.
[http://dx.doi.org/10.1093/annonc/mdy192] [PMID: 30032243]

[3]   Gradishar WJ, Moran MS, Abraham J, *et al.* Breast cancer, version 3.2022, nccn clinical practice guidelines in oncology. J Natl Compr Canc Netw 2022; 20(6): 691-722.
[http://dx.doi.org/10.6004/jnccn.2022.0030] [PMID: 35714673]

[4]   Gegechkori N, Haines L, Lin JJ. Long-term and latent side effects of specific cancer types. Med Clin North Am 2017; 101(6): 1053-73.
[http://dx.doi.org/10.1016/j.mcna.2017.06.003] [PMID: 28992854]

[5]   Collins FS, Varmus H. A new initiative on precision medicine. N Engl J Med 2015; 372(9): 793-5.
[http://dx.doi.org/10.1056/NEJMp1500523] [PMID: 25635347]

[6]   Sullivan CW, Leutwyler H, Dunn LB, *et al.* Stability of symptom clusters in patients with breast cancer receiving chemotherapy. J Pain Symptom Manage 2018; 55(1): 39-55.
[http://dx.doi.org/10.1016/j.jpainsymman.2017.08.008] [PMID: 28838866]

[7]   Klemp JR, Myers JS, Fabian CJ, *et al.* Cognitive functioning and quality of life following chemotherapy in pre- and peri-menopausal women with breast cancer. Support Care Cancer 2018; 26(2): 575-83.
[http://dx.doi.org/10.1007/s00520-017-3869-3] [PMID: 28849337]

[8]   Oh H, Seo Y, Jeong H, Seo W. The identification of multiple symptom clusters and their effects on functional performance in cancer patients. J Clin Nurs 2012; 21(19pt20): 2832-42.
[http://dx.doi.org/10.1111/j.1365-2702.2011.04057.x] [PMID: 22805185]

[9]   Boyette-Davis JA, Walters ET, Dougherty PM. Mechanisms involved in the development of chemotherapy-induced neuropathy. Pain Manag 2015; 5(4): 285-96.
[http://dx.doi.org/10.2217/pmt.15.19] [PMID: 26087973]

[10]   Leysen L, Beckwée D, Nijs J, *et al.* Risk factors of pain in breast cancer survivors: A systematic review and meta-analysis. Support Care Cancer 2017; 25(12): 3607-43.
[http://dx.doi.org/10.1007/s00520-017-3824-3] [PMID: 28799015]

[11]   Winters-Stone KM, Hilton C, Luoh SW, Jacobs P, Faithfull S, Horak FB. Comparison of physical function and falls among women with persistent symptoms of chemotherapy-induced peripheral neuropathy. J Clin Oncol 2016; 34(3_suppl): 130.
[http://dx.doi.org/10.1200/jco.2016.34.3_suppl.130]

[12]   Winters-Stone KM, Horak F, Jacobs PG, *et al.* Falls, functioning, and disability among women with persistent symptoms of chemotherapy-induced peripheral neuropathy. J Clin Oncol 2017; 35(23): 2604-12.
[http://dx.doi.org/10.1200/JCO.2016.71.3552] [PMID: 28586243]

[13]   Galley HF, McCormick B, Wilson KL, Lowes DA, Colvin L, Torsney C. Melatonin limits paclitaxel-induced mitochondrial dysfunction *in vitro* and protects against paclitaxel-induced neuropathic pain in the rat. J Pineal Res 2017; 63(4): e12444.
[http://dx.doi.org/10.1111/jpi.12444] [PMID: 28833461]

[14]   DiSipio T, Rye S, Newman B, Hayes S. Incidence of unilateral arm lymphoedema after breast cancer: A systematic review and meta-analysis. Lancet Oncol 2013; 14(6): 500-15.
[http://dx.doi.org/10.1016/S1470-2045(13)70076-7] [PMID: 23540561]

[15] Ryu E, Yim SY, Do HJ, *et al.* Risk of secondary lymphedema in breast cancer survivors is related to serum phospholipid fatty acid desaturation. Support Care Cancer 2016; 24(9): 3767-74.
[http://dx.doi.org/10.1007/s00520-016-3197-z] [PMID: 27041742]

[16] Fiorentino L, Rissling M, Liu L, Ancoli-Israel S. The symptom cluster of sleep, fatigue and depressive symptoms in breast cancer patients: Severity of the problem and treatment options. Drug Discov Today Dis Models 2011; 8(4): 167-73.
[http://dx.doi.org/10.1016/j.ddmod.2011.05.001] [PMID: 22140397]

[17] Yang H, Brand JS, Fang F, *et al.* Time-dependent risk of depression, anxiety, and stress-related disorders in patients with invasive and *in situ* breast cancer. Int J Cancer 2017; 140(4): 841-52.
[http://dx.doi.org/10.1002/ijc.30514] [PMID: 27859142]

[18] Dooley LN, Ganz PA, Cole SW, Crespi CM, Bower JE. Val66Met BDNF polymorphism as a vulnerability factor for inflammation-associated depressive symptoms in women with breast cancer. J Affect Disord 2016; 197: 43-50.
[http://dx.doi.org/10.1016/j.jad.2016.02.059] [PMID: 26967918]

[19] Von Ah D, Habermann B, Carpenter JS, Schneider BL. Impact of perceived cognitive impairment in breast cancer survivors. Eur J Oncol Nurs 2013; 17(2): 236-41.
[http://dx.doi.org/10.1016/j.ejon.2012.06.002] [PMID: 22901546]

[20] Myers JS, Koleck TA, Sereika SM, Conley YP, Bender CM. Perceived cognitive function for breast cancer survivors: Association of genetic and behaviorally related variables for inflammation. Support Care Cancer 2017; 25(8): 2475-84.
[http://dx.doi.org/10.1007/s00520-017-3654-3] [PMID: 28247126]

[21] Passildas J, Collard O, Savoye AM, *et al.* Impact of chemotherapy-induced menopause in women of childbearing age with non-metastatic breast cancer – preliminary results from the menocor study. Clin Breast Cancer 2019; 19(1): e74-84.
[http://dx.doi.org/10.1016/j.clbc.2018.10.003] [PMID: 30448088]

[22] Cordts EB, Santos AA, Peluso C, Bianco B, Barbosa CP, Christofolini DM. Risk of premature ovarian failure is associated to the PvuII polymorphism at estrogen receptor gene ESR1. J Assist Reprod Genet 2012; 29(12): 1421-5.
[http://dx.doi.org/10.1007/s10815-012-9884-x] [PMID: 23150099]

[23] Lee Chuy K, Yu AF. Cardiotoxicity of contemporary breast cancer treatments. Curr Treat Options Oncol 2019; 20(6): 51.
[http://dx.doi.org/10.1007/s11864-019-0646-1] [PMID: 31073788]

[24] Fu Z, Lin Z, Yang M, Li C. Cardiac toxicity from adjuvant targeting treatment for breast cancer post-surgery. Front Oncol 2022; 12: 706861.
[http://dx.doi.org/10.3389/fonc.2022.706861] [PMID: 35402243]

[25] Caron J, Nohria A. Cardiac toxicity from breast cancer treatment: Can we avoid this? Curr Oncol Rep 2018; 20(8): 61.
[http://dx.doi.org/10.1007/s11912-018-0710-1] [PMID: 29876677]

[26] Lyon AR, Dent S, Stanway S, *et al.* Baseline cardiovascular risk assessment in cancer patients scheduled to receive cardiotoxic cancer therapies: A position statement and new risk assessment tools from the cardio-oncology study group of the heart failure association of the european society of cardiology in collaboration with the international cardio-oncology society. Eur J Heart Fail 2020; 22(11): 1945-60.
[http://dx.doi.org/10.1002/ejhf.1920] [PMID: 32463967]

[27] Čelutkienė J, Pudil R, López-Fernández T, *et al.* Role of cardiovascular imaging in cancer patients receiving cardiotoxic therapies: A position statement on behalf of the heart failure association (hfa), the european association of cardiovascular imaging (eacvi) and the cardio-oncology council of the european society of cardiology (ESC). Eur J Heart Fail 2020; 22(9): 1504-24.
[http://dx.doi.org/10.1002/ejhf.1957] [PMID: 32621569]

[28]   Pudil R, Mueller C, Čelutkienė J, *et al.* Role of serum biomarkers in cancer patients receiving cardiotoxic cancer therapies: A position statement from the cardio-oncology study groupof the heart failure associationand the cardio-oncology council of the european society of cardiology Eur J Heart Fail 2020; 22(11): 1966-83.
[http://dx.doi.org/10.1002/ejhf.2017] [PMID: 33006257]

[29]   McDonagh TA, Metra M, Adamo M, *et al.* 2021 ESC Guidelines for the diagnosis and treatment of acute and chronic heart failure: Developed by the Task Force for the diagnosis and treatment of acute and chronic heart failure of the european society of cardiology (ESC) with the special contribution of the heart failure association (HFA) of the ESC. Rev Esp Cardiol 2022; 75(6): 523.
[http://dx.doi.org/10.1016/j.rec.2022.05.005] [PMID: 35636830]

[30]   Totzeck M, Schuler M, Stuschke M, Heusch G, Rassaf T. Cardio-oncology: Strategies for management of cancer-therapy related cardiovascular disease. Int J Cardiol 2019; 280: 163-75.
[http://dx.doi.org/10.1016/j.ijcard.2019.01.038] [PMID: 30661849]

[31]   Pituskin E, Haykowsky M, Mackey JR, *et al.* Rationale and design of the multidisciplinary approach to novel therapies in cardiology oncology research trial (manticore 101 - breast): A randomized, placebo-controlled trial to determine if conventional heart failure pharmacotherapy can prevent trastuzumab-mediated left ventricular remodeling among patients with her2+ early breast cancer using cardiac MRI. BMC Cancer 2011; 11(1): 318.
[http://dx.doi.org/10.1186/1471-2407-11-318] [PMID: 21794114]

[32]   Gulati G, Heck SL, Røsjø H, *et al.* Neurohormonal blockade and circulating cardiovascular biomarkers during anthracycline therapy in breast cancer patients: Results From the PRADA (prevention of cardiac dysfunction during adjuvant breast cancer therapy) study. J Am Heart Assoc 2017; 6(11): e006513.
[http://dx.doi.org/10.1161/JAHA.117.006513] [PMID: 29118031]

[33]   Ginzac A, Passildas J, Gadéa E, *et al.* Treatment-induced cardiotoxicity in breast cancer: A review of the interest of practicing a physical activity. Oncology 2019; 96(5): 223-34.
[http://dx.doi.org/10.1159/000499383] [PMID: 30943496]

[34]   Elad B, Habib M, Caspi O. Cardio-oncology rehabilitation—present and future perspectives. Life 2022; 12(7): 1006.
[http://dx.doi.org/10.3390/life12071006] [PMID: 35888095]

[35]   Abrams J, Conley B, Mooney M, *et al.* National cancer institute's precision medicine initiatives for the new national clinical trials network. Am Soc Clin Oncol Educ Book 2014; (34): 71-6.
[http://dx.doi.org/10.14694/EdBook_AM.2014.34.71] [PMID: 24857062]

[36]   Greenwalt I, Zaza N, Das S, Li BD. Precision medicine and targeted therapies in breast cancer. Surg Oncol Clin N Am 2020; 29(1): 51-62.
[http://dx.doi.org/10.1016/j.soc.2019.08.004] [PMID: 31757313]

CHAPTER 7

Can We Find A Noninvasive Tool of Precision Medicine That Can Always Be Used For the Individualized Treatment of Women With Breast Cancer?

Abstract: A constellation of specific personal characteristics of the patients have been described as **personomics**, which involves an individual patient's personality type, set of personal values, priorities, preferences, health-related beliefs, goals, economic status, and different life circumstances, which can affect when and how a certain disease (*e.g.*, breast cancer (BC)) can be manifested in a given woman.

As a consequence, **personomics** can be considered to be a **novel clinical instrument** that is helpful for making a **connection between the standard** and the emerging, more **individualized model of medical care**. This plays an essential role in patients diagnosed with the most aggressive and difficult-to-treat malignancies (*e.g.*, BC subtypes, such as triple-negative breast cancer (TNBC).

At present, many **biological properties** in the forms of different **"omics" platforms** (such as genomics, proteomics, transcriptomics, metabolomics, epigenomics, and pharmacogenomics) have emerged. They have been incorporated into **precision medicine**. However, to optimally tailor diagnostic and therapeutic approaches to a given patient, the biological characteristics need to be integrated with the personal ones.

This chapter aims to address some practical research ideas of personalized medicine, relevant to personomics that can incorporate individual patient issues into the comprehensive therapeutic plan.

Keywords: Breast cancer (BC), Precision medicine, Personomics, Patient-centered approach, Personalized medical care, Triple-negative breast cancer (TNBC).

INTRODUCTION

Evidence-based medicine (EBM) applies data from **randomized controlled trials (RCTs)** and formulates clinical practice guidelines for a variety of medical disciplines, including oncology [1]. Based on the EBM guidelines, the treatment of patients with breast cancer (BC) has been mostly oriented on groups of women, who shared certain BC subtypes, in similar stages of progression [1]. However, the **EBM** guidelines have not included the patient's individual variability (*e.g.*, advanced age, multiple comorbidities, life experiences, psycho-social, or personal issues). In practice, these recommendations were usually based on data obtained from large groups of patients, with similar clinical and pathological characteristics. In this situation, many of the vulnerable women with BC could potentially receive some unnecessary therapies, leading to various adverse effects, not to mention about high medical costs [1]. At present, this approach has been changed, to some degree, with the advent of **precision medicine** and **personalized medicine** [2].

This chapter aims to address some practical research ideas of personalized medicine, relevant to personomics. It also presents how the personomics may facilitate the transition from the standard treatment to personalized medical management of individual women with the most difficult to treat BC subtypes.

The Goals and Tools of Precision Medicine

Simply put, **precision medicine** is the application of **modern medical sciences** for individual patients, based on their **unique biological characteristics** [2]. By using information from different biological "omics" platforms (*e.g.*, genomics, transcriptomics, proteomics, metabolomics, epigenomics, and pharmacogenomics), precision medicine creates the most optimally targeted diagnostic and therapeutic strategies, focused on the improvement of the treatment of various medical conditions (Fig. **1**) [2].

The objective of precision medicine in the oncology area is to individualize every patient's management, according to an assessment of the risk of cancer progression or recurrence [2].

Also, the whole malignancy course, including diagnostic work-up, treatment process, monitoring, and survivorship period should be approached in an individual manner, tailored to a given patient's clinical context [2].

AN EMERGING P4 MODEL: TRANSFORMATION FOR A NEW HEALTHCARE SYSTEM

To make measurable improvements in the patients' outcomes, the data from precision medicine needs to be integrated at multiple levels (*e.g.*, starting from the molecular level, through cells, tissues, organs, systems, and whole organisms, to the population level) [3]. At this point, systems biology needs to be used, incorporating high throughput technologies to generate large data sets, which will contribute to expanding many interconnected aspects of human biology [3].

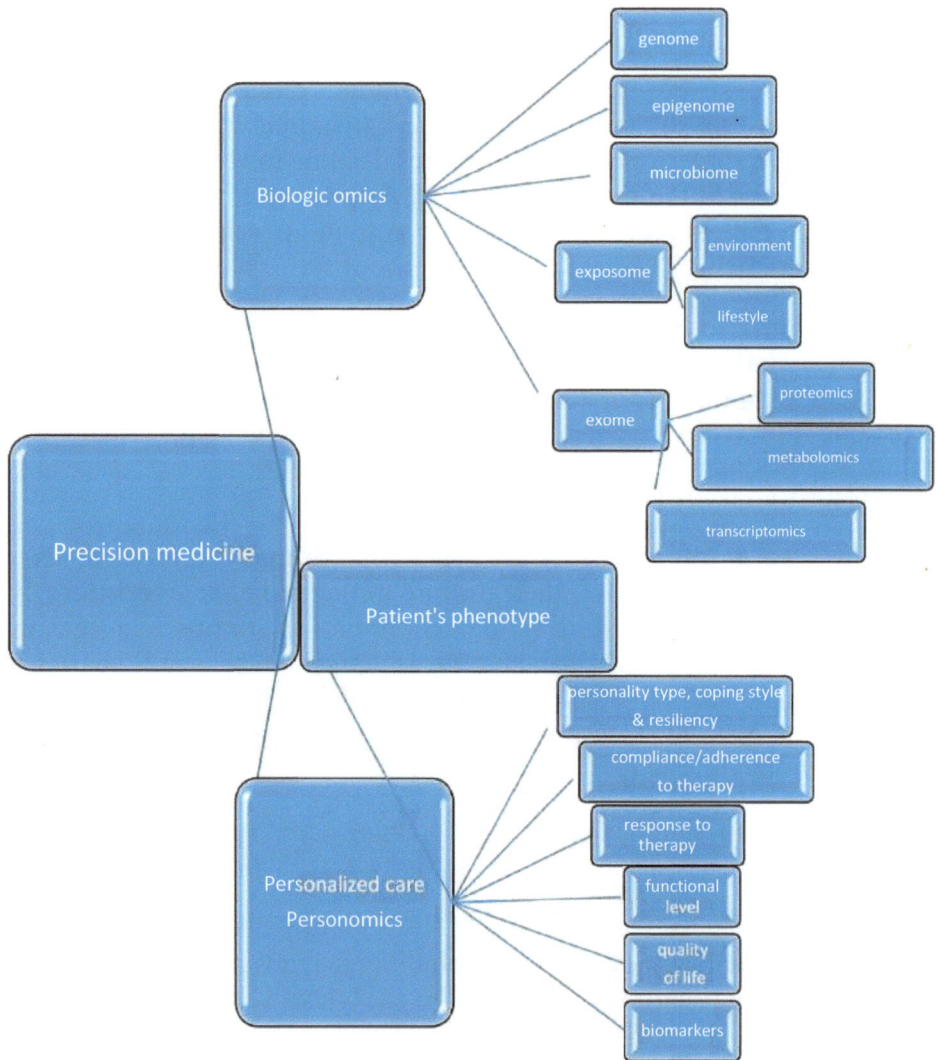

Fig. (1). Precision medicine and personalized model of care – the key interconnected components.

Furthermore, these data need to be disseminated, so that the **predictive, preventive, personalized**, and **participatory,** also known as **the P4 healthcare system,** can be developed and implemented in "real-life" circumstances, in the future (Fig. **2**) [3].

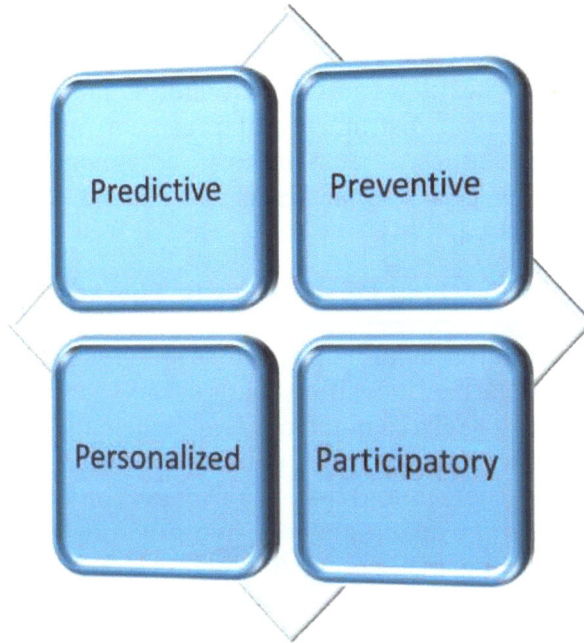

Fig. (2). Elements of the P4 healthcare system.

Some advantages of the **P4 healthcare system** for patients with BC may include the ability to determine the biological complexity of the most difficult to treat BC subtypes. In addition, possibilities for gathering, analyzing, and communicating information (*e.g.*, medical histories, diagnostic tests, and treatment results) will help integrate patient management [3]. Likewise, diseases will be diagnosed and treated in a cost-effective fashion, depending on their molecular and cellular abnormalities for individual patients (instead of the usual categories of symptoms) [3].

A Role of Personomics as A Tool to Fulfill the Unmet Healthcare Needs

In general, for improvement of the patient's management, much valuable data from "omics" have enormous potential. However, the current model of precision medicine often does not include the patient's individual variability, relevant to the life experiences, diseases, or circumstances of a given person. In fact, these issues are crucial for the composition of the most accurate patient's profile.

The term "**personomics**" includes the **psychosocial, behavioral, cultural,** and **economic factors**, which influence the **patient's health beliefs, attitude toward diseases, and potential engagement** in professional relations with healthcare providers [4]. In other words, **"personomics"** encompasses the patient's **priorities, values, goals, needs, preferences,** and **support** systems. A consideration of these personal circumstances is very helpful for a comprehensive understanding of the health conditions of individual patients [4]. Therefore, similarly to the biological instruments of precision medicine (*e.g.*, genomics, transcriptomics, proteomics, metabolomics, epigenomics, and pharmacogenomics), personomics can also serve as a valuable **tool to operationalize personalized medical care** [4].

The Aliki Initiative: Teaching Personomics In The Academic Setting

A concept of **personomics** acknowledges that individual patients present a wide spectrum of personal variabilities, life situations, and social structures, which can contribute to their health-related outcomes (*e.g.*, when and how a specific medical condition will be manifested in a given individual, or what may be the therapeutic response to a given medication) [4, 5]. The **personomics approach to the patient's medical history** taking includes five structured components, which can be addressed during the medical interview, recorded, and implemented into clinical practice (Fig. **3**) [5, 6]. As an illustration, a physicians' survey, addressing the patient's concerns, personal relationships, jobs, hobbies, and the patient's views of the patient-physician relationships, has provided some valuable details, necessary to improve patient-centered care [6, 7].

Recently, to incorporate the information from different "omics", including personomics, into patient management, the **Aliki Initiative (AI)** has been developed at Johns Hopkins Bayview Medical Center, in the U.S [8, 9]. The AI (a patient-centered curriculum for internal medicine residents) is a program that includes a focused strategy for academic teaching, addressing the main aspects of personomics. The **AI** promotes the evidence-based **diagnostic work-up, therapeutic processes tailored to a given patient**, and consistent follow-up [9]. It has been noted that patient's satisfaction has been improved, while medical care is focused on such an individualized approach [10].

Unique Values of the Patient-centered, "Humanistic" Approach to Medical Management

The concept of **treating patients as unique human beings** should be **integrated with their comprehensive management plans**. Due to rapid technological advances, the "omics" strategies can be used to individualize diagnostic work-ups and therapeutic processes [7, 8, 10]. The modern precision medicine model has been supported by the large-scale biologic databases (to characterize the patient's identity *via* molecular or cellular assays, and mobile medical devices) and the informatics infrastructure for the data analysis [2, 8, 10]. In addition to these sophisticated techniques, **the patient-centered, "humanistic" approach** seems necessary and feasible to implement. It may correspond with a decreased number of medical errors and unnecessary hospitalizations. Also, a detailed assessment of the patient's **harmful lifestyle factors** (*e.g.*, tobacco smoking, substance abuse, unhealthy nutrition, chronic stress, and insufficient physical activity) and environmental circumstances (*e.g.*, pollution) is helpful for the patient's education and potential modification or elimination of many contributors to the incidence or deteriorating course of serious diseases, including BC [5, 6, 10].

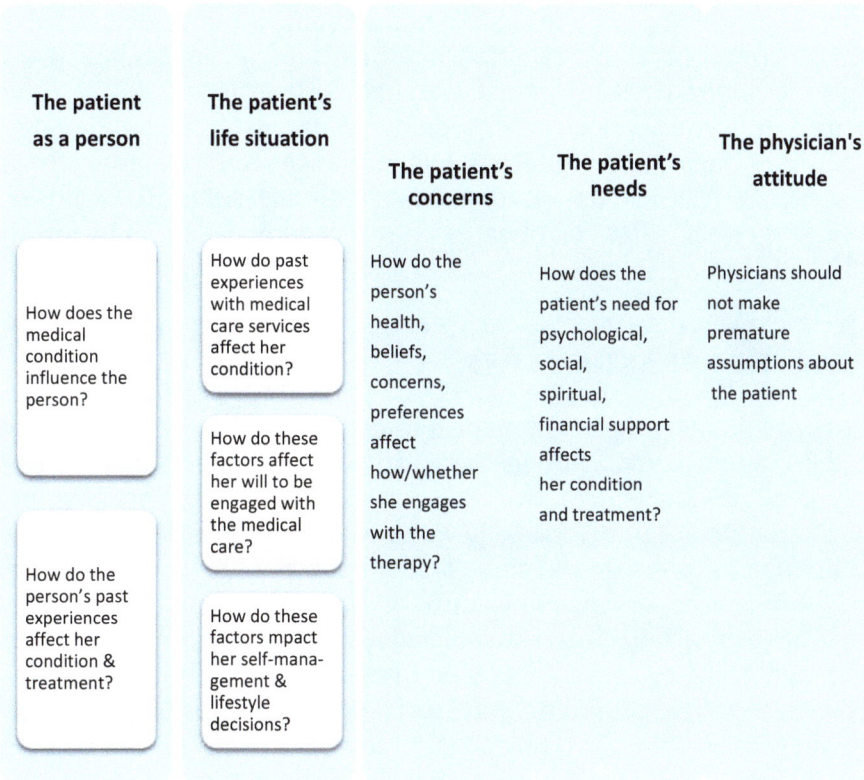

Fig. (3). Basic parts of personomics that improve the patient's medical history taking.

Current Possibilities of Personalized Medical Care for Women with Breast Cancer

It should be highlighted that the transition from standard healthcare to personalized medicine can be accelerated by asking direct questions about a patient as a person (rather than "formally" inquiring about medical symptoms). This should be helpful for providing adequate medical care, consistent with the patient's expectations, needs, and goals. Also, this approach could contribute to improved patient outcomes [11, 12]. The information about a hormone receptor

(HR) status, such as the estrogen receptor (ER), the progesterone receptor (PR), and the human epidermal growth factor receptor 2 (HER2) status allows clinicians to choose the most appropriate, molecularly targeted therapies, based on the tumor's assessment [11, 12].

The **personalized approach** can favorably change the prognosis of many women suffering from BC, especially in case of the most difficult to treat BC subtypes, such as TNBC (addressed in detail in the next section and in some other chapters) and HER2-positive BC) [11 - 14]. Approximately 15–20% of BCs overexpress HER2 which is related to aggressive tumor behavior and decreased patient survival [15, 16]. Therefore, targeted treatments with humanized monoclonal antibodies that block HER2 (*e.g.*, trastuzumab and pertuzumab) [17] have been implemented, in addition to systemic therapy, in order to improve outcomes [17, 18]. In addition, lapatinib, a small molecule that reversibly inhibits HER1 and HER2, is another treatment option for patients with metastatic HER2-positive BC, who have progressed after treatment with conventional CHT and trastuzumab therapy [19, 20].

COMMON LIMITATIONS OF PERSONALIZED MEDICAL CARE FOR WOMEN WITH BREAST CANCER

In spite of remarkable progress in precision medicine, some important limitations exist in the oncology area. For instance, some trials of anticancer treatments, guided by genetic sequencing, have revealed different safety concerns, probably due to the intratumor heterogeneity [21]. In particular, it has been reported that targeted therapies were able to (only to some degree) block the main signaling pathways, which also operate in healthy cells [21]. As a consequence, such treatments have frequently been associated with dose-limiting adverse effects. Moreover, malignant cells usually develop **resistance to different therapeutics, which target a single signaling pathway**. For this reason, **combinations of targeted therapies**, which simultaneously block various signaling pathways are necessary. Unfortunately, the **adverse effects of** such **combinations can reduce a patient's tolerability of effective therapeutic doses.**

In response to this obstacle, an application of **personomics** offers some valuable, **noninvasive tools for clinicians**, who may use additional information about a given patient, in an attempt to optimize medical management [22]. For instance, clinicians need to take into consideration the patient's age and general **health condition** (*e.g.*, **comorbidities** and the relevant **poly-pharmacotherapy, hepatic** or **renal insufficiency**) and combine these data with the molecular subtype of this patient's BC [22].

Furthermore, the physician should inquire about the **patient's goals, needs, medical insurance,** and **support system** (*e.g.*, family, friends, home and work environment). In addition, the patient's financial resources will help determine whether or not she can afford certain medications recommended for her specific BC subtype. Also, participation in a clinical trial (if available to match a patient's BC subtype) should be considered.

Selected Therapeutic Targets in Advanced or Metastatic TNBC

Estrogen receptor (ER)-negative, progesterone receptor (PR)-negative, and HER2-negative BC, called triple-negative BC (**TNBC**), is a very **heterogeneous cancer** (in comparison with other BC subtypes), with **a high risk of relapse** [23]. Due to genome-wide approaches, the following TNBC subtypes have been determined: basal-like (BL) (BL1 and BL2), immunomodulatory, mesenchymal, mesenchymal stem-like 1, luminal androgen receptor (LAR) and unstable [24]. Because of the heterogeneity, the therapy of TNBC is very difficult. In contrast to HR-positive or HER2-positive BC, TNBC does not respond to endocrine therapy or trastuzumab. CHT is the systemic therapy that improves the prognosis to a greater degree in TNBC than in HR-positive BC subtypes [25]. Recently, one of the clinical targets in TNBC is an enzyme poly adenosine diphosphate-ribose polymerase (**PARP**), which is involved in base-excision repair after DNA damage [26]. In fact, the efficacy and safety of **PARP inhibitors** (*e.g.*, **olaparib** and **talazoparib**) have been revealed in women with metastatic TNBC, harboring deleterious germline or somatic *BRCA 1* and *BRCA 2* mutations (Table **1**) [26, 27]. Similarly, favorable results of **veliparib** (another PARP inhibitor), in combination **with carboplatin** have been reported [28]. For instance, the rate of pathological complete response (pCR) in the TNBC patient population was 51% in the group receiving veliparib-carboplatin (added to the standard treatment), compared to 26% in the control group, receiving the standard treatment only (docetaxel, doxorubicin, and cyclophosphamide) [28].

In addition, some correlations between the TNBC subtypes, pCR status, and patient survival have been noted. For instance, the BL1 subtype of TNBC had the highest pCR rate (52%), compared to BL 2 (0%), and LAR (10%) subtypes [29]. Unfortunately, the mesenchymal subtype of TNBC had the worst pCR and overall survival (OS) rates [29]. According to the GeparTrio trial that assessed the androgen receptor (AR) expression in women with primary BC (who were treated with neoadjuvant docetaxel, doxorubicin, and cyclophosphamide) no significant differences between the pCR rates of women with AR-positive TNBC (29.2%) and the ones with AR-negative TNBC tumors (33.3%) were noted [30]. Similarly, it has been reported that the LAR subtype of TNBC (that has high expression of genes *LAR* and *GATA3*), is related to a more favorable prognosis than tumors, which harbor cancer stem cell markers [31]. At present, targeting specific molecules that contribute to the development of new treatment targets for TNBC is more accessible, due to the BC genome sequencing, resulting in the identification of more than two thousand somatic mutations (*e.g., p53, PIK3CA,* and *PTEN*) [32].

Table 1. Examples of targeted treatment with PARP inhibitors for patients with TNBC.

Targeted treatment with PARP inhibitors for patients with TNBC			
Parp Inhibitor	**Reference Number**	**Clinical Trial Phase**	**Treatment Arms, Clinical Implications Of The Trial & Patients' Outcomes**
Olaparib	[26]	OlympiAD Phase 3 NCT02000622	**Olaparib vs. standard CHT in patients with g*BRCA* mutations, HER2-negative metastatic BC (metastatic stage);** PFS was improved in the olaparib arm
Talazoparib	[27]	EMBRACA phase 3 NCT01945775	**Talazoparib vs. standard CHT in patients with g*BRCA* mutations, HER2-negative, advanced or metastatic BC;** PFS and QoL were improved in the talazoparib arm
Veliparib	[28]	I-SPY 2 TRIAL phase 2 NCT01042379	Veliparib-carboplatin added to standard therapy resulted in higher rates of pCR than the standard therapy alone, in patients with TNBC

BC, breast cancer; g, germline; HER2, human epidermal growth factor receptor 2; gBRCAm, germline BRCA-mutation; CHT, chemotherapy; PARP, poly (ADP-ribose) polymerase; pCR, pathological complete response; PFS, progression-free survival, QoL, quality of life; TNBC, triple-negative breast cancer; *vs., versus.*

In addition, it is important to look beyond the boundaries of scientific research that supports the modern diagnostic industry. In this way, it will be possible to achieve a more coherent strategic approach to the integration of capabilities to manage TNBC, various comorbidities, and lifestyle interventions. Introducing some personalized opportunities for the "real-life" healthcare setting should be beneficial for both the individual patients with TNBC and their treatment teams [33].

CONCLUSION

Precision medicine offers a remarkable potential for **targeted treatments** and **individualized management** plans, based on the patient's unique biological features. To accurately utilize this potential for the patients, physicians need to apply the data from the "omics" platforms, and take into account the specific information from **personomics** (focused on life circumstances of the individual patients).

In spite of the rapid progress in the characterization of some mutations and driver genes, as well as the development of innovative targeted therapies (*e.g.*, for aggressive BC subtypes, such as TNBC), many challenges still remain; for instance, the development of **resistance to treatment** that leads to **relapses**, the **adverse effects of targeted anti-BC therapies** (which are barriers to their use), and the BC heterogeneity.

To effectively address such challenges, continuous efforts are needed, aimed at novel therapeutic targets and biomarkers that can contribute to the improvement of outcomes among women with BC (*e.g.*, in advanced or metastatic stages). Simultaneously, clinicians should **approach** their **patients "as people"**, so that professional **medical care** can be more adequately **tailored to their individual's health-related needs**.

Clinical practice guidelines focus on so-called "average patients", but in reality, physicians do not treat "average patients". Therefore, the "average" recommendations are often insufficient to manage individual patients with BC.

Personomics can facilitate the transition from standard medical treatment to personalized medical management of individual women with TNBC.

• **Personomics** incorporate individual patient issues into the comprehensive therapeutic plan.

• **Personomics** may play the role of the "bridge" **connecting standard medical care with personalized medicine**.

• **Approaching women with BC "as people"** allows delivering professional medical care to fulfill their specific health-related and personal needs.

REFERENCES

[1]   Boyd CM, Darer J, Boult C, Fried LP, Boult L, Wu AW. Clinical practice guidelines and quality of care for older patients with multiple comorbid diseases: Implications for pay for performance. JAMA 2005; 294(6): 716-24.
[http://dx.doi.org/10.1001/jama.294.6.716] [PMID: 16091574]

[2]   Collins FS, Varmus H. A new initiative on precision medicine. N Engl J Med 2015; 372(9): 793-5.
[http://dx.doi.org/10.1056/NEJMp1500523] [PMID: 25635347]

[3]   Flores M, Glusman G, Brogaard K, Price ND, Hood L. P4 medicine: How systems medicine will transform the healthcare sector and society. Per Med 2013; 10(6): 565-76.
[http://dx.doi.org/10.2217/pme.13.57] [PMID: 25342952]

[4]   Ziegelstein RC. Personomics. JAMA Intern Med 2015; 175(6): 888-9.
[http://dx.doi.org/10.1001/jamainternmed.2015.0861] [PMID: 25867929]

[5]   Ziegelstein R. Personomics: The missing link in the evolution from precision medicine to personalized medicine. J Pers Med 2017; 7(4): 11.
[http://dx.doi.org/10.3390/jpm7040011] [PMID: 29035320]

[6] Hanyok LA, Hellmann DB, Rand C, Ziegelstein RC. Practicing patient-centered care: the questions clinically excellent physicians use to get to know their patients as individuals. Patient 2012; 5(3): 141-5.
[http://dx.doi.org/10.1007/BF03262487] [PMID: 22741807]

[7] Topol EJ. Individualized medicine from prewomb to tomb. Cell 2014; 157(1): 241-53.
[http://dx.doi.org/10.1016/j.cell.2014.02.012] [PMID: 24679539]

[8] Livingstone SG, Smith MJ, Silva DS, Upshur REG. Much ado about omics: Welcome to 'the permutome'. J Eval Clin Pract 2015; 21(6): 1018-21.
[http://dx.doi.org/10.1111/jep.12406] [PMID: 26149276]

[9] Hanyok L, Brandt L, Christmas C. The johns hopkins aliki initiative: A patient-centered curriculum for internal medicine residents. MedEdPORTAL 2012; 8(1).
[http://dx.doi.org/10.15766/mep_2374-8265.9098]

[10] Ratanawongsa N, Federowicz MA, Christmas C, *et al*. Effects of a focused patient-centered care curriculum on the experiences of internal medicine residents and their patients. J Gen Intern Med 2012; 27(4): 473-7.
[http://dx.doi.org/10.1007/s11606-011-1881-8] [PMID: 21948228]

[11] Bettaieb A, Paul C, Plenchette S, Shan J, Chouchane L, Ghiringhelli F. Precision medicine in breast cancer: Reality or utopia? J Transl Med 2017; 15(1): 139.
[http://dx.doi.org/10.1186/s12967-017-1239-z] [PMID: 28623955]

[12] Carels N, Spinassé LB, Tilli TM, Tuszynski JA. Toward precision medicine of breast cancer. Theor Biol Med Model 2016; 13(1): 7.
[http://dx.doi.org/10.1186/s12976-016-0035-4] [PMID: 26925829]

[13] Stover DG, Wagle N. Precision medicine in breast cancer: Genes, genomes, and the future of genomically driven treatments. Curr Oncol Rep 2015; 17(4): 15.
[http://dx.doi.org/10.1007/s11912-015-0438-0] [PMID: 25708799]

[14] Cameron D, Piccart-Gebhart MJ, Gelber RD, *et al*. 11 years' follow-up of trastuzumab after adjuvant chemotherapy in HER2-positive early breast cancer: Final analysis of the HERceptin Adjuvant (HERA) trial. Lancet 2017; 389(10075): 1195-205.
[http://dx.doi.org/10.1016/S0140-6736(16)32616-2] [PMID: 28215665]

[15] Valachis A, Nearchou A, Lind P, Mauri D. Lapatinib, trastuzumab or the combination added to preoperative chemotherapy for breast cancer: A meta-analysis of randomized evidence. Breast Cancer Res Treat 2012; 135(3): 655-62.
[http://dx.doi.org/10.1007/s10549-012-2189-z] [PMID: 22875745]

[16] Ross JS, Slodkowska EA, Symmans WF, Pusztai L, Ravdin PM, Hortobagyi GN. The HER-2 receptor and breast cancer: ten years of targeted anti-HER-2 therapy and personalized medicine. Oncologist 2009; 14(4): 320-68.
[http://dx.doi.org/10.1634/theoncologist.2008-0230] [PMID: 19346299]

[17] Slamon DJ, Leyland-Jones B, Shak S, *et al*. Use of chemotherapy plus a monoclonal antibody against HER2 for metastatic breast cancer that overexpresses HER2. N Engl J Med 2001; 344(11): 783-92.
[http://dx.doi.org/10.1056/NEJM200103153441101] [PMID: 11248153]

[18] Dawood S, Broglio K, Buzdar AU, Hortobagyi GN, Giordano SH. Prognosis of women with metastatic breast cancer by HER2 status and trastuzumab treatment: An institutional-based review. J Clin Oncol 2010; 28(1): 92-8.
[http://dx.doi.org/10.1200/JCO.2008.19.9844] [PMID: 19933921]

[19] Geyer CE, Forster J, Lindquist D, *et al*. Lapatinib plus capecitabine for HER2-positive advanced breast cancer. N Engl J Med 2006; 355(26): 2733-43.
[http://dx.doi.org/10.1056/NEJMoa064320] [PMID: 17192538]

[20] Xin Y, Guo WW, Huang Q, *et al*. Effects of lapatinib or trastuzumab, alone and in combination, in

human epidermal growth factor receptor 2-positive breast cancer: A meta-analysis of randomized controlled trials. Cancer Med 2016; 5(12): 3454-63.
[http://dx.doi.org/10.1002/cam4.963] [PMID: 27882700]

[21]   Tannock IF, Hickman JA. Limits to personalized cancer medicine. N Engl J Med 2016; 375(13): 1289-94.
[http://dx.doi.org/10.1056/NEJMsb1607705] [PMID: 27682039]

[22]   Sacristán JA, Dilla T. No big data without small data: Learning health care systems begin and end with the individual patient. J Eval Clin Pract 2015; 21(6): 1014-7.
[http://dx.doi.org/10.1111/jep.12350] [PMID: 25832820]

[23]   Bauer KR, Brown M, Cress RD, Parise CA, Caggiano V. Descriptive analysis of estrogen receptor (ER)-negative, progesterone receptor (PR)-negative, and HER2-negative invasive breast cancer, the so-called triple-negative phenotype. Cancer 2007; 109(9): 1721-8.
[http://dx.doi.org/10.1002/cncr.22618] [PMID: 17387718]

[24]   Le Du F, Eckhardt BL, Lim B, *et al.* Is the future of personalized therapy in triple-negative breast cancer based on molecular subtype? Oncotarget 2015; 6(15): 12890-908.
[http://dx.doi.org/10.18632/oncotarget.3849] [PMID: 25973541]

[25]   Colleoni M, Cole BF, Viale G, *et al.* Classical cyclophosphamide, methotrexate, and fluorouracil chemotherapy is more effective in triple-negative, node-negative breast cancer: Results from two randomized trials of adjuvant chemoendocrine therapy for node-negative breast cancer. J Clin Oncol 2010; 28(18): 2966-73.
[http://dx.doi.org/10.1200/JCO.2009.25.9549] [PMID: 20458051]

[26]   Robson M, Im SA, Senkus E, *et al.* Olaparib for metastatic breast cancer in patients with a germline *BRCA* mutation. N Engl J Med 2017; 377(6): 523-33.
[http://dx.doi.org/10.1056/NEJMoa1706450] [PMID: 28578601]

[27]   Litton JK, Rugo HS, Ettl J, *et al.* Talazoparib in patients with advanced breast cancer and a germline *brca* mutation. N Engl J Med 2018; 379(8): 753-63.
[http://dx.doi.org/10.1056/NEJMoa1802905] [PMID: 30110579]

[28]   Rugo HS, Olopade OI, DeMichele A, *et al.* Adaptive randomization of veliparib-carboplatin treatment in breast cancer. N Engl J Med 2016; 375(1): 23-34.
[http://dx.doi.org/10.1056/NEJMoa1513749] [PMID: 27406347]

[29]   Masuda H, Baggerly KA, Wang Y, *et al.* Differential response to neoadjuvant chemotherapy among 7 triple-negative breast cancer molecular subtypes. Clin Cancer Res 2013; 19(19): 5533-40.
[http://dx.doi.org/10.1158/1078-0432.CCR-13-0799] [PMID: 23948975]

[30]   Loibl S, Müller BM, von Minckwitz G, *et al.* Androgen receptor expression in primary breast cancer and its predictive and prognostic value in patients treated with neoadjuvant chemotherapy. Breast Cancer Res Treat 2011; 130(2): 477-87.
[http://dx.doi.org/10.1007/s10549-011-1715-8] [PMID: 21837479]

[31]   Yu KD, Zhu R, Zhan M, *et al.* Identification of prognosis-relevant subgroups in patients with chemoresistant triple-negative breast cancer. Clin Cancer Res 2013; 19(10): 2723-33.
[http://dx.doi.org/10.1158/1078-0432.CCR-12-2986] [PMID: 23549873]

[32]   Shah SP, Roth A, Goya R, *et al.* The clonal and mutational evolution spectrum of primary triple-negative breast cancers. Nature 2012; 486(7403): 395-9.
[http://dx.doi.org/10.1038/nature10933] [PMID: 22495314]

[33]   Riccio G, Au R, van Emmerik R, Eslami M. Situated precision healthcare in the smart medical home: Bringing nasa's research strategy down to earth. Adv Geriatr Med Res 2020; 2(3): e200017.
[PMID: 35994053]

Part 2

The Role of Patient Education, Empowerment, and Communication with Medical Teams, and Psychological or Supportive Approaches in Advanced or Metastatic Breast Cancer (BC).

"You can't stop the waves, but you can learn how to surf."

Jon Kabat-Zinn

CHAPTER 8

Distress – Our "Internal Enemy": How to "Disarm" or Lessen its Negative Impact on the Psychophysical Condition of Women with Triple-Negative Breast Cancer?

Abstract: Stress is an inevitable part of life. It constantly bombards our lives, and these explosions range from minor daily frustrations to overwhelming fear brought on by the adverse prognosis of serious diseases, like triple-negative breast cancer (**TNBC**). In patients with cancer, **distress** has been defined as "a **multifactorial unpleasant experience of a psychological** (*e.g.*, cognitive, behavioral, emotional), social, spiritual, and **physical** nature that may **interfere with the ability to cope effectively with cancer**, its physical symptoms, and its treatment. However, even in such a difficult health-related situation, it is encouraging that some consequences of **distress** are not inevitable. Some natural questions for every woman with cancer (*e.g.*, TNBC) are: "**What are the normal limits of distress?**" and "**What to do when distress becomes more serious?**"

This chapter will briefly address the above questions and will present some tools that can be used to **measure distress**. In addition, a few simple **strategies** that are easily **accessible** and **effective in Distress Management** and its complications will be suggested (*e.g.*, "**Do's** and **Don'ts**" list of recommendations).

Keywords: Cancer care team, Distress, Distress thermometer, Social services, Support.

INTRODUCTION

Women with cancer, especially as aggressive as **triple-negative breast cancer** (**TNBC**), and also, their families and friends can feel distressed after receiving a cancer diagnosis. Also, when cancer is treated and this "journey" undergoes dynamic changes, learning to cope with such a "moving target" is very difficult. Therefore, it's important to know some basic facts about the nature and manifestations of distress, and also, when, where, and how to receive help and support [1]. **Distress** is an unpleasant emotion, feeling, thought, condition, or behavior, and thus, it may influence the way how a person feels, thinks, or acts [1].

Moreover, **distress can impair a person's efforts to effectively cope with malignancy**, including managing its specific symptoms, therapies, and adverse effects [1]. In addition, distress may have a negative impact on decision-making (*e.g.*, therapeutic choices) and taking personal charge over one's health [1]. Since there are many stressful elements related to a malignant disease, some degree of distress is inevitable, and thus, considered "**normal** " (Fig. **1**) [1]. However, a transition of distress from the expected, controlled level, to the one that interferes with treatment (*e.g.*, decision-making, adherence to therapy, *etc.*) and makes it difficult to continue a usual daily functioning requires a proactive and individualized approach from the cancer care team (Fig. **2**) [2]. Furthermore, women who have limited access to health care due to language, medical insurance, or financial barriers, transportation problems, young children or elderly relatives at home, history of mental disorders, alcohol or drug abuse, usually have an increased risk for distress [2].

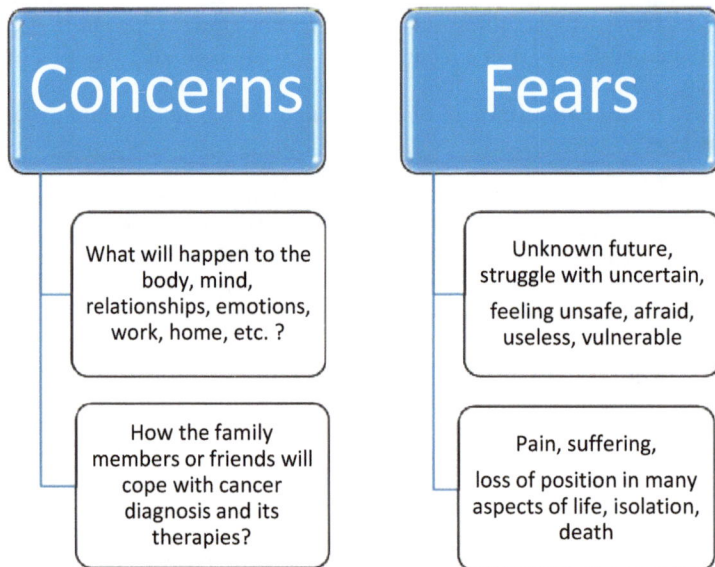

Fig. (1). Distress-related concerns and fears often experienced by patients with cancer.

Therefore, such vulnerable women should not be overlooked, since they need to receive immediate attention and help to be able to cope with different adversities [2]. This chapter will briefly address the issues linked with cancer-related distress and will present some tools that can be used **to measure the distress levels**. In addition, a few simple **strategies** that are easily **accessible** and **effective in distress management** and its complications will be suggested (*e.g.*, in the form of "**Do's** and **Don'ts**" recommendations).

Feeling

Overwhelmed, sad, irritable, anxious, fearful, hopeless, angry, in panic

Unable to cope with pain or side effects of therapies

Experiencing

Difficulties with making treatment decisions, poor concentration, memory problems

Trouble sleeping, eating, coping with fatigue, vomiting, diarrhea

Thinking

About being worthless, 'burden' to others, family conflicts, issues 'impossible' to resolve

Questioning faith, beliefs, values, wondering if there's any point in going on

Diagnosis of an aggressive cancer (e. g., TNBC)

Return or progression of cancer despite the treatment

Advanced or metastatic cancer

Waiting for tests results (e.g., biopsy, laboratory, imaging, genetic, etc.)	Admission/discharge from the hospital	Serious side effects or complications of treatment
starting treatment course	finishing ineffective treatment course	decline of general status
enrolling into a clinical trial	starting another type of treatment	loss of independence
	deterioration of comorbidities	the end of life period

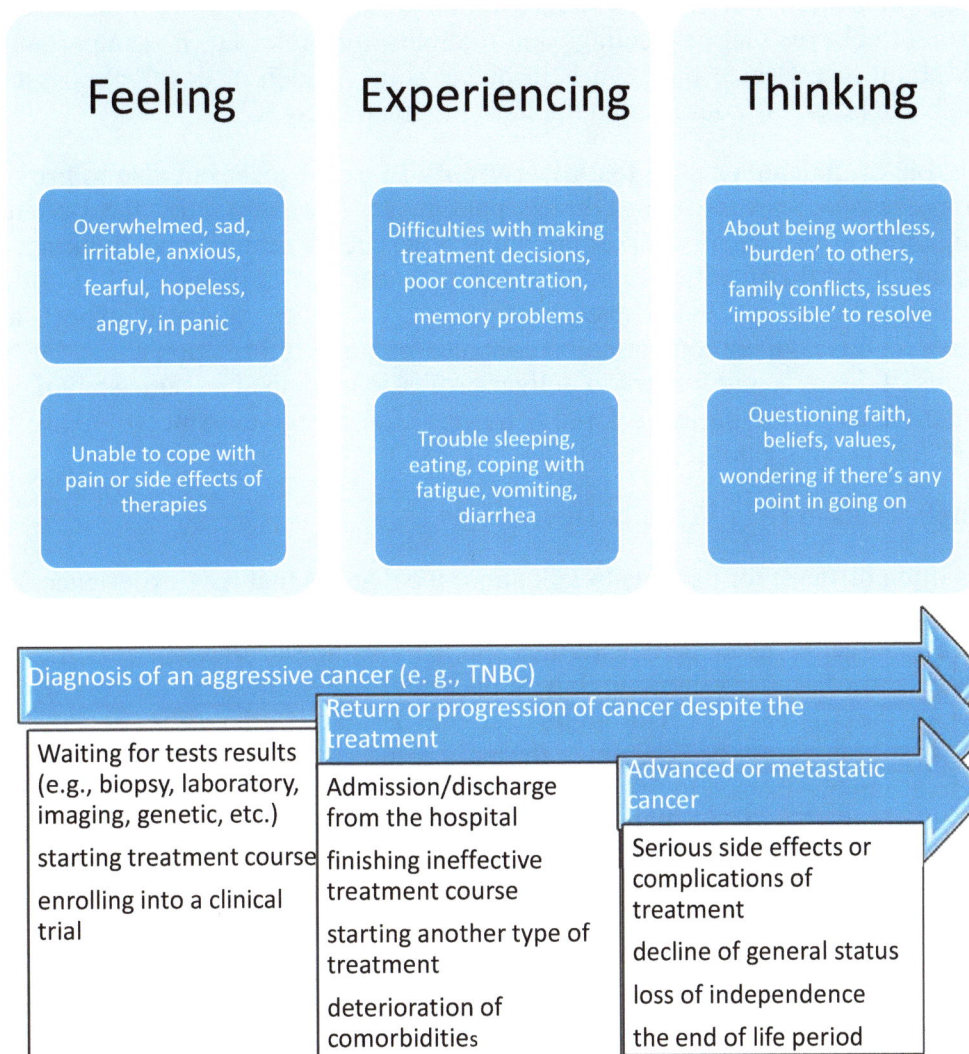

Fig. (2). Common challenging moments of the cancer journey, when the distress becomes very serious; TNBC, triple-negative breast cancer.

WHAT CAN PATIENTS WITH CANCER, CANCER CARE TEAMS, AND CAREGIVERS DO WHEN THE DISTRESS BECOMES VERY SERIOUS?

The distress can be particularly aggravated during some periods of the cancer journey. Since serious distress affects many key areas of one's life (*e.g.*, a patient has trouble sleeping, eating, or concentrating), it is critical to prepare the first line of defense as soon as possible. This means an ability to cope with distress, which can be triggered by various factors, together with **a cancer care team,**

caregivers, family, or friends, with whom a woman feels comfortable. Even if a patient believes that her feelings and thoughts are irrelevant, it is important to talk about them, since they can help detect some hidden or developing issues, which can be timely addressed in the most pragmatic way [2].

The role of the **cancer care team is not only to** treat cancer but also to provide comprehensive care to the "whole" patient. In line with this, the patient's obligation is to honestly report to them how she is feeling and thinking, in addition to all the specific issues relevant to cancer and its therapies (Fig. **2**) [2]. Of course, no one can do that except the patient. The cancer care team expects and counts on this cooperation, based on concrete, ongoing information about various origins of distress, and will try to deliver professional help. The same should also be beneficial to the patient's family, friends, and caregivers since they are the main "circle" of support.

Simple Tools to Help Measure Distress

It is often difficult for patients to talk about the distress that they experience, in a manner that helps the cancer care team understand what is the distress level and how it's affecting usual daily activities and therapeutic schedules. Therefore, two simple and easily accessible tools can be used to help measure distress levels, namely the **Distress Thermometer** and the **Problem List** (Fig. **3**) [3]. The **Distress Thermometer** resembles the pain scale (0-10). A patient is asked to circle a number from 0 to 10, which reflects how much distress she feels today and how much she has felt over the last week (10 - means the highest level of distress that one can imagine, and 0 means no distress [3]. The main goal is to use this scale to accurately rate and monitor individual distress levels, in a way that helps the cancer care team provide the necessary care and support, in a timely fashion. If a patient's response is 4 or above, she probably suffers from a moderate-to-high degree of distress. This should be a "red flag" for the cancer care team that should investigate possible reasons for distress and immediately offer some helpful strategies [3]. Another tool in the distress assessment armamentarium is the **Problem List**, which contains possible causes of distress. A patient needs to go through a list of typical problems and check the most likely reasons for her distress [3]. This aids the cancer care team understand what kind of help is primarily needed.

HOW TO TAKE AN ACTIVE ROLE IN PERSONAL MANAGEMENT OF THE CANCER-RELATED DISTRESS AND COOPERATE WITH THE CANCER CARE TEAM? – THE ART OF "DO'S" AND "DON'TS"

Since every woman with TNBC is different, she can work with her cancer care team to choose the best action to take, based on her individual situation. Here are some general ideas from a multidisciplinary group of experts about counteracting distress or anxiety feelings, often associated with cancer [3, 4]. The lists presented below include some tips, which might be helpful (the Do's list), and some attitudes or actions that could be harmful (the Don'ts list) (Tables **1** and **2**) [3, 4].

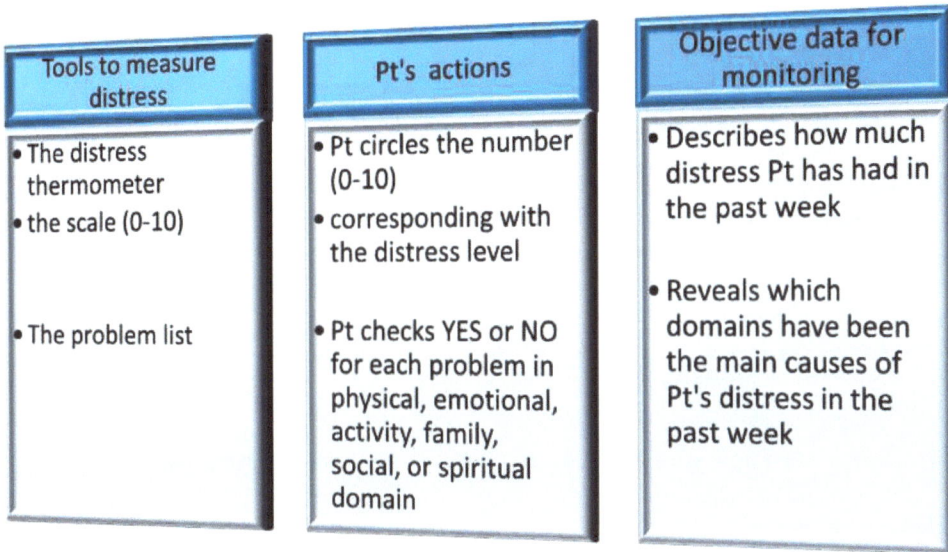

Tools to measure distress	Pt's actions	Objective data for monitoring
• The distress thermometer • the scale (0-10) • The problem list	• Pt circles the number (0-10) • corresponding with the distress level • Pt checks YES or NO for each problem in physical, emotional, activity, family, social, or spiritual domain	• Describes how much distress Pt has had in the past week • Reveals which domains have been the main causes of Pt's distress in the past week

Fig. (3). Simple tools to help measure the distress level: the Distress Thermometer and Problem List; Pt, patient.

Table 1. The Do's list illustrated with practical examples and suggested actions.

Apply Reasonable Coping Strategies	Practical Approaches That Were Helpful In Solving Previous Problems	Use Any Proven Way To Cope, Which Has Worked Before; Tell The Cancer Care Team About Any Changes Or Concerns
Take "one day at a time"	*e.g.*, focus on getting the most out of each day despite the serious disease.	If you divide big problems into "small pieces," it will be easier to manage them.
Accept a support	*e.g.*, self-help, help from someone (or a group) you feel comfortable talking about your cancer.	A friend or caretaker can help you with transportation to & from medical visits or procedures.
Find a respectful doctor & care team, real partners in the care, ready to answer your questions	*e.g.*, ask what side effects of a given therapy are expected & how to prepare for them or how to avoid them.	Anticipating what problems may come makes it easier to deal with them when they actually happen.

Apply Reasonable Coping Strategies	Practical Approaches That Were Helpful In Solving Previous Problems	Use Any Proven Way To Cope, Which Has Worked Before; Tell The Cancer Care Team About Any Changes Or Concerns
Keep well-organized personal medical records	*e.g.*, doctors' phone numbers, emails, addresses, dates of visits, treatments, lab values, x-rays, USG, CT, MRI, or PET scans, symptoms, prescribed medications (with start & stop dates), side effects, allergies, general medical and mental status.	Concise, calendar-based, information about the cancer, its treatment & other personal medical records are crucial for the most adequate care & no one can keep them better than you.
Keep a journal to express yourself	It can help you survive the most difficult moments during the cancer journey.	Try relaxation, meditation, music, art, pet therapy, or other activities that can comfort you.
Explore spiritual practices or get support from valuable belief systems	This may comfort you or help you find meaning in the experience of your illness.	Find a professional help if what you're doing isn't working.

Table 2. The Don'ts list illustrated with common examples and recommended actions.

Don't blame yourself for causing cancer	Even if your unhealthy lifestyle could have increased your cancer risk, it's not helpful to blame yourself.	Encourage your family or friends to go for cancer screening or diagnostic tests early & to stop harmful habits.
Don't feel guilty if you are sometimes unable to comply with med. advice	"Bad days" may come, but waiting for "better times" is always a good attitude.	If 'low periods" become more frequent, call for medical help.
Don't suffer alone	Don't be isolated, but try to connect with someone, who understands what you're going through.	Get support from your family, friends, doctors, nurses, or members of support/community group.
Don't be embarrassed to ask for help from mental health services	Distress, anxiety, depression - can disrupt your sleep, concentration, eating, moving, or other abilities.	If you feel that your distress is getting out of control & interfere with a daily functioning ask for help.
Don't conceal your disease symptoms (physical or psychological) or concerns from the medical team members, caretakers, family, or other close persons	Ask the caretaker (whom you really trust) to go with you to medical appointments and talk about treatment, prognosis, different management options, or plans for the future.	Since patients may not hear or absorb information when they are anxious, a family member or friend may help correctly recall or interpret medical recommendations, tests results, & treatments.

(Table 2) cont.....

Don't blame yourself for causing cancer	Even if your unhealthy lifestyle could have increased your cancer risk, it's not helpful to blame yourself.	Encourage your family or friends to go for cancer screening or diagnostic tests early & to stop harmful habits.
Don't self-stop any recommended oncology treatment for an alternative therapy	Ask if any nutritional supplement or medication can be safely used along with your regular anticancer medical therapies (*e.g.*, as a complementary therapy)	Discuss the pros & cons of alternative/complementary therapies with a trustworthy expert to objectively evaluate their risks & benefits, prior to any potential use, upon the agreement from your doctor/care team

HELPFUL OPTIONS TO MANAGE CANCER-RELATED DISTRESS AND ITS COMPLICATIONS

In addition to applying in practice some well-known, useful suggestions, attending a **support group** or using **social services** can help ease feelings of distress by providing comfort, education, or resources for patients, their families, and caregivers. If a support group is not available or does not appear suitable to someone, a social worker or individual counseling may offer helpful options, depending on the type of problems, generating feelings of distress.

Since having cancer affects usual, daily needs, social workers may practically connect many patients with various needs to community organizations. In addition, **mental health services** are available to assess and manage moderate or severe distress levels (*e.g.*, frequently caused or aggravated by previous psychological or psychiatric disorders that the person had before the TNBC diagnosis) [5]. Psychology and psychiatry experts apply a spectrum of strategies, aimed at helping a given patient to figure out what has worked well for her, in the past most difficult situations [5, 6]. In this way, by connecting previous problems with current experiences, an individual coping style can be evaluated, and potentially reinforced. This may be done in form of practical education, by introducing the basic techniques, such as relaxation and meditation to alleviate distress or anxiety feelings [6].

In addition, in some instances, **pharmacologic interventions** are needed to reduce severe distress levels, associated with cancer or its therapies. For instance, steroids (*e.g.*, prednisone) can cause mood swings, and opioid analgesics (*e.g.*, morphine or fentanyl) can cause constipation, confusion, or lethargy. To address these undesirable symptoms, it is necessary to work closely with the cancer care team and mental health professionals, to decide whether certain medications may be helpful (*e.g.*, anti-depressants) as possible therapeutic options [7]. Some specific areas, in which support groups, social services, mental health services, or individual counseling can be particularly helpful for patients with cancer are briefly presented (Fig. **4**) [5 - 7]. The most frequently employed scales to assess psychological distress and interventions to alleviate this distress include the **Profile of Mood States-Short Form (POMS-SF), Hospital Anxiety and Depression (HADS)**, and **Distress Thermometer (DT)** (described in detail in another section) [8].

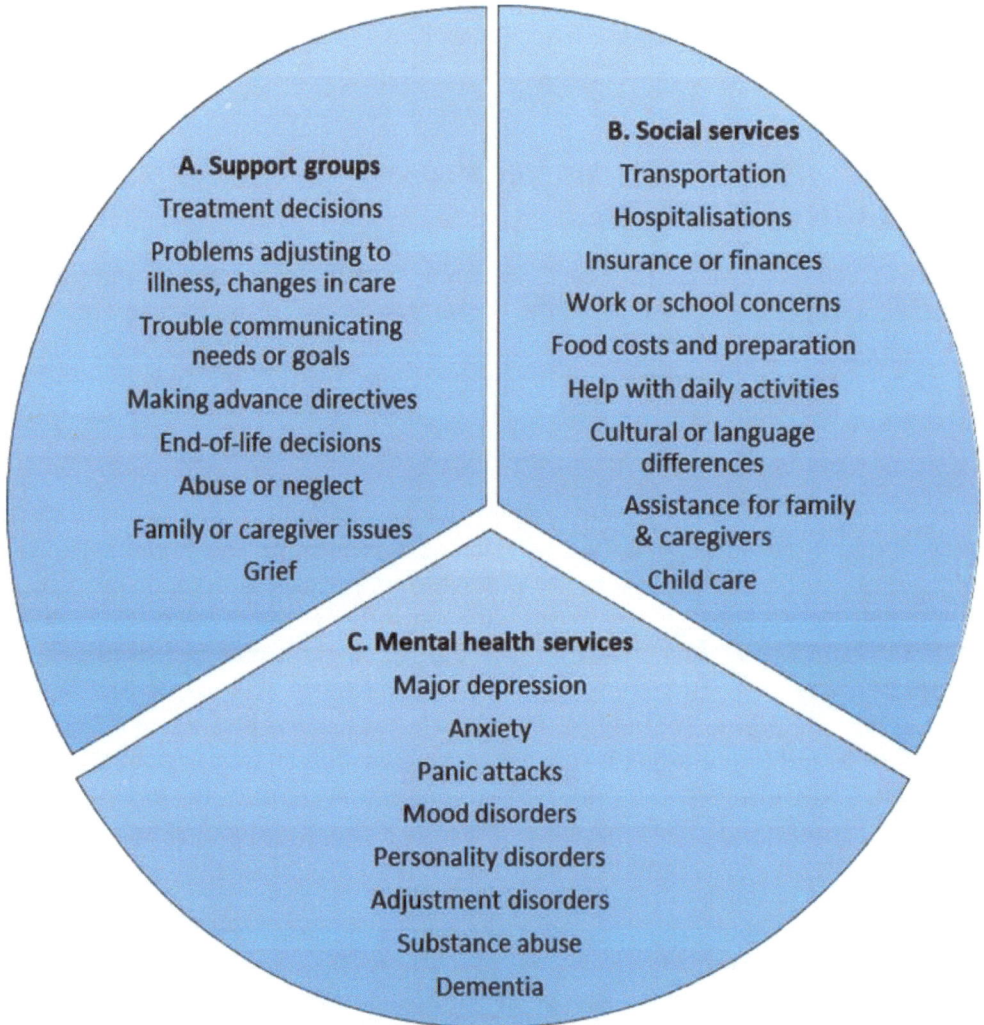

A. Support groups

Treatment decisions

Problems adjusting to illness, changes in care

Trouble communicating needs or goals

Making advance directives

End-of-life decisions

Abuse or neglect

Family or caregiver issues

Grief

B. Social services

Transportation

Hospitalisations

Insurance or finances

Work or school concerns

Food costs and preparation

Help with daily activities

Cultural or language differences

Assistance for family & caregivers

Child care

C. Mental health services

Major depression

Anxiety

Panic attacks

Mood disorders

Personality disorders

Adjustment disorders

Substance abuse

Dementia

Fig. (4). Specific areas, in which the support groups, social services, or mental health services can be helpful to lower feelings of distress or anxiety for patients with cancer, their families, and caregivers.

CONCLUSION

The majority of **patients with cancer experience serious psychological distress** at some periods of the malignancy course. Such patients, as well as their caregivers, families, and friends, can feel particularly stressed out shortly after receiving a cancer diagnosis, unfavorable test results, lack of response to treatment, or poor prognosis. Such distress can be manifested in different ways. When the situation suddenly changes, or remains uncertain, learning how to cope can be very difficult. At that point, it's always important to be **"armed" in practical knowledge** or resources, and to be able to get the necessary help and support on time. Numerous reports have shown that interventions like moderate **exercise training, cognitive behavioral therapy,** and **scientifically verified complementary therapies** can assist oncology personnel in alleviating the distress among patients. Future studies should consider optimizing such interventions in various patient groups, and measuring the effects of psychological distress, might be incorporated into screening programs for checking unmet needs, clinical responses, and longitudinal outcomes.

There are some **simple, easily accessible strategies to manage distress** and **reclaim** a more **comfortable life**. Therefore, **it is strongly suggested that a woman with TNBC should:**

• Use support and self-help groups if they make her feel better.

• Explore spiritual beliefs and practices, that were helpful in the past.

• Keep records of her doctors' phone numbers, dates of tests & treatments, laboratory tests, x-rays, scan results, a list of currently used medicines, their side effects, allergies, and symptoms, or changes in general medical status.

• Keep a journal if she needs to express her emotions, moods, or thoughts.

Also, it is recommended that a woman with TNBC should not:

• Believe in the harmful slogan that "cancer equals death".

• Blame herself for causing cancer.

• Feel guilty if she can't keep a positive attitude all the time.

• Suffer in silence.

• Be embarrassed or ashamed to get help from a mental health expert.

• Keep her worries or symptoms (physical or psychological) secret from the person closest to her.

• Abandon her regular treatment for any unproven therapy.

REFERENCES

[1]   National comprehensive cancer network (NCCN). Available at: https://www.nccn.org/patients/ resources/life_with_cancer/distress.aspx (Accessed on January 31, 2020).

[2]   Grassi L. Psychiatric and psychosocial implications in cancer care: The agenda of psycho-oncology. Epidemiol Psychiatr Sci 2020; 29: e89.
[http://dx.doi.org/10.1017/S2045796019000829] [PMID: 31915101]

[3]   Hammelef KJ, Tavernier SS. Distress.A Guide to Oncolo Symptom Manag. 2nd ed. Pittsburgh, PA: Oncology Nursing Society 2015; pp. 265-81.

[4]   Oncology nursing society (ONS), Symptom interventions: Anxiety. Available at: https://www. ons.org/pep/anxiety (January on: January 31, 2022).

[5]   Mehta RD, Roth AJ. Psychiatric considerations in the oncology setting. CA Cancer J Clin 2015; 65(4): 299-314.
[http://dx.doi.org/10.3322/caac.21285] [PMID: 26012508]

[6]   National institute of mental health. Anxiety. Disorders. Available at: https://www.nimh. nih.gov/health/topics/anxiety-disorders/index.shtml (Accessed on: January 31, 2020).

[7]   Pitman A, Suleman S, Hyde N, Hodgkiss A. Depression and anxiety in patients with cancer. BMJ 2018; 361: k1415.
[http://dx.doi.org/10.1136/bmj.k1415] [PMID: 29695476]

[8]   Yeh ML, Chung YC, Hsu MYF, Hsu CC. Quantifying psychological distress among cancer patients in interventions and scales: A systematic review. Curr Pain Headache Rep 2014; 18(3): 399.
[http://dx.doi.org/10.1007/s11916-013-0399-7] [PMID: 24500637]

CHAPTER 9

Teaching the Brain How to Counteract Distress: Practical Lessons About the Stress and Relaxation Responses for Women with Triple-Negative Breast Cancer

Abstract: In spite of a very difficult situation, women with triple-negative breast cancer (TNBC) need to realize that some consequences of the cancer-related **distress** can be alleviated. Moreover, it is possible to counteract, to some degree, the damaging effects of this distress. In particular, the **relaxation response**, as the opposite, "**calming version**" of the "**typical**" **stress response** can be achieved by a given patient with cancer, with some simple, intentional, and conscious efforts.

In fact, modern s**tress management** offers a whole armamentarium of **tools** and **strategies** that are necessary to reduce negative results of stress-related reactions. Since many warning signs of stress are connected with certain activities of the **autonomic nervous system (ANS),** it should be beneficial to patients to learn some basic information about the ANS functions.

This chapter will explain how to elicit the **relaxation response** as the "**common denominator**" to counterbalance the "typical" stress response. It will also teach how to use **diaphragmatic breathing**, and the most **feasible to adopt elements of the mindfulness-based interventions,** as well as **cognitive-behavioral approaches,** to more effectively combat distress daily.

Keywords: Relaxation response, Stress response, Autonomic nervous system (ANS), Parasympathetic nervous system (PNS), Sympathetic nervous system (SNS), Diaphragmatic breathing, Cognitive-behavioral therapy (CBT), Acceptance and commitment therapy (ACT), Mindfulness-based interventions (MBI), Meditation.

INTRODUCTION

Despite an extremely difficult situation, women with triple-negative breast cancer (TNBC) should realize that some consequences of the cancer-related **distress** can be alleviated, to some degree. In fact, it is possible to counteract the damaging effects of this distress by calling upon the body's inherited potential for natural controlling mechanisms and healing processes [1].

In particular, the beneficial **relaxation response**, as the "**calming response**", which is opposite to the "**typical" stress-related response** can be achieved, with some intentional, conscious efforts of any woman with cancer, including TNBC. However, this pattern is not intuitive, and unfortunately, it is not on the front line of the therapeutic process. Therefore, it is necessary to educate both the patients in need and their cancer care teams about simple and easily accessible steps to prevent or combat some destructive consequences of undesirable **"stress response"** [1]. Moreover, the main goal of stress management is to help a person timely and correctly identify and interpret the warning signs of stress, which are manifested by certain activities of the **autonomic nervous system (ANS).** That's why this is of great importance to teach patients about ANS functions, so that they are able to recognize subtle changes, which may have a substantial impact on their overall psychophysical condition. Such a vigilant and noninvasive approach can bring some balance to an unstable, malignancy-related stressful situation. Since such distress can diminish a person's efforts to successfully cope with cancer, including managing its symptoms, therapies, and their adverse effects, as well as can impair decision-making abilities, it is crucial to explain what exact factors or behaviors can make some women more "stress-resistant", at least to some degree. Moreover, the simple and insightful s**tress management techniques** will help acquire skills, which are needed to neutralize the detrimental effects of distress and restore inner peace, stability, and confidence, especially for women with TNBC, who subjectively experience distress, such as feeling anxious, fearful, hopeless, concerned about cancer and also, about lost roles *(e.g.*, as a mother, wife, grandmother, coworker, colleague, friend, *etc.)*, which they played at home, family, workplace, or a social group.

This chapter will explain how to elicit the **relaxation response** as the "**common denominator**" to counteract the "typical" stress response [1]. It will teach how to apply **slow, diaphragmatic breathing,** to more effectively combat distress on a daily basis. Furthermore, this chapter will encourage moderate **exercise, rest, relaxation,** and **social connections**. It will also provide some tips for the "informal" applications of **mindfulness-based interventions (MBI), cognitive and behavioral therapy (CBT),** and **acceptance and commitment therapy (ACT)** [2]. In essence, it will explore the key elements of these approaches, allowing making constructive changes to the "routine ways", in which many women with TNBC think, feel, and react to the stressful demands of the surrounding reality.

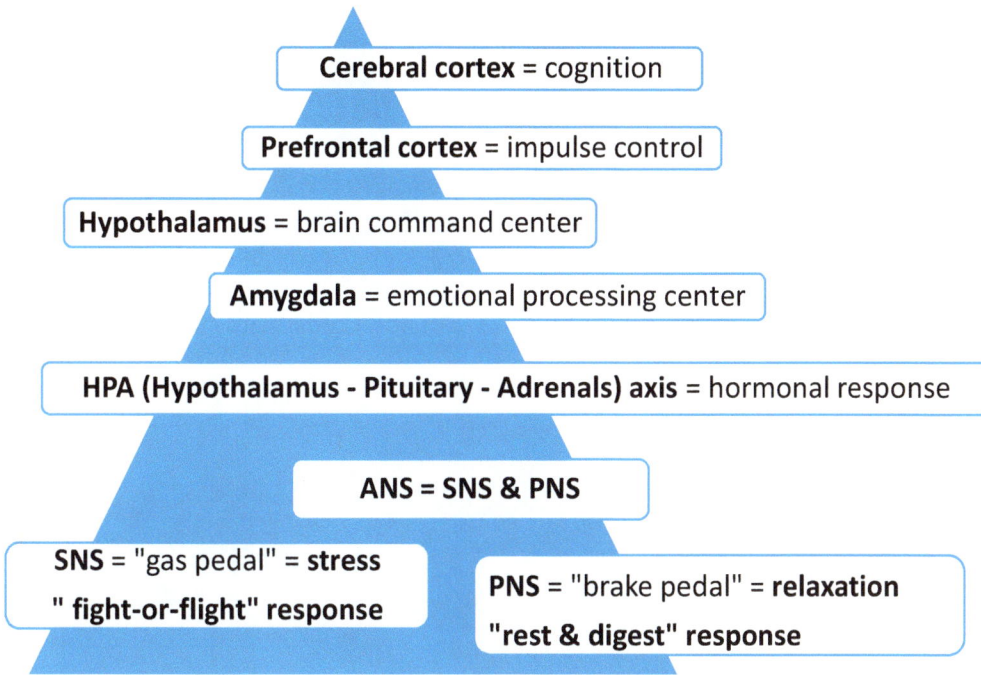

Fig. (1). Central, autonomic nervous system, and HPA axis - their roles in the perception or reaction to stress; ANS, autonomic nervous system; HPA, Hypothalamus - Pituitary -Adrenals; PNS, the parasympathetic nervous system; SNS, the sympathetic nervous system.

OPPOSITE PHYSIOLOGIC ACTIONS OF TWO PARTS OF THE AUTONOMIC NERVOUS SYSTEM (ANS) – THE SYMPATHETIC NERVOUS SYSTEM (SNS) AND THE PARASYMPATHETIC NERVOUS SYSTEM (PNS)

The nervous system consists of the **central nervous system (CNS)** which contains the brain and spinal cord, and **the peripheral nervous system** which contains all the neurons outside of the **CNS** (Fig. 1).

The **autonomic nervous system (ANS)** is part of the **peripheral nervous system** that consists of a collection of neurons, which affect the activity of various internal organs. The ANS has two parts: **the sympathetic nervous system (SNS)** which prepares the body to actively respond to changes or perceived threats (*e.g., via* activation of the "fight or flight" response), and **the parasympathetic nervous system (PNS)** is responsible for bodily functions at rest (*e.g., via* activation of the repair mechanisms) (Fig. **2**) [3]. Regulation of the internal environment is critical for maintaining homeostasis (*e.g.*, relatively stable blood pressure, heart rate, respiratory rate, metabolism, temperature, *etc.*). The main function of the ANS is to prepare the body for confronting a threat in the environment) *via* regulation of various physiologic processes *(e.g.,* the fight or flight response of the SNS evolved to protect the body from dangers around it) (Fig. **2**) [3]. However, many stressful events related to every step of malignancy management, such as BC, can also trigger these automatic responses, especially when the mind perceives a threat or distress, even without a real reason. In particular, chronic stress related to BC can often cause the SNS to trigger the fight, flight, or freeze response. Although this is a "false alarm", such activation of SNS can eventually exhaust the body. To protect patients from this "avoidable harm", simple psychoeducation about ANS can be very helpful (Fig. **2**) [3].

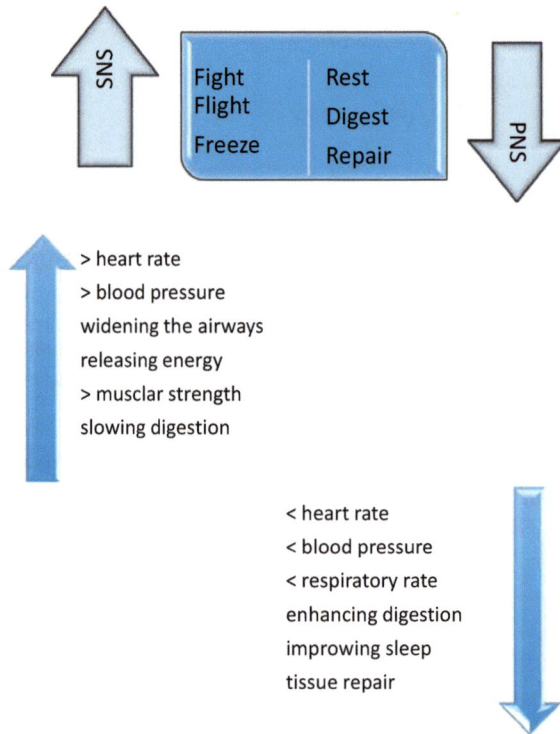

Fig. (2). The autonomic nervous system (ANS) – regulation of the main physiologic processes; SNS, the sympathetic nervous system; PNS, the parasympathetic nervous system.

HOW THE PARASYMPATHETIC NERVOUS SYSTEM (PNS) ACTIVATION CAN BE APPLIED TO BENEFIT WOMEN WITH TNBC?

Learning how to elicit the relaxation response is essential to restoring a calming balance or comfort, and stimulating numerous **psychosomatic healing processes.** Some easily-accessible **practices** *(e.g.,* diaphragmatic breathing**) can improve the QoL, at any moment of the cancer journey of women with**

TNBC, without any side effects. This sounds simple, but it is not easy. However, it becomes easier with time, proper guidance *(e.g.,* online resources), personal experience, and repetitions, even if one has struggled to calm the mind and slow down some physiological activities *(e.g.,* heart rate and respiratory rate) in the past.

Unquestionably, some **distress is inevitable**, especially when a person has been repeatedly exposed to serious external or internal stressors, which generate stress responses that have adverse consequences. In this way, daily distress can exacerbate various health problems, often associated with TNBC. However, it's still possible to "**disassemble**" some negative cycles of **stress responses**, using simple and easily-accessible methods. For instance, **diaphragmatic breathing** can help relax and reduce distress and anxiety. In fact, slowing the breathing rate can reduce arousal in the **sympathetic nervous system (SNS)** [3].

COMBINING THE AWARENESS ABOUT AUTONOMIC NERVOUS SYSTEM (ANS) SIGNALS WITH INFORMAL APPLICATIONS OF COGNITIVE AND BEHAVIORAL INTERVENTIONS: HOW TO MAKE A POSITIVE TRANSFORMATION?

How to teach ANS to be our "allay"? Since the **autonomic nervous system (ANS)** regulates various physiologic processes, often beyond a person's conscious will or awareness, it is important to **combine awareness about ANS signals with cognitive and behavioral interventions**.

The goal of **cognitive and behavioral** interventions is to change some specific *(e.g.,* pessimistic or destructive) thoughts and behaviors and teach constructive coping skills, such as cognitive restructuring, positive behavioral modification, or relaxation, which can be flexibly incorporated into an individual plan for a given patient. This approach can be coordinated with any therapeutic strategies, during the entire spectrum of the cancer journey, and the patient is "in charge" of every step (Fig. **3**) [4].

ELICITING RELAXATION RESPONSE TO RESTORE A CALMING BALANCE OF THE MIND AND A HEALING POTENTIAL OF THE BODY

Based on many research studies, it was found that **meditation** can be useful for alleviating numerous health problems, often encountered by patients with TNBC *(e.g.,* chronic pain, insomnia, gastrointestinal symptoms, *etc.)* and associated, common comorbidities *(e.g.,* HTN, CVD, CHD, *etc.),* due to the lowering of the stress response. Moreover, with regular practice, **meditation** may also help a woman gain a deeper **awareness of her inner self** [5].

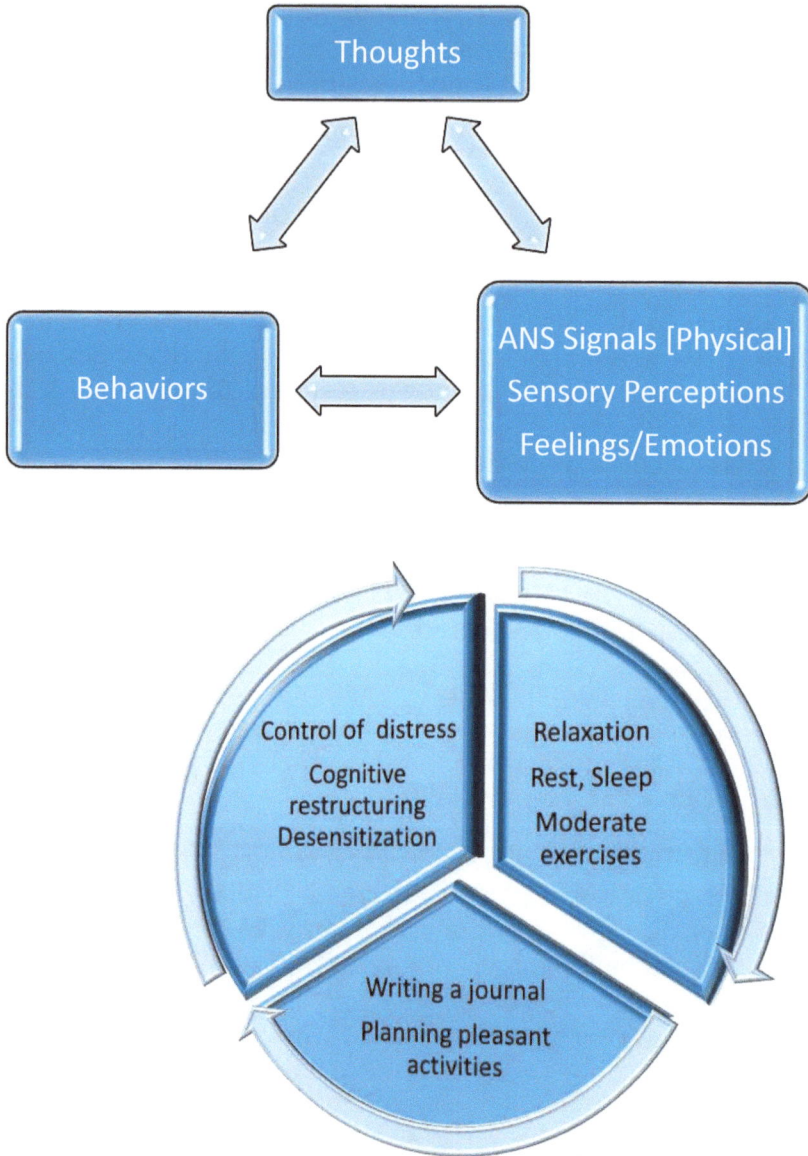

Fig. (3).   Combining the awareness about ANS signals with "informal" cognitive and behavioral interventions; ANS, autonomic nervous system.

Meditation contributes to some biological changes in the brain *(e.g.,* augmenting certain areas, which are responsible for thinking, learning, and impulse control, such as the **left prefrontal cortex**, and reducing other areas, which that are related to excessive arousal, anxiety, fear, anger, and response to stress, such as

amygdala) [5]. Focusing the attention on breathing or a chosen object *(e.g.,* a sound, a word, *etc.)* can induce the **"relaxation response"**, which is a unique state of a calm mind, characterized by reduced heart rate and blood pressure, experienced by those, who meditate (meditators). Moreover, according to recent studies, in the field of modern neuroscience, some specific patterns of electrical activity have been found in the brains of longtime meditators, compared to the study participants from the control group (non-meditators). Such a significant difference between the two study groups is very encouraging because it means that entering the state of relaxation *(e.g., via* diaphragmatic breathing or meditation practice) could really induce measurable changes in the brain that can subsequently be translated into favorable physical and mental health effects.

HOW TO TEACH THE BRAIN TO REENGAGE IN THE REPAIR OF SOME STRESS-RELATED DAMAGES? – A THERAPEUTIC "MENU" TO CHOOSE FROM, FOR WOMEN WITH TNBC

Numerous health benefits of regular meditation or diaphragmatic breathing practice, including improvements in cardiovascular diseases, gastrointestinal disorders, chronic pain, fatigue, insomnia, anxiety, and depression, should encourage women with TNBC to learn these safe and friendly practices, and then, apply them systematically, whenever possible. (Fig. **4**). In fact, **diaphragmatic breathing** and **meditation** should be at the top of the activity list, together with the **recommended anticancer therapies** [6].

Similarly, **spiritual support** may bring consolation, especially during crisis, uncertainty, or emotional turbulence. Such counseling could be available during a women's cancer journey since it might reinforce her emotional stability or QoL. Likewise, **creative therapies** or **pet therapy** represent activities, which are usually useful for reducing distress, among patients with cancer, as well as light or moderate levels of **physical exercise** are generally safe for many patients with cancer [7].

Moreover, such exercises can help alleviate anxiety, and improve muscle strength and cardiovascular status *(e.g.,* walking). However, any exercise plans need to be discussed with a doctor, physical therapist, or cancer care team, before their initiation. Women with TNBC may use different safe and pleasant therapeutic activities, depending on their personal preferences, needs, and possibilities (Fig. **4**).

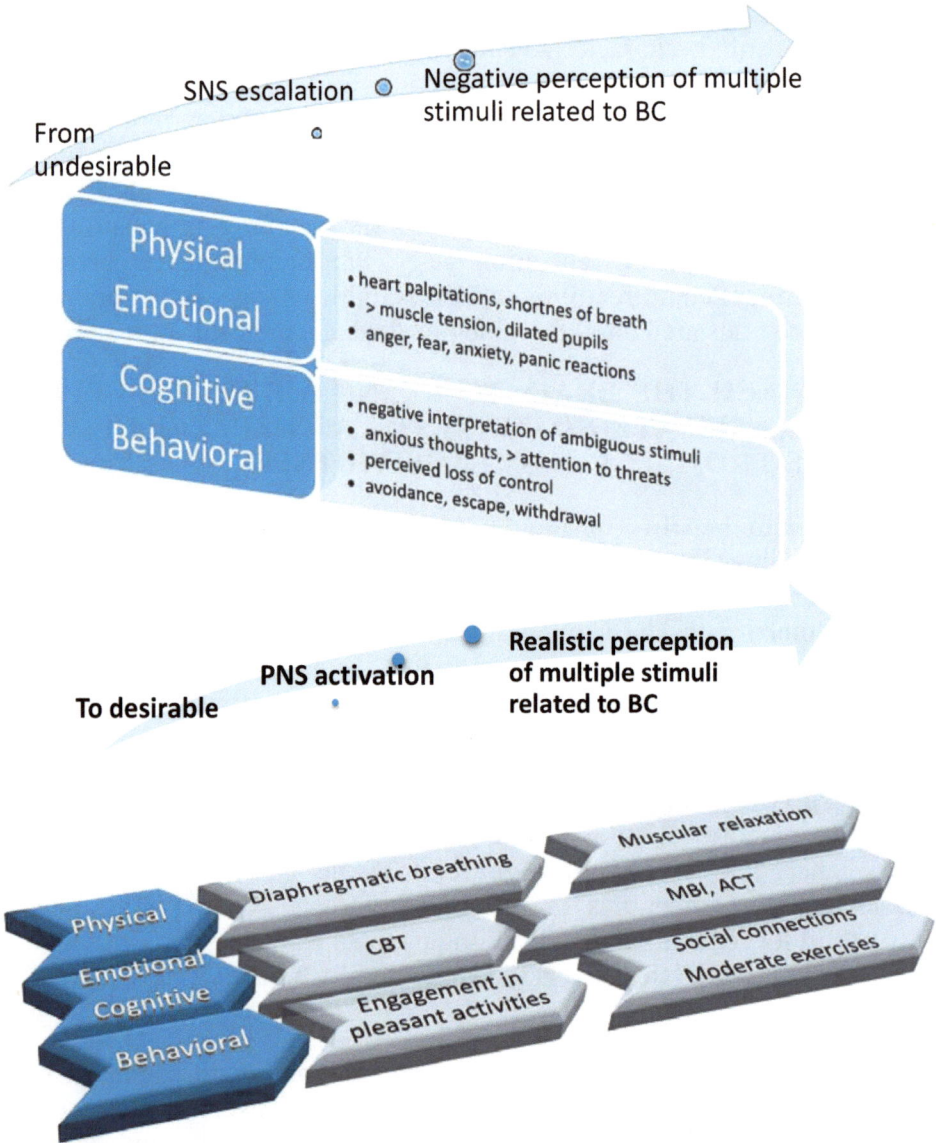

Fig. (4). A major transformation - How to train the brain to stay away from danger and come closer to safety? ACT, acceptance and commitment therapy; CBT, cognitive behavioral therapy; MBI, mindfulness-based interventions; PNS, parasympathetic nervous system; SNS, the sympathetic nervous system.

CONCLUSION

Meditation activates various parts of the brain, and the main goal of meditation is to elicit the "relaxation response", which is opposite to stress response.

During meditation, the sympathetic nervous system (SNS) (responsible for distress feelings and **stress responses**) is turned down, while the parasympathetic nervous system (PNS), contributing to the **relaxation response,** is turned up. As a consequence, t**he relaxation response can restore a calming balance of the mind and activate a healing potential of the body** *(e.g.,* return the heart rate, blood pressure, and breathing rate to normal ranges.

Learning how to elicit the relaxation response (*e.g., via* simple techniques, such as diaphragmatic breathing or focused attention) **is essential to meditating effectively, and obtaining health-related benefits.**

Furthermore, an important purpose of **meditation** and **cognitive-behavioral** interventions is to **change some specific thoughts, emotional perceptions,** and **behaviors**, and to **teach** selective **coping skills**, such as cognitive restructuring, desensitization, acceptance, or positive behavioral modifications. In addition, these interventions will help design an individual **activity plan**, fully compatible with any medical therapy, during the cancer journey of women with TNBC.

• When a woman meditates, she turns down her sympathetic nervous system (SNS), responsible for distress feelings and **stress responses**) and turns up her parasympathetic nervous system (PNS), which is "in charge of" the **"relaxation response"** (returns the heart rate, blood pressure, and breathing to normal ranges).

• Fortunately, some approaches **to meditation** *(e.g.,* **focused attention, breathing,** or **movement-based practices**) are really simple, so one can pick the one that is the most suitable for her to use regularly.

• It is critical to learn some specific "**warning signals**", especially for negative emotions, which one might not wish to act on automatically, with a cascade of destructive thoughts and behaviors, which can not only make every problem worse but also aggravate health condition.

• However, when a woman examines her emotions carefully, she will see that they consist of bodily sensations, accompanied by thoughts, images, or both. The more accurately one can recognize emotions in the body, the more clearly one knows when a certain feeling is arising within her. By this token, sensations can serve as "early warning signals" for emotions.

• If she imagines that a doctor will give her the bad news about BC on the next visit, she can create an intentional **"shift" of attitude**. For instance, she can take a moment to feel the sensations of anger in her body, but will not react or say anything automatically right away. Rather she will wait a few moments silently until she can think clearly before responding with self-confidence.

• Another helpful practice is to write a **journal**, to memorize how specific events or personal interactions *(e.g.*, with cancer care team members) one had during the day made her feel. Talking with trusted friends, family, or a therapist can also help explore various emotions, and then, gradually re-program the negative ones, in more positive and rational directions.

• Two simple components, necessary to **elicit the relaxation response** include:

1. **Choosing a calming focus** - one needs to pick a sound, a word ("peace"), or a simple phrase ("I am calm"). Repeat this sound or word out loud or silently, while breathing in deeply and breathing out. Exhaling (breathing out) should be longer than inhaling (breathing in) *(e.g.*, two times longer). Target respiratory rate should be between 6 and 10 per minute.

2. **"Letting go" and relaxing** - it is natural that the mind wanders (*e.g.*, "travels" to the future or to the past). Whenever this happens, one should take a deep breath, and then, gently return the attention back to the focus. Staying focused on the calming word, image, or sound is crucial.

• **Exercises "without borders" – an example of an exercise that focuses on emotions:**

1. Sit quietly in a comfortable position and close your eyes.

2. Bring to mind something a little sad, but not overwhelming.

3. Notice where in your body you feel that sadness.

4. Put one of your hands on that part of your body in a caring, soothing manner.

5. Repeat these steps, but substitute different emotions for sadness *(e.g.*, fear, anger, joy).

REFERENCES

[1]   Dusek JA, Benson H. Mind-body medicine: A model of the comparative clinical impact of the acute stress and relaxation responses. Minn Med 2009; 92(5): 47-50.
        [PMID: 19552264]

[2]   Oberoi S, Yang J, Woodgate RL, *et al.* Association of mindfulness-based interventions with anxiety severity in adults with cancer. JAMA Netw Open 2020; 3(8): e2012598.
        [http://dx.doi.org/10.1001/jamanetworkopen.2020.12598] [PMID: 32766801]

[3]   Goldstein DS. Stress and the "extended" autonomic system. Auton Neurosci 2021; 236: 102889.
        [http://dx.doi.org/10.1016/j.autneu.2021.102889] [PMID: 34656967]

[4]   Smith T, Panfil K, Bailey C, Kirkpatrick K. Cognitive and behavioral training interventions to promote self-control. J Exp Psychol Anim Learn Cogn 2019; 45(3): 259-79.
        [http://dx.doi.org/10.1037/xan0000208] [PMID: 31070430]

[5]   Tang YY, Hölzel BK, Posner MI. The neuroscience of mindfulness meditation. Nat Rev Neurosci 2015; 16(4): 213-25.
[http://dx.doi.org/10.1038/nrn3916] [PMID: 25783612]

[6]   Hopper SI, Murray SL, Ferrara LR, Singleton JK. Effectiveness of diaphragmatic breathing for reducing physiological and psychological stress in adults. JBI Database Syst Rev Implement Reports 2019; 17(9): 1855-76.
[http://dx.doi.org/10.11124/JBISRIR-2017-003848] [PMID: 31436595]

[7]   National comprehensive cancer network (NCCN), Patient and family resources: Managing stress and distress.   Available   at: https://www.nccn.org/patients/resources/life_with_cancer/distress.aspx (Accessed on: January 31, 2020).

CHAPTER 10

An Intersectional Neuroscience Approach for Disadvantageous Populations: Meditation Practice as a Possible Support Option for Women with Breast Cancer?

Abstract: Mindfulness and **compassion meditation** have a positive impact on cognition, mood, behavior, and general health, based on recent studies in neuroscience. However, the research methodology is still insufficient to **determine and measure different mental states during meditation**, especially **in minority populations**.

Intersectional Neuroscience, which is an innovative research model, may provide some solutions since it adapts modern research procedures to include **disadvantageous groups of participants** (*e.g.*, **ethnic minorities,** patients with **chronic diseases**, like **cancer, heart disease,** or **depression**). **Evaluating Multivariate Maps of BODY Awareness (EMBODY)** is a task designed to accommodate diverse neural structures and functions, using the **multi-voxel pattern analysis (MVPA)** classifiers, with **functional magnetic resonance imaging (fMRI)**. The **EMBODY** task applies individualized **artificial intelligence** algorithms to the **fMRI** data, in order to identify mental states during **breath-focused meditation**, a **basic skill that stabilizes attention**.

This chapter describes a potential application of the Intersectional Neuroscience (IN) approach to developing useful metrics of meditation practice, including participants from disadvantageous groups. Hopefully, these findings can be explored in-depth, and possibly applied to **patients with triple-negative breast cancer** (**TNBC**), in the future.

Keywords: Breath-focused meditation, Community-based participatory research (CBPR), Compassion meditation, Functional magnetic resonance imaging (fMRI), Intersectional neuroscience (IN), Mindfulness, Mindfulness-based interventions (MBI).

INTRODUCTION

Meditation is considered to be a part of **integrative medicine** since it connects the traditional, 7,000-year-old practice of **mindfulness** that is focused on paying close attention to the present moment ("**here and now**"). Nonjudgmental acceptance of whatever arises in the awareness is a cornerstone of **mindfulness,** according to modern neuroscience and psychology (Fig. **1**) [1]. **The main approaches to meditation practice** include focused attention, breath-focused, compassion, and movement-based practices so that a patient can choose the one that is most convenient for her [1].

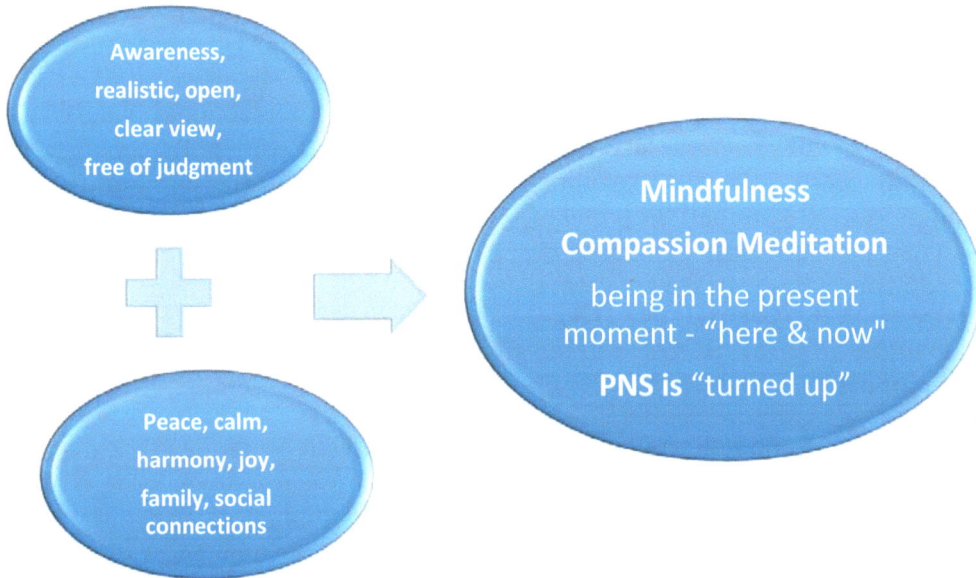

Fig. (1).   Important Components of Mindfulness and Compassion Meditation; PNS, parasympathetic nervous system.

During meditation, a **sympathetic nervous system** (**SNS**) (responsible for arousal, stress-response, and stressful feelings) is "turned down". Simultaneously, a parasympathetic nervous system (**PNS**) (responsible for the relaxation response, rest, and repair) is "turned up" [2]. This allows the heart rate, blood pressure, and respiratory rate to return to physiological ranges [2].

Mindfulness and **compassion meditation** represent **contemplative practices** that may increase [3] the **neuroplasticity of cerebral communication pathways,** relevant to **emotional regulation** and **empathy** [3, 4]. The roots of contemplative research originate from a dynamic exchange between meditation practitioners and scientists, and this interaction has a unique potential for promoting social and behavioral skills in a multicultural environment.

Moreover, in the face of suffering due to common somatic and mental health problems (*e.g.*, a chronic disease, such as TNBC with comorbidities), especially in the ethnic minority groups of women, contemplative interventions (*e.g.*, mindfulness or compassion training) may decrease stress-related reactions to these adversities [5]. Unfortunately, in the contemplative research field, many ethnic minorities are under-represented in the studies of **mindfulness-based interventions (MBI)** [6] Moreover, participation rates of patients from minority groups in neuroscience studies focused on meditation and using **functional magnetic resonance imaging (fMRI)** methodologies, still remain low. As an attempt to address this challenge, an **Intersectional Neuroscience** model has been designed, to be used in the context of contemplative neuroscience [7].

This chapter describes a potential application of the Intersectional Neuroscience approach to developing useful metrics of meditation practice, including disadvantageous groups of participants. Perhaps, after further exploration, these findings may be applied to patients with aggressive subtypes of breast cancer (BC) (*e.g.*, triple-negative breast cancer (TNBC)).

Intersectional Neuroscience (IN) - A Novel Research Model That Can Help Determine Mental States during Meditation in Diverse Populations of Participants

A new research model, known as **Intersectional Neuroscience (IN)**, may offer some helpful solutions to this challenge. **IN** adapts research procedures to include some minority or disadvantageous groups of participants, so that, they can be properly represented [7]. Moreover, **IN** incorporates some inclusive processes into research study designs, based on community engagement with diverse populations of participants [7]. Simultaneously, some individualized multivariate neuroscience methods to accommodate individual neural diversity are also introduced [7].

Recently, the feasibility of this framework was tested with a meditation center, in the US, using a small focus group [7]. The **functional magnetic resonance imaging (fMRI)** screening and recruitment procedures were adapted to be inclusive of participants from various under-represented groups, including ethnic minorities, people with disabilities, neuropsychiatric disorders, and low-income [7].

EVALUATING MULTIVARIATE MAPS OF BODY AWARENESS (EMBODY) - THE INNOVATIVE TASK TO "DECIPHER" MENTAL STATES DURING THE BREATH-FOCUSED MEDITATION

In a recent study, the participants completed the **Evaluating Multivariate Maps of BODY Awareness (EMBODY)** task, which applies individualized machine learning algorithms to fMRI data, in order to identify mental states during **breath-focused meditation**, a **basic skill that stabilizes attention** to support **interoception** and **compassion** [7].

To decode the internal focus of attention during a **breath-focused meditation** episode (specific to every meditating person), the individualized brain patterns were analyzed [7]. Based on these findings, individual-level attention profiles during meditation (*e.g.*, the percentage (%) of time attending to the breath, mind wandering, or engaging in self-referential processing) were recorded [7]. The study has revealed the feasibility of employing an IN approach, which allows inclusion of diverse groups of participants and permits the development of **individualized neural metrics of meditation practice** [7].

In most of the study participants (including experienced meditators and inexperienced controls), it was possible to recognize some unique brain patterns for each of the above conditions. These **brain patterns were subsequently used to decode the presence of various mental states, during 10 min. of breath-focused meditation**. This was the first attempt to obtain brain-derived estimates of **attentional focus during meditation**, **at the individual level** (in the form of the % of time focused on breath) [8]. Such an individualized approach is helpful for studying diverse patient populations since it allows an **individual variability of neural representations** and **characteristics of distinct mental states**. Moreover, the study procedures were appropriate for different ethnic minorities, and people from lower socioeconomic groups [7, 8].

Moreover, the study has explored whether the individualized nature of the EMBODY task would be feasible in the diverse samples, where **artificial intelligence** classifiers can be used to recognize participant-specific brain patterns, relevant to breath-focused meditation (attention on the breath, mind wandering, or self-referential processing), decode these mental states that fluctuate during meditation practice for each meditator, and quantify individual-level attention measures (*e.g.*, % of time attending to the breath) [7, 8]. Since the study was using individualized neuroscientific methods, inclusion/exclusion criteria can be modified (*e.g.*, by adding present medical or mental diseases).

A POSSIBLE APPLICATION OF THE COMMUNITY-BASED PARTICIPATORY RESEARCH (CBPR) TO INTRODUCE INTERSECTIONAL METHODOLOGY TO BRIDGE THE GAP BETWEEN RESEARCH AND PRACTICE

An **intersectional methodology** that is applied in neuroscience research, creates a diversified spectrum of participants, including those from various marginalized social groups (*e.g.*, women of color) [9]. In this model, individualized fMRI techniques, which include neural diversity, create subject-specific brain maps that reflect mental states during practicing breath-focused meditation [10]. Moreover, the **IN** approach uses the analytic system, which recognizes that various life experiences involve several aspects of personal identity, which may be related to socio-economical disadvantages [9, 10].

It should be noted that **community-based participatory research (CBPR)** represents a suitable methodology to implement the above-mentioned intersectional principles, as a possibility to bridge the gap between research and practice *via* community engagement and social efforts to achieve health equity [11]. In brief, **CBPR** is a strategy geared toward equalizing relationships between academic and community research, including bilateral learning exchange and long-term partnership [11]. Moreover, in the **CBPR,** a research process attempts to address multiple cross-cultural aspects of various applied interventions [11]. In this way, the **CBPR** approach can bring helpful solutions to many groups of patients, acting as valuable research partners [11].

HOW THE DIFFERENT ATTENTIONAL STATES DURING THE BREATH-FOCUSED MEDITATION CAN BE MEASURED?

To integrate intersectional approaches with neuroscience, individualized neuroscientific methods to accommodate neural diversity and extend participation need to be used. Unfortunately, serious obstacles to enrolment into different fMRI studies have been related to participants, who have some abnormalities in their brain structure and function (*e.g.*, elderly, individuals diagnosed with mental or neurological diseases, *etc.*).

A simple assumption that the brain structure and function are similar across the population, and thus, can serve as a basis for brain maps, which can be generalized is inadequate. It should be underscored that in neuroscience and psychology, strategies which reflect within-subjects designs are often more appropriate for creating brain maps [12]. Group averages can also be useful, but there are some important limitations related to such designs (*e.g.*, small study samples) [12].

EMPLOYING AN INTERSECTIONAL NEUROSCIENCE APPROACH TO DEVELOP METRICS OF MEDITATION PRACTICE IN DISADVANTAGEOUS GROUPS OF PARTICIPANTS: A POSSIBLE FUTURE STRATEGY FOR WOMEN WITH BREAST CANCER

It should be highlighted that in the **MyConnectome** project, certain characteristics of brain connectivity, gene expression, and metabolism were gathered, and these data were analyzed within one person, over many time points [13]. Similarly, in the **EMBODY** task, the individualized multivariate neuroimaging analytic methods (**multi-voxel pattern analysis, MVPA**) were applied to characterize structural and functional neural diversity [7, 10, 14]. Moreover, the EMBODY task uses the **MVPA in connection with the fMRI data**, in order to decode distinct mental states, which occur in meditation, *via* creating novel, **individualized metrics of internal attention during meditation**, for each participant (*e.g.*, the % of time attending to the breath) [7, 8, 14]. Notably, this approach could reveal fluctuations in attention, for which the novel metrics of attention during meditation sessions included estimating the % of time attending to the breath or engaging in mind wandering, or self-referential processing, specifically for each participant [8, 14].

In addition, **the MVPA** is particularly suitable in the **IN** model. In short, the **MVPA** uses **artificial intelligence (machine learning)** algorithms to detect unique brain patterns for each distinct mental state, in every individual study participant. Subsequently, these detected brain patterns can be used to assess the presence of specific mental states in separate tasks (*e.g.*, whether or not empathic care or distress can be activated in response to visions of suffering [10, 14]. As a result, the obtained information can serve as an **estimate of the presence of certain mental states**, which are based on brain maps. By creating brain maps related to mental states, data from these brain patterns can be learned *via* **artificial intelligence** to make possible connections about certain mental states, which are present and can oscillate [10, 14].

Notably, the **MVPA** that uses neural variability as an advanced technique to find within-subject patterns, may be feasible to measure different mental states during meditation [15]. For example, in **breath-focused meditation** (an essential meditation skill that promotes stability of attention), attention is focused on sensations of the breath (until distracted by other internal or external stimuli, and then, the attention is returned to the breath again). Although this practice is simple, it is not easy. Even during this simple practice, the **focus of attention may fluctuate between attention to the breath, mind wandering,** and **engaging in self-referential processes** [15, 16].

In the **EMBODY task,** the **MVPA classifiers**, together with **the fMRI** data were programmed to distinguish the following **foci of internal attention states:** breath, feet, mind wandering, self-referential processing, and sounds, according to given verbal instructions [7, 8, 16].

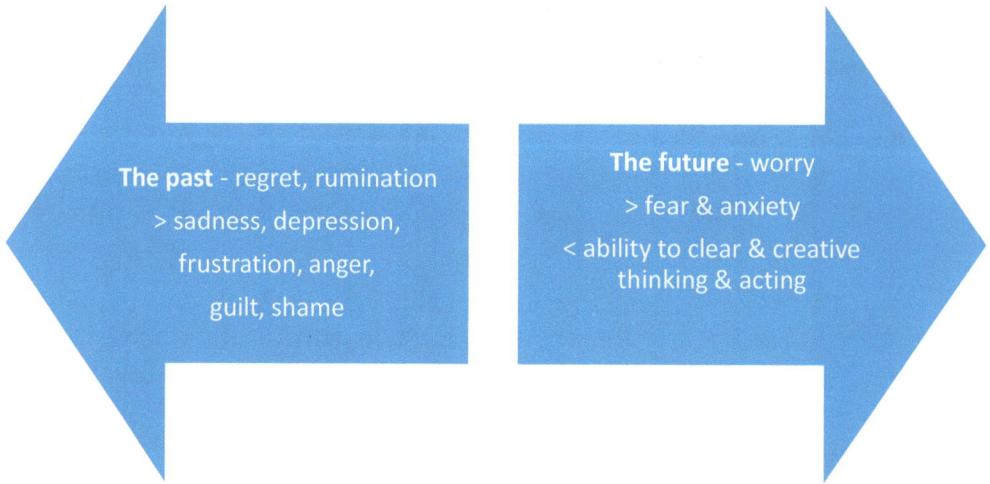

Fig. (2). Different coping styles and their emotional consequences: mindfulness vs. worrying about the future or regretting the past.

CONCLUSION

Meditation is considered to be a part of **integrative medicine** since it connects the traditional, 7,000-year-old practice (focused on paying close attention to the present moment) with modern neuroscience, medicine, and psychology. **The main approaches to meditation practice** include **focused attention** (*e.g.*, on the breath), **open monitoring, loving-kindness, and movement-based practices** so that a woman can choose the one that is most convenient for her.

EMBODY is a specific task designed to accommodate diverse neural structures and functions, in which, the IN model creates person-specific attention metrics using individualized brain signals. It appears that the individualized nature of the EMBODY task would be feasible in the diverse research study samples, where the **artificial intelligence** classifiers can be employed to recognize participant-specific brain patterns, link to **breath-focused meditation** (attention on the breath), and decode the meditation-related mental states, which often oscillate during meditation practice, specifically for every meditator.

Due to the application of individualized neuroscientific methods in the IN studies, the inclusion/exclusion criteria can be modified, depending on the study sample (*e.g.*, patients with cancer, by adding current medical conditions or mental diseases, which they suffer from). It is conceivable that in future research studies in this area, it will be possible to include different ethnic minority groups of patients with chronic diseases (*e.g.*, women with advanced or metastatic TNBC and comorbidities), to explore the effects of practicing **mindfulness** and **compassion meditation,** and their possible contribution to the patient clinical outcomes.

• **Mindfulness is the ability to be present "here and now"** with an open and curious mind.

• **Meditation** helps patients with various diseases and healthy individuals focus on the present moment.

• It also stops annoying self-talk (often containing negative thoughts and emotions).

• Just 15 minutes of mindfulness a day promotes positive emotions and creative thinking, while it increases patience, decreases frustrations, as well as helps alleviate common symptoms of cancer (*e.g.*, chronic pain, poor sleep, depressed mood, anxiety, distress, and fatigue).

• That is so important because if a woman with TNBC is not in the present moment, she is probably caught up inside of her mind, either worrying about the unknown future or regretting some impossible-to-change events from her past (Fig. **2**).

• A patient with TNBC She may also be planning future actions or reviewing some important life events from the past. Of course, this is necessary to either constructively move forward, or to look objectively at what worked and what didn't work in the past.

• However, this should be done in a way that is free of judgment, negative thoughts, or emotions, which often lead to destructive behaviors. Otherwise, these negative elements will "automatically" and unnecessarily deteriorate a patient's condition, and decrease her QoL.

• Some patients, can aggravate their distress. However, this can be good news, because they can also create resilience to stress, with a calm mind, achieved due to regular mindfulness practice.

• Mindfulness should be recommended to many patients, as a "friendly" part of their care plan. Simply put, this concept is somewhat similar to requiring a car to engage another gear.

REFERENCES

[1]   Carmody J. Evolving conceptions of mindfulness in clinical settings. J Cogn Psychother 2009; 23(3): 270-80.
[http://dx.doi.org/10.1891/0889-8391.23.3.270]

[2]   Wu SD, Lo PC. Inward-attention meditation increases parasympathetic activity: A study based on heart rate variability. Biomed Res 2008; 29(5): 245-50.
[http://dx.doi.org/10.2220/biomedres.29.245] [PMID: 18997439]

[3]   Ashar YK, Andrews-Hanna JR, Dimidjian S, Wager TD. Empathic care and distress: Predictive brain markers and dissociable brain systems. Neuron 2017; 94(6): 1263-1273.e4.
[http://dx.doi.org/10.1016/j.neuron.2017.05.014] [PMID: 28602689]

[4]   Klimecki OM, Leiberg S, Ricard M, Singer T. Differential pattern of functional brain plasticity after compassion and empathy training. Soc Cogn Affect Neurosci 2014; 9(6): 873-9.
[http://dx.doi.org/10.1093/scan/nst060] [PMID: 23576808]

[5]   Weng HY, Fox AS, Shackman AJ, *et al.* Compassion training alters altruism and neural responses to suffering. Psychol Sci 2013; 24(7): 1171-80.
[http://dx.doi.org/10.1177/0956797612469537] [PMID: 23696200]

[6]   Waldron EM, Hong S, Moskowitz JT, Burnett-Zeigler I. A systematic review of the demographic characteristics of participants in US-based randomized controlled trials of mindfulness-based interventions. Mindfulness 2018; 9(6): 1671-92.
[http://dx.doi.org/10.1007/s12671-018-0920-5]

[7]   Weng HY, Ikeda MP, Lewis-Peacock JA, *et al.* Toward a compassionate intersectional neuroscience: Increasing diversity and equity in contemplative neuroscience. Front Psychol 2020; 11: 573134.
[http://dx.doi.org/10.3389/fpsyg.2020.573134] [PMID: 33329215]

[8]   Weng HY, Lewis-Peacock JA, Hecht FM, *et al.* Focus on the breath: Brain decoding reveals internal states of attention during meditation. Front Hum Neurosci 2020; 14: 336.
[http://dx.doi.org/10.3389/fnhum.2020.00336] [PMID: 33005138]

[9]   Cho S, Crenshaw KW, McCall L. Toward a field of intersectionality studies: Theory, applications, and praxis. Signs 2013; 38(4): 785-810.
[http://dx.doi.org/10.1086/669608]

[10]   Norman KA, Polyn SM, Detre GJ, Haxby JV. Beyond mind-reading: Multi-voxel pattern analysis of fMRI data. Trends Cogn Sci 2006; 10(9): 424-30.
[http://dx.doi.org/10.1016/j.tics.2006.07.005] [PMID: 16899397]

[11]   Wallerstein N, Duran B. Community-based participatory research contributions to intervention research: The intersection of science and practice to improve health equity. Am J Public Health 2010; 100(S1) (1): S40-6.
[http://dx.doi.org/10.2105/AJPH.2009.184036] [PMID: 20147663]

[12]   Smith PL, Little DR. Small is beautiful: In defense of the small-N design. Psychon Bull Rev 2018; 25(6): 2083-101.
[http://dx.doi.org/10.3758/s13423-018-1451-8] [PMID: 29557067]

[13]   Poldrack RA, Laumann TO, Koyejo O, *et al.* Long-term neural and physiological phenotyping of a single human. Nat Commun 2015; 6(1): 8885.
[http://dx.doi.org/10.1038/ncomms9885] [PMID: 26648521]

[14]   Haxby JV, Connolly AC, Guntupalli JS. Decoding neural representational spaces using multivariate pattern analysis. Annu Rev Neurosci 2014; 37(1): 435-56.
[http://dx.doi.org/10.1146/annurev-neuro-062012-170325] [PMID: 25002277]

[15]   Hasenkamp W, Wilson-Mendenhall CD, Duncan E, Barsalou LW. Mind wandering and attention during focused meditation: A fine-grained temporal analysis of fluctuating cognitive states. Neuroimage 2012; 59(1): 750-60.

[http://dx.doi.org/10.1016/j.neuroimage.2011.07.008] [PMID: 21782031]

[16]   Lutz A, Jha AP, Dunne JD, Saron CD. Investigating the phenomenological matrix of mindfulness-related practices from a neurocognitive perspective. Am Psychol 2015; 70(7): 632-58.
[http://dx.doi.org/10.1037/a0039585] [PMID: 26436313]

CHAPTER 11

May We Adjust the "Third Wave" of Cognitive and Behavioral Therapies (CBT) and Psychological Processes of Change for Women with Breast Cancer?

Abstract: To emphasize on the suffering of women with breast cancer (BC), it is necessary to identify and deeply understand many aspects of BC etiology, development, and complex management. However, the strategies for achieving these goals for individual patients often need to be refocused, or redirected, based on personal expectations, needs, and circumstances that can differ considerably among women with very aggressive BC, such as triple-negative breast cancer (TNBC). The main goal of cognitive-behavioral interventions is to change some specific thoughts, emotions, and behaviors and teach constructive coping skills and behavioral modifications, which will aid in building an individual activity plan, coordinated with cancer-related therapies.

This chapter will present the concept of the **"third-wave" cognitive and behavioral therapies (CBT)** and the importance of **psychological processes of change**, in supportive care interventions, for patients with TNBC. Adding such processes of change should facilitate the development of personalized care solutions for better outcomes for many patients suffering from BC, despite their poor prognosis. This should encourage the patients, caregivers, and their medical care teams to learn, and then, apply these safe interventions in their individualized contexts.

Keywords: Acceptance and commitment therapy (ACT), Cognitive and behavioral therapies (CBT), Psychological processes of change, Psychological flexibility, Mindfulness-based cognitive therapy (MBCT).

INTRODUCTION

Traditionally, **cognitive and behavioral therapies (CBTs)** have been studied in **randomized controlled trials (RCTs)** for specific psychiatric syndromes. However, the **RCTs** have often failed to pay attention to the **processes of change**, which play a critical role in the survival of many women, who struggle with breast cancer (BC). In order to rectify this problem and to effectively help individual patients with BC achieve their functional goals (often in the face of adverse prognosis) a new solution is needed, in which, person-oriented, feasible, and effective methods should be applied [1]. It appears that the **"third-wave" CBTs** attempts to offer a reasonable solution to this challenge. It should be highlighted that in the **"third wave" of CBTs**, the cognitive and behavioral components began with **a person-oriented focus**, which represents a **transition** from rather "static" classical therapeutic models to much more dynamic **processes of change** [1]. Since many mental disorders or psychosomatic diseases (*e.g.*, BC associated with distress or depression) cannot be simply classified into predefined, "formal" categories, the new CBT methods may be more suitable to target some processes of change [1].

This chapter will briefly describe the concept of the **"third-wave" CBT** and the **psychological processes of change**, and their role in supportive interventions, for patients with triple-negative breast cancer (TNBC). This should encourage the patients, their caregivers, and medical care teams to learn and then apply these safe interventions in their individualized contexts.

AN ADVENT OF THE "THIRD-WAVE" COGNITIVE AND BEHAVIORAL THERAPIES AND PROCESS-BASED APPROACHES TO PATIENTS WITH BREAST CANCER

The main innovative features of the **"third-wave" CBTs** involve **focusing on the context and function**, as well as on applying a concept of **psychological processes of change** to the patients and their clinicians or care teams [1]. In this way, such new CBT methods can be considered as a well-organized approach to process-based functional analysis [1]. **Psychological processes of change** can be structured in six domains, including cognition, affect, attention, self, motivation, and behavior (Fig. **1**) [1].

Moreover, the **"third-wave" processes** are characterized by **psychological flexibility**, which combines the concepts in each of the above six dimensions, and enriched them by adding a perspective-taking sense of self, and personal values as motivating factors [1].

In addition, the **psychological processes of change** are adaptable and can harmoniously blend two or more of the six domains. Subsequently, matching the safe, simple, and accessible psychological intervention strategies, to target the appropriate goals for individual women with TNBC, may represent an important step forward in the direction of personalized care (Fig. **2**) [2].

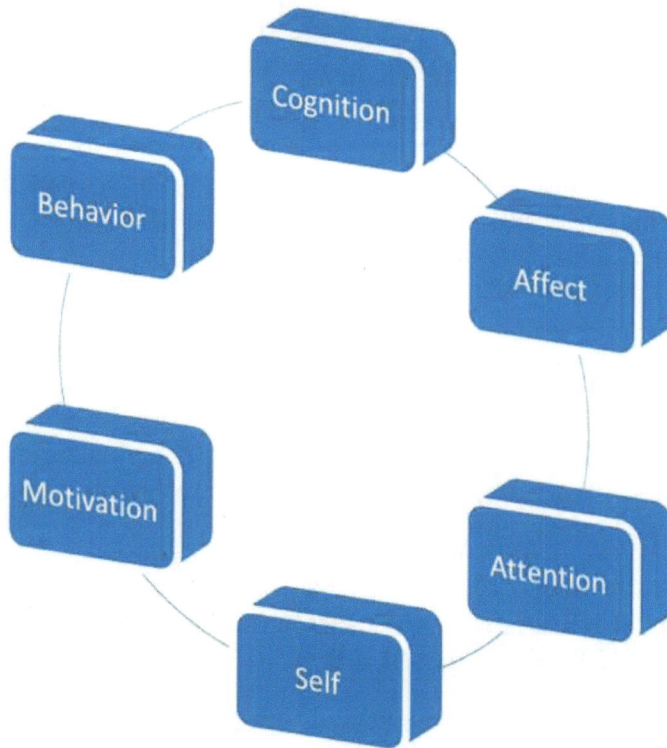

Fig. (1). The "third-wave" CBT - psychological processes of change organized in six domains; CBT, cognitive and behavioral therapy.

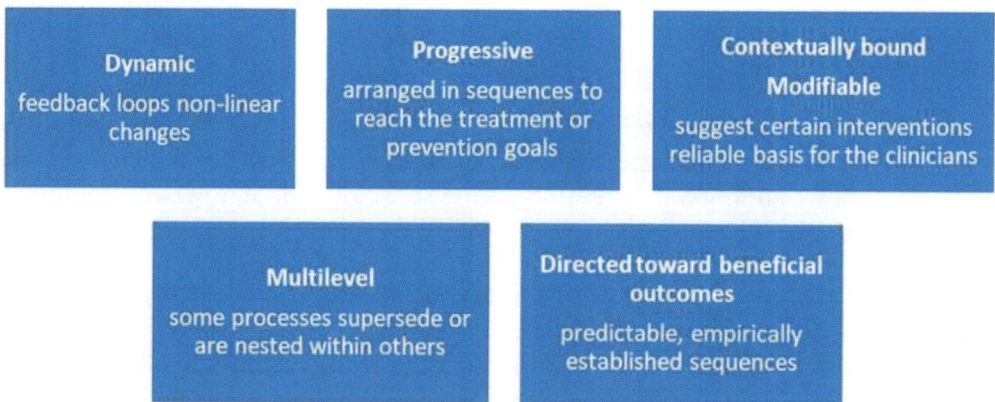

Fig. (2). Common mechanisms involved in the psychological processes of change in the new cognitive and behavioral therapy (CBT).

A FOCUS ON CONTEXT AND FUNCTION: A COMBINED APPROACH FROM THE COGNITIVE AND BEHAVIORAL DIRECTIONS

The new methods of CBT are focused on principles of change, mostly related to the context and function of psychological events (*e.g.*, thoughts, feelings, perceptions, and actions). From a **cognitive** direction, some examples of methods that can be applied in a simple, even "informal" manner include **mindfulness-based cognitive therapy (MBCT), cognitive and behavioral therapy (CBT),** and **meta-cognitive therapy (MCT),** while from a **behavioral** direction, they involve the **acceptance and commitment therapy (ACT)** and **modern behavioral activation (MBA)** (Fig. **3**) [1, 3].

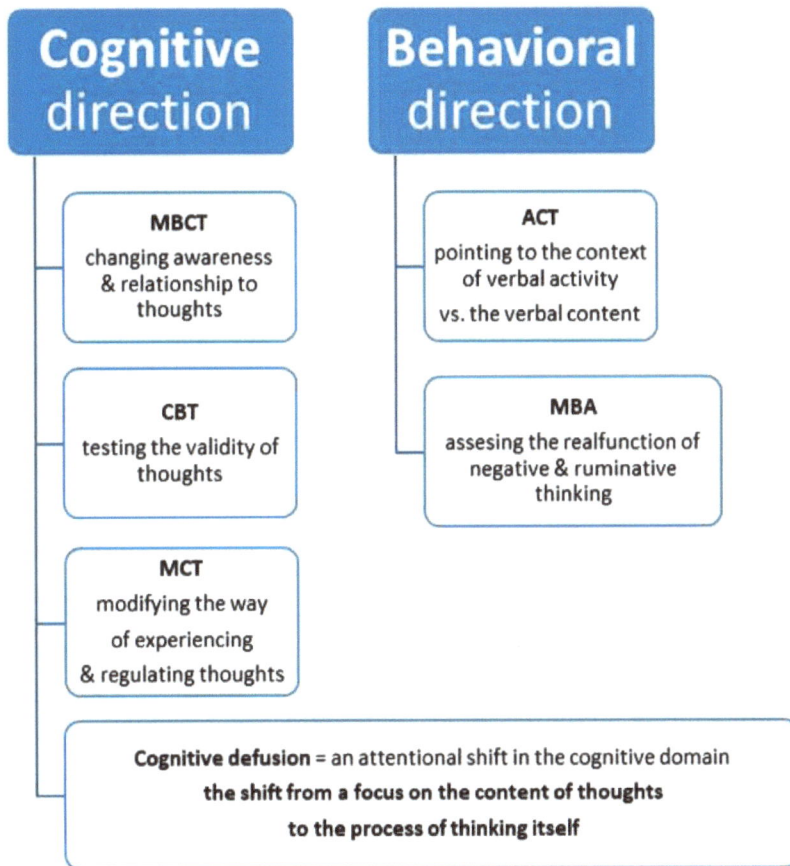

Fig. (3). A combination of the "third-wave" CBT models; MBCT, mindfulness-based cognitive therapy; CBT, cognitive and behavioral therapy; MCT, meta-cognitive therapy; ACT, acceptance and commitment therapy; MBA, modern behavioral activation.

It should be highlighted that in the **MBCT,** there is a little emphasis on changing the content of thoughts, while the main focus is on changing the awareness and relationship to arriving thoughts. Similarly, **CBT** is mostly concerned with testing the validity of thoughts, while **MCT** is concentrated on modifying the way, in which thoughts are experienced and processed. In agreement with that, the **ACT** points out the context of verbal activity as the key element, *vs.* the verbal content itself, and **MBA** evaluates the practical impact of negative or ruminative thinking [3, 4].

In an attempt to adequately address these concepts, a **shift from focusing on the content of thoughts to the process of thinking itself,** known as **cognitive defusion**, was introduced. This **attentional shift in the "third-wave" CBT** models represents a transformation from the earlier CBT waves to the newer ones, which can be more suitable for many patients, who struggle with BC and relevant psychological problems (Fig. **3**) [1, 3, 4].

HOW CAN WE ACCOMMODATE THE KEY PSYCHOLOGICAL PROCESSES OF CHANGE TO HELP ACHIEVE THE PATIENT'S PERSONALIZED GOALS MORE EFFECTIVELY?

At first, some of these new concepts may appear difficult to grasp. However, after their clear explanation, these **psychological processes of change** should be easily introduced and naturally "assimilated" by both the medical practitioners and their patients, as "partners" involved in this mutual journey of care [2, 4]. Some universal steps leading to long-term goals should be precisely explained, so that they can always guide the processes of change, even at the most challenging moments [5]. In particular, it is critical to realize that the **exposure** to many difficult aspects of reality should predominantly serve the value-based new learning, and thus, it should not be avoided [5]. In fact, some potential benefits of learning from different, sometimes unexpected, or unpleasant exposures can be even more valuable than the commonly encountered emotional habituation [5].

Similarly, **acknowledging thoughts** serves the reduction of their automatic and often harmful impact, while **thought recording** (*e.g.*, in the form of writing a journal) should help the **decentering** or **defusion** of **goals**, especially those, which are not beneficial, or even dysfunctional. In this way, **cognitive reappraisal** aids in achieving **cognitive flexibility** (*vs.* only noticing or eliminating some obvious cognitive errors), while the exposure to **values-based learning** is definitely superior to emotional habituation (Fig. **4**) [1, 5].

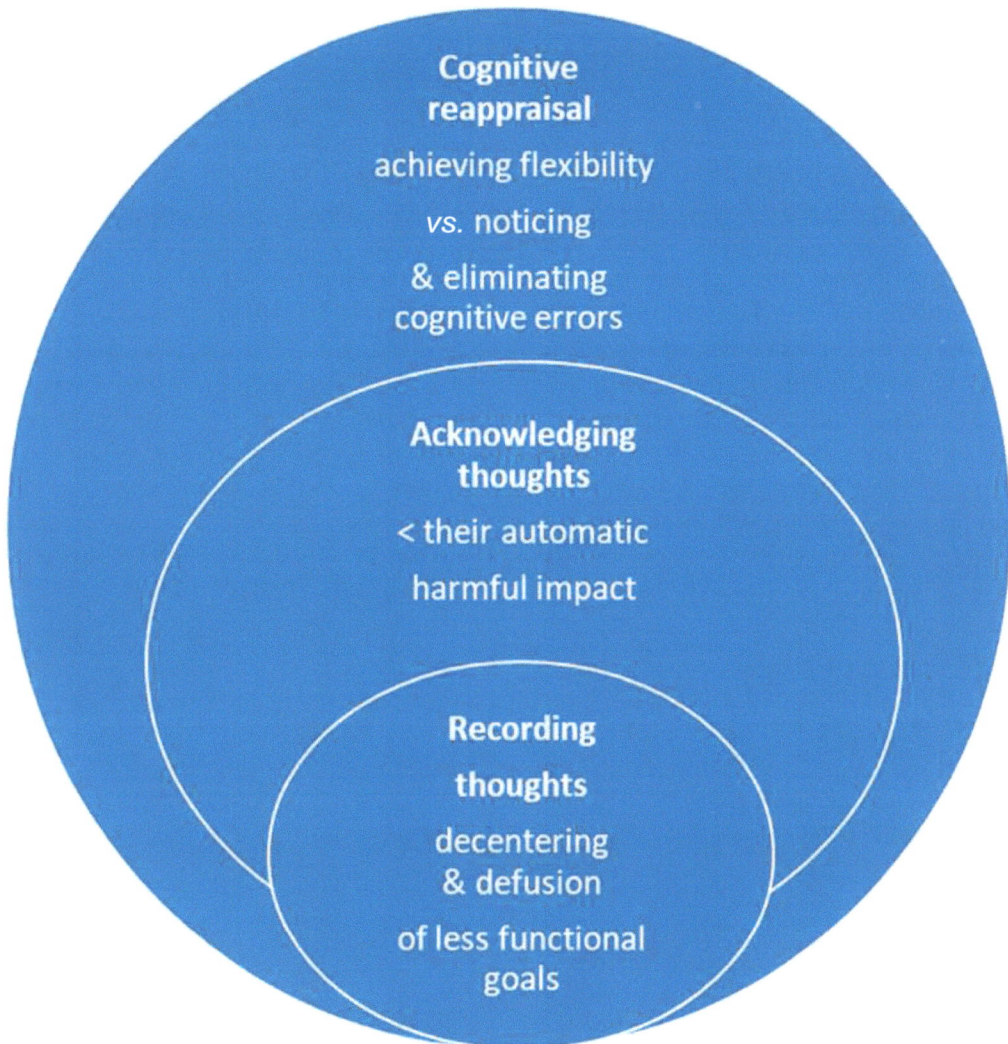

Fig. (4). Some universal steps applied in the "third-wave" CBT models – focus on the exposure that reinforces the values-based learning processes; CBT, cognitive and behavioral therapy.

PSYCHOLOGICAL PROCESSES OF CHANGE IN SIX BASIC DOMAINS: A FOCUS ON FLEXIBLE THERAPEUTIC OPTIONS *VS.* TRADITIONAL SIGNS OR SYMPTOMS ANALYSIS IN THE SCOPE OF THEIR APPLICATIONS

Currently, new and more flexible CBT methods, aimed at the psychological processes of change can be applied to any life situation, including the most challenging ones, often encountered by patients with TNBC. As a result, the "third-wave" CBT should be very appropriate for introducing simple techniques for constructive coping with challenging situations and building psychological resilience to overcome distress [1, 5].

Cognition

The new forms of CBT have added some processes of change in the domain of cognition, focusing on altering the relationship between a thinker and a thought. In this scenario, **cognitive defusion** practically means the **ability to experience thoughts** with a sense of keeping **distance from them**, in order to **attenuate their automatic**, often suboptimal, or harmful **behavioral impact** [5, 6]. Similarly, **non-reactivity** means allowing cognitive or other experiences to come and go without reacting with an intentional effort to change them [5, 6]. In consequence, these processes alter the ultimate impact of cognition, *via* **changing the person's relationship to her own thoughts** (Fig. **5**) [6]. This is often more effective than attempting to change the content or frequency of thoughts. In addition, **cognitive flexibility** allows a person in any given situation to select from a variety of thoughts the most suitable ones, to find the best solution, even in the most difficult circumstances (*e.g.*, advanced or metastatic TNBC) [6, 7].

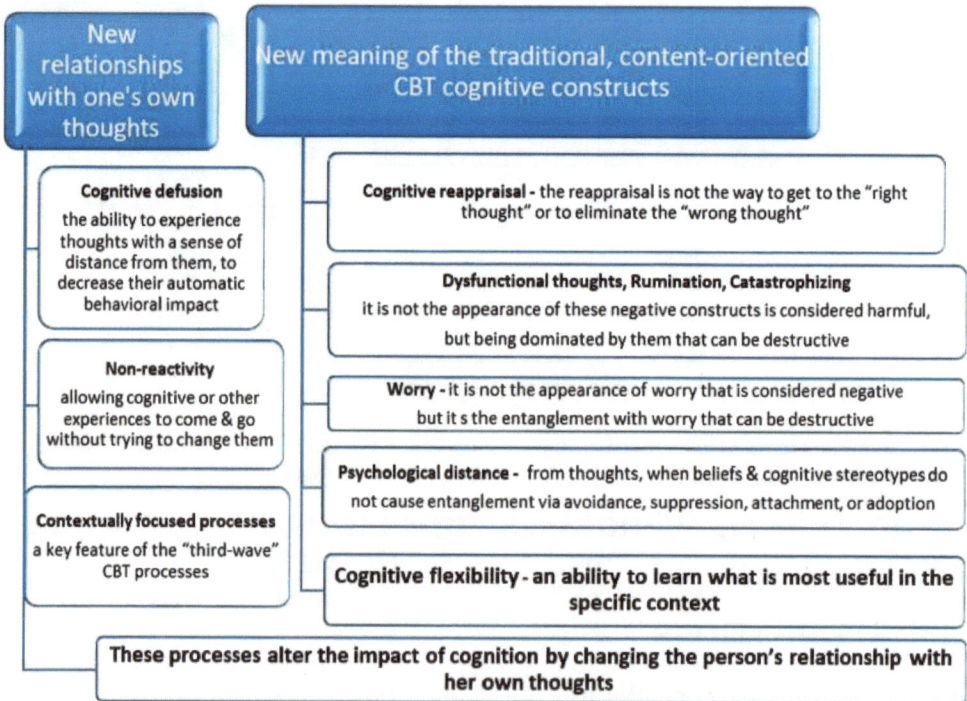

New relationships with one's own thoughts	New meaning of the traditional, content-oriented CBT cognitive constructs
Cognitive defusion the ability to experience thoughts with a sense of distance from them, to decrease their automatic behavioral impact	**Cognitive reappraisal -** the reappraisal is not the way to get to the "right thought" or to eliminate the "wrong thought"
	Dysfunctional thoughts, Rumination, Catastrophizing it is not the appearance of these negative constructs is considered harmful, but being dominated by them that can be destructive
Non-reactivity allowing cognitive or other experiences to come & go without trying to change them	**Worry -** it is not the appearance of worry that is considered negative but it s the entanglement with worry that can be destructive
	Psychological distance - from thoughts, when beliefs & cognitive stereotypes do not cause entanglement via avoidance, suppression, attachment, or adoption
Contextually focused processes a key feature of the "third-wave" CBT processes	**Cognitive flexibility -** an ability to learn what is most useful in the specific context
	These processes alter the impact of cognition by changing the person's relationship with her own thoughts

Fig. (5). Psychological processes of change in cognition – the main focus is on changing the relationship between the thinker and the thought; CBT, cognitive and behavioral therapy.

Affect

The newer forms of CBT have added some affective processes to those, which were previously targeted *via* more traditional methods. In particular, these new CBT concepts mainly focused on how the person relates to emotions (*e.g.*, *via* openness and willingness to deepen some experiences and ongoing learning from different emotional experiences) [7, 8]. As a consequence, **acceptance** simply translates to embracing various effects, without unnecessary escape, avoidance, or constraint [3, 9].

In fact, such an open attitude is far from resignation or some other popular, negative connotations, such as a loss or depletion of something. On the contrary, **acceptance** implies active learning from the content of affective events, and thus, can serve as a basis for desirable **self-compassion** or **self-kindness,** and **distress tolerance** abilities [3, 9]. Notably, some **content-focused concepts** from traditional CBT, such as **loneliness** and **hopelessness** may also play the role of important clinical guides, for both the patients and their clinicians or care teams (Fig. **6**) [8, 9]. It should be underscored that the ability to notice and correctly characterize negative emotional experiences may help design some positive coping approaches, or reduce the impact of negative affects, in the individual medical and psychological context of any patient suffering from malignancy (*e.g.*, advanced or metastatic TNBC) [8, 9].

Attention

In the "third-wave" CBT, processes of change incorporate **attention, affect, sense of self, motivation,** and **behavioral abilities**, as a cluster of interrelated domains. The common origin of psychological processes of change in these domains is a **shift from focusing on the content of thoughts to the process of thinking itself** (as in cognitive defusion).The methods of "third-wave" CBT are influenced by different forms of **mindfulness-based interventions (MBI)**, which consist of training and practice in attentional control (*e.g.*, shifting or maintaining the attention span, and broadening or narrowing the spectrum of attention, depending on the demands of a given situation) (Fig. **7**) [10 - 12]. This can be accomplished *via* guided imagery, or other techniques that help focus on the " here and now", without making any **judgment**.

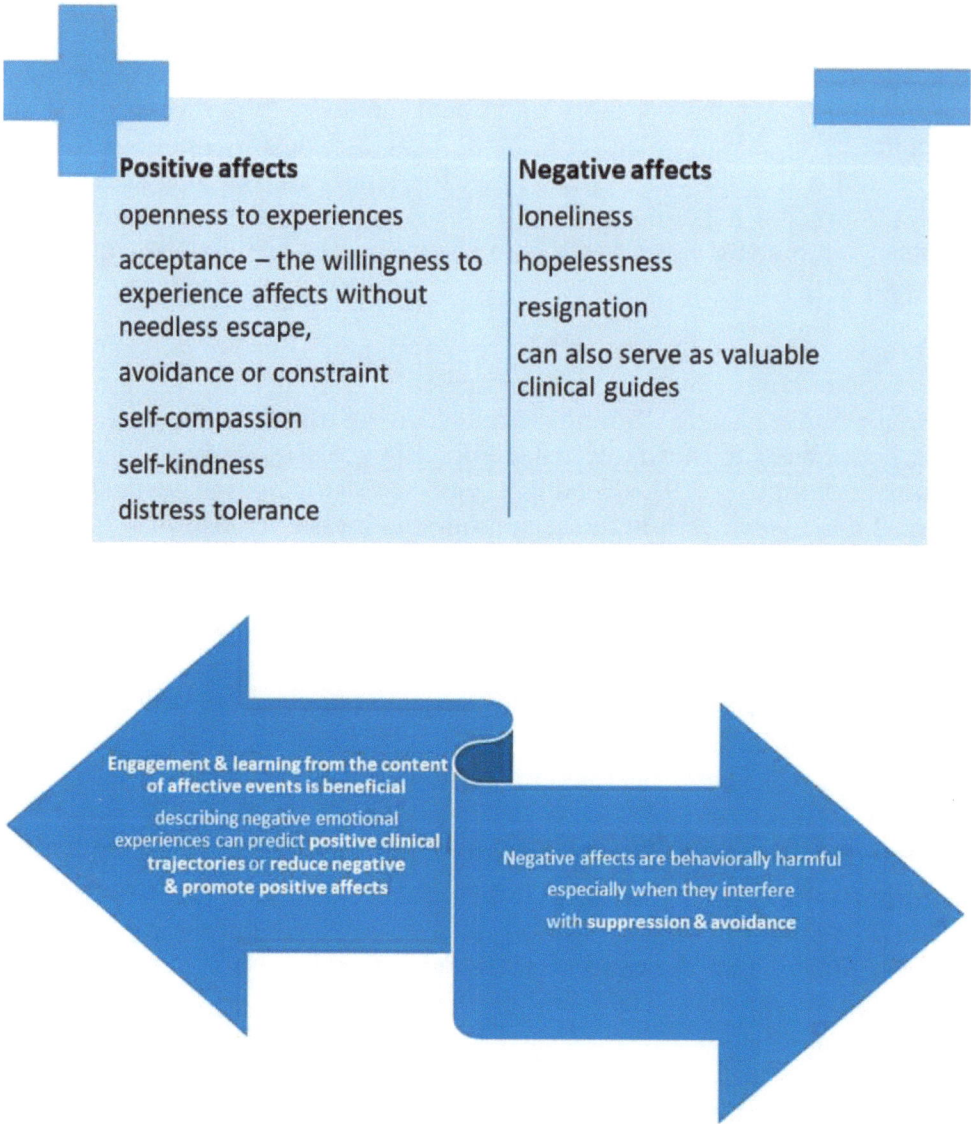

Positive affects

openness to experiences

acceptance – the willingness to experience affects without needless escape,

avoidance or constraint

self-compassion

self-kindness

distress tolerance

Negative affects

loneliness

hopelessness

resignation

can also serve as valuable clinical guides

Engagement & learning from the content of affective events is beneficial

describing negative emotional experiences can predict **positive clinical trajectories or reduce negative & promote positive affects**

Negative affects are behaviorally harmful especially when they interfere with **suppression & avoidance**

Fig. (6). Common examples of positive and negative effects, as content-focused concepts in traditional CBT & their transformation into the newer forms of CBT; CBT, cognitive and behavioral therapy.

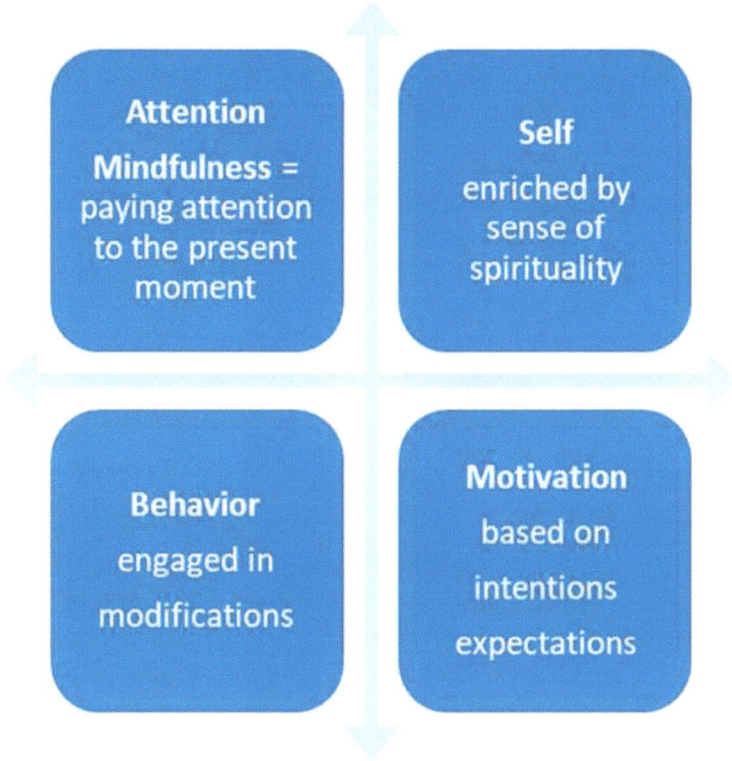

Fig. (7). The "third-wave" CBT processes of change in attention, sense of self, behavior, and motivation.

Self

In the "third-wave" CBT approaches, the self is presented as a sense of **awareness** or **perspective taking**, including **conscious experience** [1, 12]. However, the self is not defined by its content. Furthermore, the "third wave" CBT added some **spiritual dimensions of self**, involving new concepts, such as an **observing self** or **"self-as-context"**, **self-distancing,**, **decentering**, or a **sense of spirituality** [1, 12]. These new concepts create a well-balanced collection with some traditional CBT concepts, such as **self-efficacy, self-regulation,** and **self-management** [1, 12]. Simply put, the deep insight into multiple dimensions of self is clinically valuable, but it is difficult to measure by self-report, and thus, it requires some time for careful observation and assessment from the afflicted patients and their medical care team.

Motivation

Motivation is one of the key elements of CBT, mostly in the form of **goal setting** and **reinforcement**. The "third-wave" CBT (*e.g.*, ACT) has added an emphasis on chosen values as the main mediator of changes [1, 13]. In this way, greater emotional awareness can guide certain valuable choices, which are convergent with the **motivational intentions** and **expectations** of many patients with BC. Such an approach to the motivational processes of change requires various components of context, together with cognitive flexibility.

Behavior

A number of targeted skills have emerged in modern CBT, but these are often focused on other processes. The main traditional behavioral targets include safety behaviors, behavioral activation, problem-solving, social skills, planning, or reductions in impulsivity [1, 14].

PSYCHOLOGICAL FLEXIBILITY – THE COURAGE OF OVERCOMING BARRIERS BY USING CROSS-DIMENSIONAL CONCEPTS

It should be highlighted that the psychological processes of change often combine two or more interrelated dimensions. For instance, mindfulness combines attention, affect, and a sense of self. Similarly, self-regulation involves behavior and a sense of self. In these circumstances, **psychological flexibility** allows the construction of individual **behavioral patterns,** according to values-based habits, depending on the patient's beliefs and needs [1, 15]. Moreover, changes in brain connectivity have been shown to influence some cognitive interventions, and thus, the psychological processes of change, like acceptance can be mediated by the connectivity strength between different cerebral areas, which are often related to different emotional responses (Fig. **8**) [15, 16].

Similarly, various positive behavioral changes, relevant to nutrition, exercises, rest, and sleep patterns may be accomplished by motivated patients [17]. Moreover, well-directed modifications of some behavioral processes at the socio-cultural level, which can vary between different patient groups (*e.g.*, forms of social support or styles of family communication) can favorably influence patients' daily functioning or outcomes, even in the face of malignant disease [18]. In this way, **psychological flexibility** by blending various approaches and overcoming barriers is moving toward supporting and improving the comfort of any individual patient, such as a woman with advanced or metastatic TNBC [1, 15, 18]. Hopefully, a deeper understanding of the process-based complexity of the psychosomatic oncology problems allows for using more personalized interventions, in line with the patient's current needs and goals.

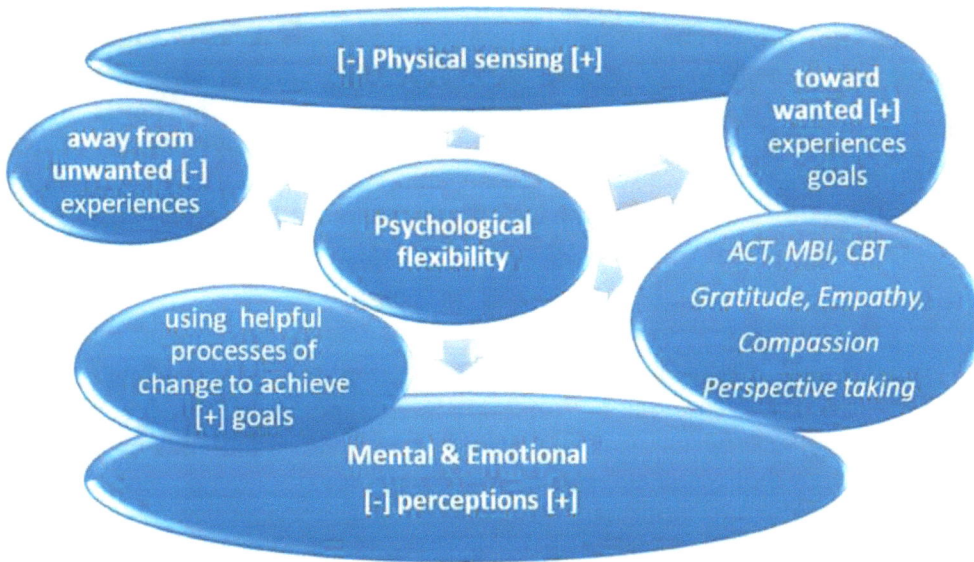

Fig. (8). Psychological flexibility - The concept of moving toward treating the individual patient *via* understanding the process-based complexity of her problems and using personalized interventions; [-], negative; [+]; positive; ACT, acceptance and commitment therapy; CBT, cognitive behavioral therapy; MBI, mindfulness-based interventions.

FUNCTIONAL ANALYTIC PSYCHOTHERAPY (FAP) – POTENTIAL VALUES TO THE PATIENTS AND THEIR CLINICAL/CANCER CARE TEAMS

Functional analytic psychotherapy (FAP) focuses on the qualities of the therapeutic alliance, and the possibilities of using them, in order to build more supportive relationships between patients and their care teams [19]. For instance, the application of **FAP** combined with an empirical approach, based on ongoing assessment of a given clinical situation represents a **process-based strategy**, which can provide a practical **therapeutic model** [19]. The steps needed in this process-based form of functional analysis begin with a detailed assessment of the given patient's case. Subsequently, the relevant management steps should target the key elements of the patient's experiences and actions, as well as her psycho-physical, socio-cultural, or environmental features. If the processes are being altered in an expected, positive direction, then the outcomes should be evaluated, and the management would be continued in the same fashion [19].

However, if such processes do not change in a desirable manner, or the expected, beneficial outcomes do not follow, then the cycle of process-based **functional analysis (FAP)** should be re-directed or restarted. In other words, it may be useful if the physicians and other care team members would pay attention to the functional links between common problems that the women with TNBC experience and the circumstances, in which they happen. Although it appears time-consuming, in the long run, such an approach can possibly serve as a flexible way to alleviate some unnecessary patient suffering. Overall, **experiential** models for targeting patient-specific processes of change are **superior to the traditional** ones, which are focused only on disease symptoms, without considering the dynamic impact of the multi-level psychological aspects on the patient's clinical condition and functional level [1, 19, 20].

CONCLUSION

The **"third-wave" CBT** has addressed some complex issues, which are more characteristic of the existential, cultural, or social domains than the medical ones. Nevertheless, some benefits of these **methods** are universal and may contribute to more positive psychological and medical outcomes for both the patients and their care teams of medical practitioners. This is particularly valuable in the context of the dramatic situation of women with advanced or metastatic stages of TNBC and the demanding and difficult work circumstances for the medical staff members, who take care of them.

• The new methods of **cognitive and behavioral therapy (CBT)** are focused on principles of change, relevant to the context and function of psychological events (*e.g.*, thoughts, feelings, perceptions, and actions).

• Accessible techniques that can be applied in a simple or even "informal" way include **mindfulness-based cognitive therapy (MBCT)** and **acceptance and commitment therapy (ACT).**

• In practical terms, a **shift from focusing on the content of thoughts to the process of thinking itself (cognitive defusion)** is necessary to alleviate some psychological problems for many patients, who struggle with TNBC.

• The simple habit of **acknowledging thoughts** helps in the reduction of their automatic and often harmful impact while **recording thoughts** (*e.g.*, by writing a journal) should be useful in the **decentering** or **defusion** of **goals** (*e.g.*, which are not constructive).

• **Cognitive reappraisal** aids in achieving **cognitive flexibility** and exposure to **values-based learning** that is superior to emotional habituation.

• **Flexible CBT methods,** based on the **psychological processes of change** can be applied to any real-life situations, including the most challenging ones (*e.g.*, for constructive coping with distress or to build psychological resilience) often encountered by patients with TNBC.

• New **experiential CBT methods** could be easily introduced to both the medical practitioners and their patients, as "partners" involved in the mutual journey of care.

REFERENCES

[1]   Hayes SC, Hofmann SG. *Third-wave* cognitive and behavioral therapies and the emergence of a process-based approach to intervention in psychiatry. W Psychiatry 2021; 20(3): 363-75.
      [http://dx.doi.org/10.1002/wps.20884] [PMID: 34505370]

[2]   Ciarrochi J, Hayes SC, Oades LG, Hofmann SG. Toward a unified framework for positive psychology interventions: Evidence-based processes of change in coaching, prevention, and training. Front Psychol 2022; 12: 809362.
      [http://dx.doi.org/10.3389/fpsyg.2021.809362] [PMID: 35222161]

[3]   Yovel I. Acceptance and commitment therapy and the new generation of cognitive behavioral treatments. Isr J Psychiatry Relat Sci 2009; 46(4): 304-9.
      [PMID: 20635779]

[4]   Hayes SC, Luoma JB, Bond FW, Masuda A, Lillis J. Acceptance and commitment therapy: Model, processes and outcomes. Behav Res Ther 2006; 44(1): 1-25.
      [http://dx.doi.org/10.1016/j.brat.2005.06.006] [PMID: 16300724]

[5]   Hofmann SG, Curtiss JE, Hayes SC. Beyond linear mediation: Toward a dynamic network approach to study treatment processes. Clin Psychol Rev 2020; 76: 101824.
      [http://dx.doi.org/10.1016/j.cpr.2020.101824] [PMID: 32035297]

[6]   Zou Y, Li P, Hofmann SG, Liu X. The mediating role of non-reactivity to mindfulness training and cognitive flexibility: A randomized controlled trial. Front Psychol 2020; 11: 1053.
      [http://dx.doi.org/10.3389/fpsyg.2020.01053] [PMID: 32670135]

[7]   Kashdan TB, Barrios V, Forsyth JP, Steger MF. Experiential avoidance as a generalized psychological vulnerability: Comparisons with coping and emotion regulation strategies. Behav Res Ther 2006; 44(9): 1301-20.
      [http://dx.doi.org/10.1016/j.brat.2005.10.003] [PMID: 16321362]

[8]   Arch JJ, Craske MG. First-line treatment: A critical appraisal of cognitive behavioral therapy developments and alternatives. Psychiatr Clin North Am 2009; 32(3): 525-47.
      [http://dx.doi.org/10.1016/j.psc.2009.05.001] [PMID: 19716989]

[9]   Harris VW, Anderson J, Visconti B. Social emotional ability development (SEAD): An integrated model of practical emotion-based competencies. Motiv Emot 2022; 46(2): 226-53.
      [http://dx.doi.org/10.1007/s11031-021-09922-1] [PMID: 35034996]

[10] Hayes SC, Villatte M, Levin M, Hildebrandt M. Open, aware, and active: Contextual approaches as an emerging trend in the behavioral and cognitive therapies. Annu Rev Clin Psychol 2011; 7(1): 141-68.
      [http://dx.doi.org/10.1146/annurev-clinpsy-032210-104449] [PMID: 21219193]

[11] Duarte J, Pinto-Gouveia J. Mindfulness, self-compassion and psychological inflexibility mediate the effects of a mindfulness-based intervention in a sample of oncology nurs`es. J Contextu Behav Sci 2017; 6(2): 125-33.
      [http://dx.doi.org/10.1016/j.jcbs.2017.03.002]

[12] Petrova K, Nevarez MD, Waldinger RJ, Preacher KJ, Schulz MS. Self-distancing and avoidance mediate the links between trait mindfulness and responses to emotional challenges. Mindfulness 2021; 12(4): 947-58.

[http://dx.doi.org/10.1007/s12671-020-01559-4] [PMID: 34149956]

[13]   Viskovich S, Pakenham KI. Randomized controlled trial of a web-based Acceptance and Commitment Therapy (ACT) program to promote mental health in university students. J Clin Psychol 2020; 76(6): 929-51.
[http://dx.doi.org/10.1002/jclp.22848] [PMID: 31468528]

[14]   Bordieri MJ. Acceptance: A research overview and application of this core act process in ABA. Behav Anal Pract 2022; 15(1): 90-103.
[http://dx.doi.org/10.1007/s40617-021-00575-7] [PMID: 35340386]

[15]   Stockton D, Kellett S, Berrios R, Sirois F, Wilkinson N, Miles G. Identifying the underlying mechanisms of change during acceptance and commitment therapy (ACT): A systematic review of contemporary mediation studies. Behav Cogn Psychother 2019; 47(3): 332-62.
[http://dx.doi.org/10.1017/S1352465818000553] [PMID: 30284528]

[16]   Falletta-Cowden N, Smith P, Hayes SC, Georgescu S, Kolahdouzan SA. What the body reveals about lay knowledge of psychological flexibility. J Clin Med 2022; 11(10): 2848.
[http://dx.doi.org/10.3390/jcm11102848] [PMID: 35628974]

[17]   Firth J, Solmi M, Wootton RE, *et al.* A meta-review of *lifestyle psychiatry* : The role of exercise, smoking, diet and sleep in the prevention and treatment of mental disorders. W Psychiatry 2020; 19(3): 360-80.
[http://dx.doi.org/10.1002/wps.20773] [PMID: 32931092]

[18]   Tarbox J, Szabo TG, Aclan M. Acceptance and commitment training within the scope of practice of applied behavior analysis. Behav Anal Pract 2022; 15(1): 11-32.
[http://dx.doi.org/10.1007/s40617-020-00466-3] [PMID: 35340381]

[19]   Hofmann SG, Hayes SC. The future of intervention science: Process-based therapy. Clin Psychol Sci 2019; 7(1): 37-50.
[http://dx.doi.org/10.1177/2167702618772296] [PMID: 30713811]

[20]   Hayes SC. Acceptance and commitment therapy: Towards a unified model of behavior change. W Psychiatry 2019; 18(2): 226-7.
[http://dx.doi.org/10.1002/wps.20626] [PMID: 31059616]

CHAPTER 12

Exceptional Responders: Exploring the Molecular "Make-up" of Patients with Cancer Who Experienced Recovery

Abstract: Patients with cancer, who have achieved an unexpectedly **favorable** and long-term clinical **response** are commonly known as **exceptional responders (ER)**. Such patients have often experienced extraordinary responses to some oncology therapies, which have been ineffective for other individuals with similar malignancies.

These unusually positive responses may be partially due to some unique genetic and molecular mechanisms, which can be further studied. This, in turn, could provide some directions to a better understanding of why the specific therapy works for only a small number of patients with cancer, but not for everybody. To further elucidate these issues, the **National Cancer Institute (NCI)** has been conducting various research projects to explain biological processes, which can be responsible for these remarkable responses.

A recent pilot study, known as the **Exceptional Responders Initiative (ERI),** has evaluated the feasibility of identifying exceptional responders retrospectively, by obtaining pre-exceptional response treatment tumor tissues and analyzing them with modern molecular tools. The promising findings of this study can inspire many women with breast cancer (BC) and their medical teams.

This chapter presents a synopsis of the **ERI**. It suggests some possibilities to adjust this concept for patients with breast cancer (BC) (*e.g.*, advanced or metastatic triple-negative breast cancer (TNBC)).

Keywords: Actionable mutations, Exceptional responders, Exceptional responses, Integrated studies, Next-generation sequencing (NGS), Precision oncology.

INTRODUCTION

Patients with cancer, who have achieved **unexpectedly beneficial** and **long-standing clinical responses to therapy** are commonly known as **exceptional responders (ER)** [1]. Such patients have demonstrated an extraordinary response to some anticancer treatments, which have been ineffective for others with similar types of cancers [1].

These **exceptional patient cases** are very interesting and challenging to many researchers and clinicians, who want to find out what exactly they have been doing to recover from cancer, despite the adverse prognosis. Initially, casual examples of remarkable outcomes of chemotherapy (CHT) or targeted therapy were rather informal observations, because the clinicians' ability to identify the molecular mechanisms underlying relatively rare responses has been limited. However, currently, with a growing interest in this area, the situation has changed. It is conceivable that such unusual responses can be attributed, to some degree, to individual genetic and molecular mechanisms, which may offer valuable directions to a better understanding of why the specific therapy works for only a small number of patients, but not for a majority of them. Recently, the **National Cancer Institute (NCI)** has been conducting research projects, trying to explain complex biological processes that are potentially responsible for these unusually positive clinical responses [1, 2].

This chapter briefly presents a synopsis of the **Exceptional Responders Initiative (ERI).** It suggests some possibilities to adjust this concept to patients with breast cancer (BC), in particular with aggressive subtypes (*e.g.*, triple-negative breast cancer (TNBC)).

The Exceptional Responders Initiative (ERI) – New Hopes and Challenges Uncovered by a Pilot Study

The **exceptional response** has been defined as a **partial response (PR)** or **complete (CR) response** to systemic anticancer treatment with a population PR or CR rate less than 10% or an unusually lengthy response (*e.g.*, duration three times higher than the median) [2].

The **NCI** has recently conducted a **pilot study** that retrospectively evaluated **clinical data** and **tumor samples** from over one hundred cases of patients with cancer [2]. To test the feasibility of collecting the archival tissues from **exceptional patients** and conducting subsequent molecular profiling, **NCI** introduced a protocol for the **Exceptional Responder Initiative (ERI)** study [2].

Molecular profiling technology, including **next-generation sequencing (NGS)**, has transformed the development of oncology therapies, especially in the early phases of clinical trials, with efforts to select patients, depending on molecular aberrations. The **ERI** tumor material, collected from several cancer types, provided by the participated oncologists, was profiled [2]. These cancer cases usually involved patients undergoing targeted therapies. However, these **patients were treated without knowing their tumor's genomic alterations**. Post-treatment, when it was revealed that some of them had specific genomic changes, which could have made their tumor particularly sensitive to blocking of a driving pathway by a given targeted agent, this "puzzle" of better clinical effects (than expected initially) was at least partially solved [2].

The next step to elucidate this topic was to determine the exact molecular causes and precise reasons why some tumors responded to targeted therapies or to standard chemotherapies (CHT). Finding correct answers to this question would potentially allow adjusting the therapeutic options to patients, who have the highest probability to respond to certain therapies. For instance, in the **ERI** pilot study, including over one hundred cases of exceptional responders, about 70% of participants were treated with combination CHT regimens, almost 30% had received anti-angiogenesis agents, and a few patients had been treated with immune checkpoint inhibitors (ICI) [2]. Moreover, clinically relevant germline mutations were identified in six tumors, including pathogenic *BRCA1* or *BRCA2* mutations, which were found in two women with BC. For instance, one patient with BC had a pathogenic *BRCA1* germline mutation, and another had a germline mutation in *CHEK2*. In addition, a patient with lung cancer, who had a history of BC, had also a *PALB2* mutation [2].

Molecular mechanisms are crucial, but other factors (*e.g.*, comorbidities, use of medications, complementary approaches, and lifestyle components) can also contribute, often in unpredictable ways, to eliciting an **exceptional response** [2]. Therefore, a future gathering of such variables would allow adequately presenting the findings, in order to design concepts about molecular and other reliable predictors of response or resistance to anticancer treatment.

In summary, in the **ERI** pilot study, **ER cases** represented different types of cancers and treatment strategies, such as standard cytotoxic chemotherapy (*e.g.*, single or multi-agent CHT), CHT/radiation combinations, or investigational therapeutics (*e.g.*, modern targeted therapies) [2]. Several cases with exceptionally durable PRs (*e.g.*, over 100 months) may represent actual CRs or tumors with an indolent clinical course. Prolonged responses may suggest favorable immune system influence. In this analysis, creating clusters of patients, who were treated with medications, which have similar mechanisms of action could increase confidence in reported associations between molecular alterations and responses to anticancer agents within a particular pharmaceutical class [2].

Unfortunately, the **ERI study was limited**, since there was no molecular analysis of tumors from patients, who responded poorly to the same treatment that was administered to the ER patients. In fact, for an adequate comparison, clinical characteristics of non-responders to the same therapy regimen would have to be matched (*e.g.*, primary tumor, performance status, medications for comorbidities, and line of treatment) to those in the **ER** group [2].

AN IMPACT OF PRECISION ONCOLOGY ON THE EXCEPTIONAL RESPONDERS INITIATIVE (ERI)

Precision oncology is an approach to **personalized medicine** that applies innovative genomic and molecular technologies to achieve particular profiles of tumors, in order to develop targeted therapeutics to improve patient outcomes. Advancing these profiles from the histology basic examination and moving towards a genomic and molecular examination has caused many novel approaches, linked to targetable driver mutations, innovative study designs for genomically targeted agents, and large datasets to develop new recommendations for patient management [3]. A possible approach to using the **NGS** for the discovery of targeted anticancer therapeutic agents has been matching it to evaluations of tissue specimens derived from **ER cases** [3].

The **ERI** study has been using **NGS** to explore the molecular "make-up" of **exceptional responders** to different therapies. Notably, in **the ERI**, one of the key objectives was to collect tumor tissue samples from patients who displayed unusually beneficial responses in early-phase studies of new therapeutics. This was an attempt to "**rescue**" such agents, which otherwise could have been considered as a failure [1, 3]. In addition, future studies on **exceptional responders** should include a comparison of the data from **exceptional** patients with those from individuals who had poor outcomes, despite undergoing the same treatment [4]. Moreover, prospective studies of tumors from exceptional responders, linked with the novel, **genomically targeted agents**, may provide a powerful approach to cancer treatment.

It should be noted that **precision oncology** is also a term describing cancer care that is optimally adjusted for an individual patient. In fact, communicating this innovative concept to patients and their families or caregivers can be difficult for many physicians. To shed some light on this topic, a qualitative study has been completed, in which clinicians shared their opinions about communication, as one of the "pillars" of precision oncology [5]. Overcoming communication barriers and building helpful strategies, so that patients and clinicians can make the most optimal decisions are critical to achieving the best effects in precision oncology.

SELECTED TOOLS OF PRECISION ONCOLOGY APPLIED IN THE EXCEPTIONAL RESPONDERS INITIATIVE (ERI)

Recently, modern molecular profiling technology, such as **NGS** has expanded the therapeutic horizons in oncology. At present, in many clinical trials, in early drug development, it is mandatory to include (or exclude) patients, with certain molecular alterations. Concurrently, efforts to identify molecular alterations in tumors that exhibited exceptional response after systemic treatment with standard or investigational agents have been in progress. These discoveries may ultimately serve as predictive markers or "**actionable mutations**" for future therapies [6]. In recent years, biotechnological breakthroughs have led to the identification of complex and unique biologic features associated with carcinogenesis. Tumor and cell-free DNA profiling, immune markers, and proteomic and RNA analyses are used to identify these characteristics for the optimization of anticancer therapy in individual patients. Recently, many clinical trials have changed their designs from tumor type-oriented to gene-targeted and patient-centered and introduced novel, more flexible strategies, aimed at improving the patient QoL and survival [7].

Many **precision medicine** studies have shown that targeted or matched therapy is related to improved outcomes compared to non-matched therapy, in cases of various tumor types and in certain malignancies. To expand the impact of precision medicine, this strategy should be used early in the course of the malignancy. Moreover, some patients with particularly high recurrence risk should undergo tumor profiling and possibly receive matched therapy. To explore the complexity of tumor biology, clinical trials with combinations of gene-targeted therapy with immune-targeted approaches (*e.g.*, **checkpoint blockade, personalized vaccines,** and/or **chimeric antigen receptor T-cells**), hormonal therapy, CHT, and/or novel agents should be considered. These studies should target dynamic changes in tumor biological abnormalities, eliminating minimal residual disease, and eradicating significant subclones that confer resistance to treatment [7].

THE NCI-MATCH TRIAL - A MOLECULAR ANALYSIS FACILITATING THE CHOICE OF OPTIMAL ONCOLOGIC THERAPY

Since the proportion of tumors with various histologies, which may respond to drugs targeted to molecular alterations remains unclear, the **NCI-MATCH** trial was designed to explore the efficacy signals. This was accomplished by matching patients with refractory cancers to therapies, which were targeted to potential tumor molecular drivers, irrelevant to cancer histology. The findings of the NCI-MATCH study have suggested that profiling from tumor biopsies and applying treatment accordingly can be done successfully in a large patient population [8, 9]. Due to multiple factors involved in clinical responses (*e.g.*, host and tumor properties), gathering tumor samples, correlated with clinical data, similar to the **NCI-MATCH** trial, represents a helpful model for designing future genomic trials in this area [9].

CHALLENGES IN INVESTIGATING THE EXCEPTIONAL RESPONDERS AND EXCEPTIONAL RESPONSES

As previously mentioned, an **exceptional responder** has been considered the patient, who had experienced a complete response to one or more therapeutics, to which complete responses were seen in fewer than 10% of patients, who received a similar therapy, or partial response lasting at least six months, during which, such a response has been seen in fewer than 10% of patients, who received a similar treatment, or complete or partial response of a duration that is three times the median response duration, described in the medical literature for a given treatment (Fig. **1**) [10]. It should be underscored that a formal definition of an **exceptional response** is complicated, since, such a definition relies on the existence of data that a particular therapy will achieve specific responses in groups of patients with similar tumors, as defined by an organ of origin. In addition, it is necessary to gather tumor tissue samples, and comprehensive medical records (*e.g.*, previous treatments, the patient's responses to these treatments, and molecular test results). Unfortunately, an absence of data relevant to other risk factors for malignancy, and a lack of molecular analyses of tumors (*e.g.*, since they were unavailable in the past) create some serious obstacles (Fig. **2**) [10].

FUTURE STEPS TO UNLOCK THE DOOR TO NOVEL ANTICANCER TREATMENTS

In the future, studies may utilize data from completed clinical trials, in which tumors and normal tissue samples were collected before the oncology therapy, and clinical variables can be analyzed in both responders and non-responders.

Clinical trials randomizing patients to different treatments would inform about molecular alterations correlating with a more indolent or more aggressive disease course (prognostic alterations) as well as alterations that predict a very good or very poor response (predictive alterations). In addition, sharing these data among multidisciplinary, international treatment teams will allow us to discern predictive molecular markers that can guide treatment choices [10].

Also, findings from studies of **exceptional responses**, who had particularly beneficial or adverse responses to treatment may inspire researchers to continue their search to be able to predict real chances for survival in the most vulnerable patients with cancer.

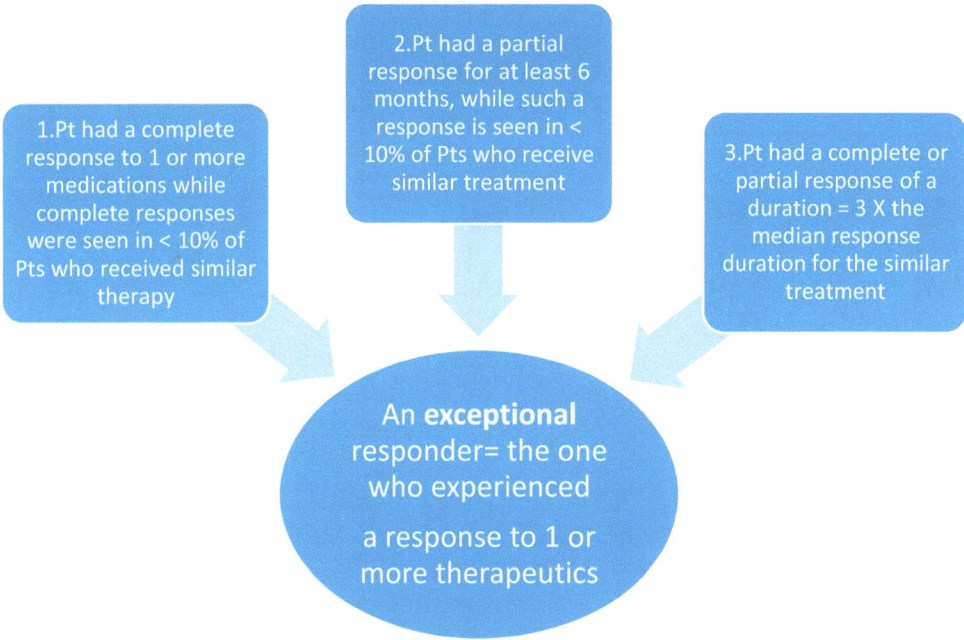

Fig. (1). Patient's Criteria for the Exceptional Responder; Pts, patients;

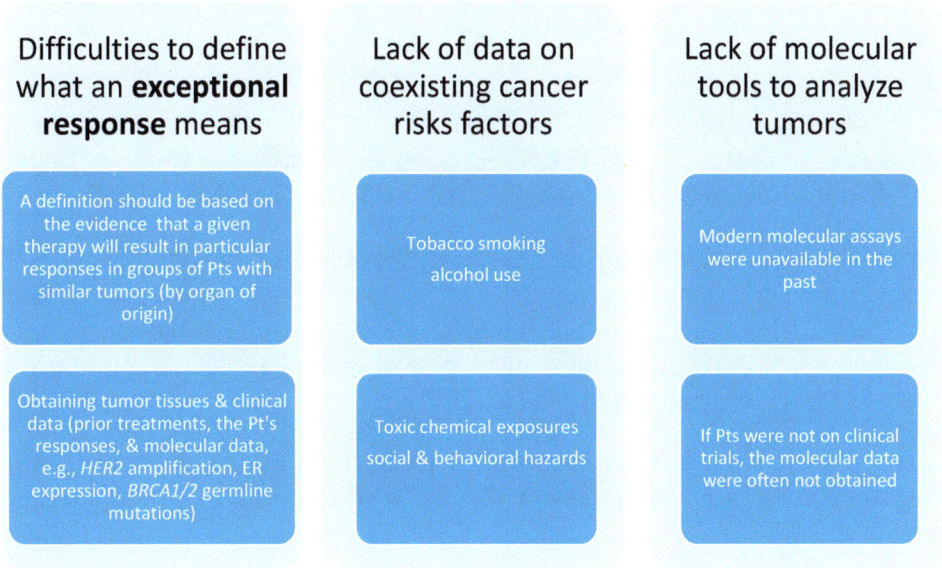

Fig. (2). Examples of the Challenges in Studying Exceptional Responses; ER, estrogen-receptor; Pts, patients; *vs, versus*.

It should be underscored that a close collaboration within the **ERI** is necessary to provide a special **registry,** based on international **standard operating procedures (SOP)** for the storage of data before analysis, harmonized policies and procedures, and a secured system of medical records [10]. It should be highlighted that some patients with cancer, who responded exceptionally well to certain treatments may have molecular changes in their tumors, which can possibly explain their favorable responses and "open the gate" to innovative targeted therapies [11]. Since it has been indicated that the genomic "make-up" of cancer may help uncover genetic alterations, which contribute to unexpected or long-term responses to given treatments, a detailed assessment of the groups of patients with the detected genetic changes can accelerate the development of novel therapies [12]. For instance, in the ERI, various genomic approaches to assess the tumor and normal tissue, were applied (*e.g.*, DNA mutations, RNA expression levels, DNA copy number alterations, and DNA methylation). Also, the immune cells in the tumor microenvironment were investigated [12]. According to the ERI, some mechanisms related to exceptional responses included the patient's internal ability to repair DNA damage and the immune system's possibility to generate a response against tumors. Simultaneously, synthetic lethality is a rare combination of genomic changes, which contributes to tumor cell death during treatment and can potentially create new therapeutic horizons [12]. In addition, examining patients with cancer for tumor alterations, as well as exploring the vulnerabilities or defects, identified in the tumor cells of exceptional responders, can offer possible targeted anticancer treatments, in the future [12].

THE POWER OF INTEGRATED STUDIES –THE INTERFACE BETWEEN THE PATIENTS, TUMORS, AND SOCIO-EPIDEMIOLOGICAL RISK FACTORS FOR MALIGNANCIES

Integrated studies, which analyze a dynamic combination of genetic and immune characteristics of a patient's tumor with clinical, and socio-epidemiological factors can shed some light on the interrelations between a patient's biology, lifestyle, and molecular alterations in the tumor, as well as the ability to generate an immune response against malignancy [13].

For instance, the **Exceptional Responder Initiative (ERI)** and the **Network of Enigmatic Exceptional Responders (NEER)** reflect an idea of integrated, long-term studies.

In essence, the **Network of Enigmatic Exceptional Responders (NEER)** contains a registry of patients with various types of cancer, who had **exceptional**

responses to treatment [14]. The goal of the **NEER** study has been to profile blood, tumor, and gut microbiome samples, as well as to include epidemiological data, such as environmental factors, physical activity, sleeping patterns, detailed medical records, and information on the personality type, communication style, and social interactions of exceptional responders [14]. Moreover, the **NEER** has been focused on the contributions of lifestyle and genetic factors and the exploration of whether the individual factors act separately or interact together to influence a patient's survival [14]. Gathering such multidimensional datasets is an enormous challenge, in which, interdisciplinary expertise is mandatory (Fig. 3). Similarly, the **ERI** offers the potential to connect clinically important insights with molecular features related to exceptional responses or beneficial outcomes from specific treatments. In the ERI, a complete analysis of every case, followed by a subsequent grouping of similar treatments or similar tumors is a priority [2, 12].

A SPOTLIGHT ON THE NETWORK OF ENIGMATIC EXCEPTIONAL RESPONDERS (NEER)

The **Network of Enigmatic Exceptional Responders** (**NEER**) program has been created to detect **exceptional responders** and to perform molecular profiles of their tumors, in order to determine molecular correlates with exceptional responses. In this way, **exceptional responder molecular analysis** may contribute to the discovery of new biomarkers and targeted anticancer therapeutics, in the future. The **NEER** is searching for patients who have had unique responses to cancer treatments that were not effective for most other oncology patients, who had identical diagnoses. Previously, these patients were often dismissed, assuming that no valuable data could be obtained from them. However, this point of view has recently changed. Since the **NEER** is reflecting new findings of cancer biology, in early studies of exceptional responders, some details about tumor heterogeneity and ways to circumvent heterogeneity-imposed therapeutic barriers can be determined. This, in turn, may allow more accurate pre-trial patient screening [14]. In addition, various tumors and their standard or experimental treatments were analyzed. Both the tumor and normal tissue samples were **profiled** with whole exome sequencing, and potentially actionable germline mutations were tracked for relevance to the neoplastic disease. For instance, several mutations in *BRCA1* and *BRCA2* genes have been noted. This creates some hope that certain medications, which target the DNA repair pathways (*e.g.*, **PARP-inhibitors** and platinum CHT agents) can be effective, even in the most challenging cases. Moreover, it has been suggested that genetic predictors of anticancer therapies may be identified by examining the exceptional responders' cases [2, 14]. Also, tumor **molecular profiling from patients, who revealed exceptional responses** to systemic therapy may provide valuable insights into their tumor biology, as well as refine personalized treatment options for many patients with the most aggressive and resistant malignancies, in the future.

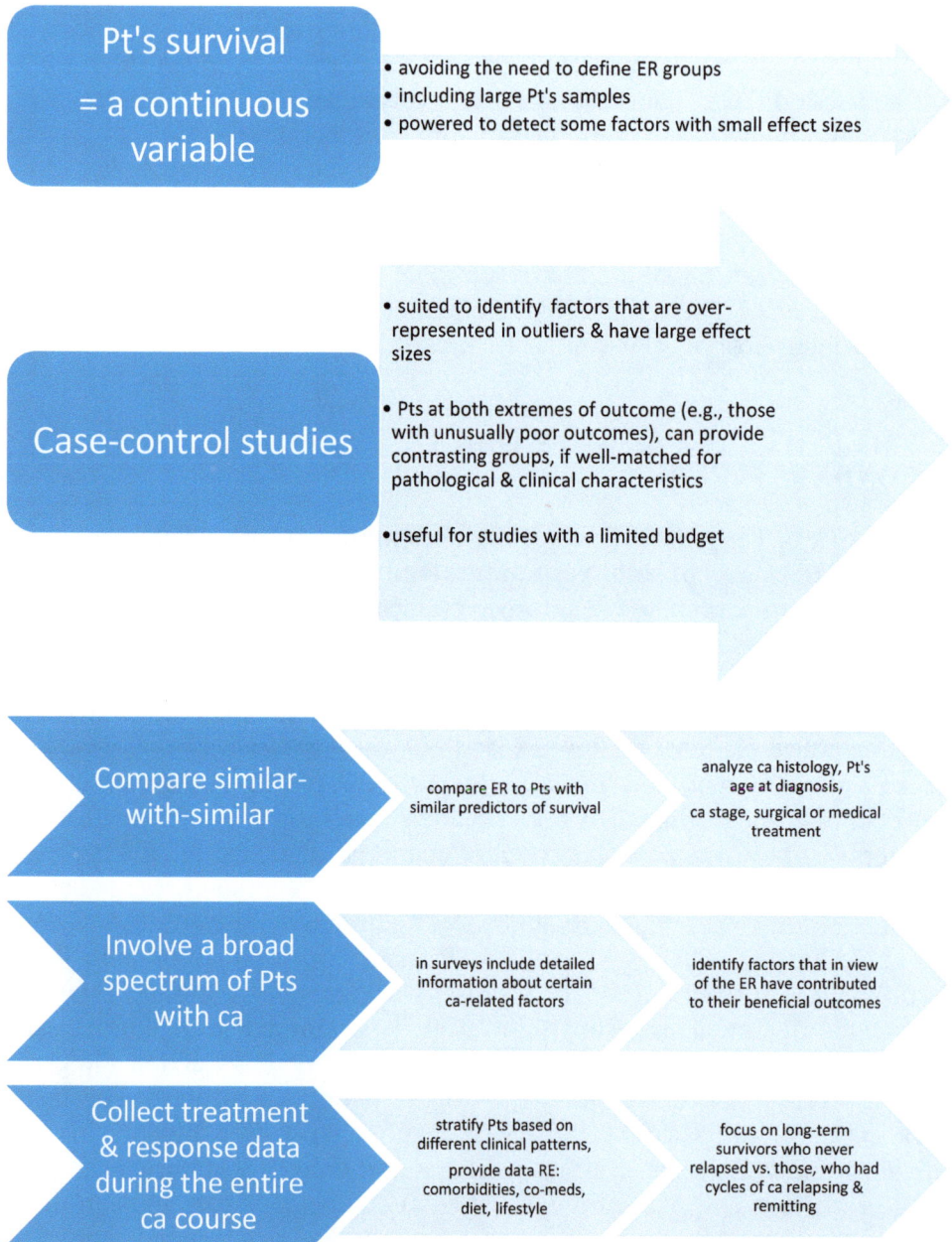

Pt's survival = a continuous variable
- avoiding the need to define ER groups
- including large Pt's samples
- powered to detect some factors with small effect sizes

Case-control studies
- suited to identify factors that are over-represented in outliers & have large effect sizes
- Pts at both extremes of outcome (e.g., those with unusually poor outcomes), can provide contrasting groups, if well-matched for pathological & clinical characteristics
- useful for studies with a limited budget

Compare similar-with-similar — compare ER to Pts with similar predictors of survival — analyze ca histology, Pt's age at diagnosis, ca stage, surgical or medical treatment

Involve a broad spectrum of Pts with ca — in surveys include detailed information about certain ca-related factors — identify factors that in view of the ER have contributed to their beneficial outcomes

Collect treatment & response data during the entire ca course — stratify Pts based on different clinical patterns, provide data RE: comorbidities, co-meds, diet, lifestyle — focus on long-term survivors who never relapsed vs. those, who had cycles of ca relapsing & remitting

Fig. (3). Examples of Helpful Study Designs and Recommendations for Detecting and Analyzing Exceptional Responders (ER) to Cancer; ca, cancer; Pts, patients;

CONCLUSION

There are multiple factors, which impact **exceptional responses** and survival among **exceptional patients** with malignancies. **Exceptional response**s are most probably due to combinations of clinical, genetic, epigenetic, immune, psychological, and socio-epidemiological factors, and thus, studies that simultaneously consider these elements may uncover complex interactions between the tumor, host, and environment. To explore this fascinating area, future large-scale studies are merited. In this way, exceptional patients with cancer can provide the most valuable "pearls", which would be applicable to the broader oncology patient population.

Examples of such **integrated studies include** the **Network of Enigmatic Exceptional Responders (NEER)** program (which detects exceptional responders with molecular profiling of their tumors to determine molecular and clinical correlates with exceptional responses) and the **Exceptional Responder Initiative (ERI)** (which was designed to investigate the feasibility of collecting and evaluating exceptional responders' medical records, and biospecimens to learn about their responses to anticancer therapies).

Likewise, in the **NCI-MATCH** trial, various tumors were sequenced and targeted treatment was given to participants, revealing the feasibility of detecting both frequent and rare actionable genetic mutations.

Hopefully, in the future, prospective studies of tumors and clinical data from **exceptional responders** can offer novel strategies (*e.g.*, genomically-targeted agents) to solve some "dilemmas" relevant to the most difficult cases in cancer care.

In the oncology practice, **exceptional responses** can occur with both standard and investigational treatments.

How this knowledge can be linked to the real-life scenarios of patients with the most aggressive cancers (*e.g.*, advanced or metastatic TNBC)?

• Most probably, **tumor molecular analyses** from patients, who revealed exceptional responses to systemic therapy may provide **valuable insights into cancer biology** and effective **treatment interventions**;

• **Combining molecular data of the aggressive tumors with clinical records from patients**, who received certain similar treatment regimens, might shed some light on the **molecular background of the exceptional responders**;

• This, in turn, can **refine potential personalized treatment options among the most vulnerable oncology patients**, in the future.

REFERENCES

[1]   Ford JM, Mitchell BS. One step further toward defining the exceptional cancer responder. J Natl Cancer Inst 2021; 113(1): 3-4.
[http://dx.doi.org/10.1093/jnci/djaa062] [PMID: 32339239]

[2]   Conley BA, Staudt L, Takebe N, *et al.* Exceptional responders initiative: A national cancer institute pilot study. J Natl Cancer Inst 2021; 113(1): 27-37.
[http://dx.doi.org/10.1093/jnci/djaa061] [PMID: 32339229]

[3]   Ford JM. Precision oncology: A new forum for an emerging field. JCO Precis Oncol 2017; 1(1): 1-2.
[http://dx.doi.org/10.1200/PO.16.00048] [PMID: 35172478]

[4]   Printz C. NCI launches exceptional responders initiative: Researchers will attempt to identify why some patients respond to treatment so much better than others. Cancer 2015; 121(6): 803-4.
[http://dx.doi.org/10.1002/cncr.29311] [PMID: 25739575]

[5]   Hamilton JG, Banerjee SC, Carlsson SV, *et al.* Clinician perspectives on communication and implementation challenges in precision oncology. Per Med 2021; 18(6): 559-72.
[http://dx.doi.org/10.2217/pme-2021-0048] [PMID: 34674550]

[6]   Tsimberidou AM, Said R, Staudt LM, Conley BA, Takebe N. Defining, identifying, and understanding *exceptional responders* in oncology using the tools of precision medicine. Cancer J 2019; 25(4): 296-9.
[http://dx.doi.org/10.1097/PPO.0000000000000392] [PMID: 31335394]

[7]   Tsimberidou AM, Fountzilas E, Nikanjam M, Kurzrock R. Review of precision cancer medicine: Evolution of the treatment paradigm. Cancer Treat Rev 2020; 86: 102019.
[http://dx.doi.org/10.1016/j.ctrv.2020.102019] [PMID: 32251926]

[8]   Flaherty KT, Gray R, Chen A, *et al.* The molecular analysis for therapy choice (NCI-MATCH) trial: Lessons for genomic trial design. J Natl Cancer Inst 2020; 112(10): 1021-9.
[http://dx.doi.org/10.1093/jnci/djz245] [PMID: 31922567]

[9]   Murciano-Goroff YR, Drilon A, Stadler ZK. The NCI-MATCH: A national, collaborative precision oncology trial for diverse tumor histologies. Cancer Cell 2021; 39(1): 22-4.
[http://dx.doi.org/10.1016/j.ccell.2020.12.021] [PMID: 33434511]

[10] Saner FAM, Herschtal A, Nelson BH, *et al.* Going to extremes: Determinants of extraordinary response and survival in patients with cancer. Nat Rev Cancer 2019; 19(6): 339-48.
[http://dx.doi.org/10.1038/s41568-019-0145-5] [PMID: 31076661]

[11] Wheeler DA, Takebe N, Hinoue T, *et al.* Molecular features of cancers exhibiting exceptional responses to treatment. Cancer Cell 2021; 39(1): 38-53.e7.
[http://dx.doi.org/10.1016/j.ccell.2020.10.015] [PMID: 33217343]

[12] Printz C. Exceptional responders may be key to new cancer treatments. Cancer 2021; 127(9): 1359.
[http://dx.doi.org/10.1002/cncr.33579] [PMID: 33900617]

[13] Pearce CL, Rossing MA, Lee AW, *et al.* Combined and interactive effects of environmental and GWAS-identified risk factors in ovarian cancer. Cancer Epidemiol Biomarkers Prev 2013; 22(5): 880-90.
[http://dx.doi.org/10.1158/1055-9965.EPI-12-1030-T] [PMID: 23462924]

[14] Harvard medical school department of biomedical informatics. Available at: https://people poweredmedicine.org/neer(2018) (Accessed on: 1 July 2022).

Radical Remissions: Unique Lessons from Patients with Cancer Who Were Able to Defy the Odds and Recover

Abstract: Many women with aggressive BC subtypes are devastated, due to metastatic spread, resistance to therapy, and poor prognosis. However, there is a growing body of scientific evidence that some patients have been able to defy the odds of advanced malignancy and recover, in spite of their fatal prognosis and dismal oncology statistics. Also, these **"better than expected" clinical effects** were not totally rare.

To explore this fascinating subject, future research is undoubtedly necessary. In line with this challenge, the innovative **"Radical Remission Project"** was created, which allows collecting cases of Radical Remissions for research studies. It also connects survivors with patients, who actually struggle with aggressive cancers. Since there is a **concern about giving false hope** to patients with advanced malignancies, they need to be professionally informed that the cases of Radical Remissions must be first explored in detailed research studies, before making any conclusions about their potential applicability to patients with similar prognoses. This is necessary to protect the most vulnerable patients, who must not be given any false expectations, and the practical **communication** skills of the cancer care teams are crucial to accomplish it.

In addition, **Complementary** and **Integrative Medicine (CIM)**, which manages the physical, mental, emotional, and spiritual needs of patients with cancer, **regardless of their prognosis**, appears to be helpful in an attempt to meet these needs. CIM is gradually becoming a part of each stage of the cancer journey, from active to supportive and palliative oncology care. Similarly, **integrative oncology** that uses **evidence-based**, lifestyle modifications, mind-body techniques, and specific natural products in combination with conventional anticancer treatments is in line with patients' safety.

This chapter briefly addresses some universal factors, which can make a genuine difference to help in recovery from cancer, based on the **Radical Remission Project** and **CIM**-related research. It focuses on the role of open and precise **communication** between patients and cancer care teams. The ongoing **Radical Remission Project** can inspire many women with breast cancer (BC) and their medical teams to consider introducing some safe and useful approaches to their standard oncology management.

Keywords: Complementary and integrative medicine (CIM), Communication, Decision-making, Integrative oncology, Radical remissions, Supportive care.

INTRODUCTION

It should sound optimistic for some women with aggressive BC subtypes, who are often overwhelmed, due to metastatic spread and poor prognosis) that there is a growing body of research evidence that some patients were able to defy the odds, and recover, in spite of their adverse prognosis and dismal oncology statistics [1]. These individuals have often been diagnosed with incurable malignancies, but their experiences have been atypical or uncommon, in a positive sense. Moreover, these **"better than expected" clinical outcomes** were not totally rare. In fact, there are numerous patients with cancer, who have extended their survival far beyond the upper limits of the median, or who recovered, after having received a terminal prognosis, based on the standard oncology approach [1, 2].

On the other hand, however, there is a real **concern about giving false hopes** to patients with advanced malignancies [2]. It should be underscored that such patients need to be clearly informed that the cases of **remissions** must be first explored in detail, according to strict research procedures, before making any conclusions about their potential applicability to patients with similar prognoses. Also, it should be emphasized that navigating through false hope (often promoted in the media) is very difficult, and the patients should be protected, and not be given false expectations. Therefore, any extraordinary remissions cases need to be discussed with caution and analyzed in the individual patient's context. Of course, studying long-term survivors should be a high priority, for both clinicians and researchers [2].

In line with these goals is **Complementary** and **Integrative Medicine** (**CIM**), which gradually becomes a part of each stage of the cancer journey, and in particular, supportive and palliative oncology care [3]. **CIM** manages the physical, psychological, emotional, and spiritual needs of patients with cancer, **regardless of their prognosis** [3]. Similarly, **integrative oncology** uses **evidence-based**, safe lifestyle modifications, mind-body practices, and specific natural products in conjunction with conventional anticancer treatments [4]. Effective **communication** about applying the most appropriate **CIM** or **integrative oncology** interventions requires multidisciplinary skills from the cancer care team members.

This chapter briefly addresses some universal factors, which can make an actual difference to help with recovery from cancer, based on the **Radical Remission Project** and **CIM**-related research. It also focuses on the remarkable role of **communication** between patients and providers. Recent reports of the ongoing **Radical Remission Project** can inspire many women with breast cancer (BC) and their medical teams to consider incorporating some safe and useful approaches to their standard oncology management.

"The Radical Remission Project"-Directions for Future Research and Navigation Through the Labyrinth of False Hope

"The Radical Remission Project" offers an innovative website (www.RadicalRemission.com) that allows collecting cases of Radical Remissions for research studies [5]. In addition, this project connects Radical Remission survivors with patients, who actually struggle with various types of aggressive cancers [5]. According to a detailed analysis of numerous cases, documented in this project, some common factors that can make a real difference to help achieve recovery from cancer were reported, involving universal psychosocial (mental or emotional) and nutritionally-related domains (Fig. **1**) [5].

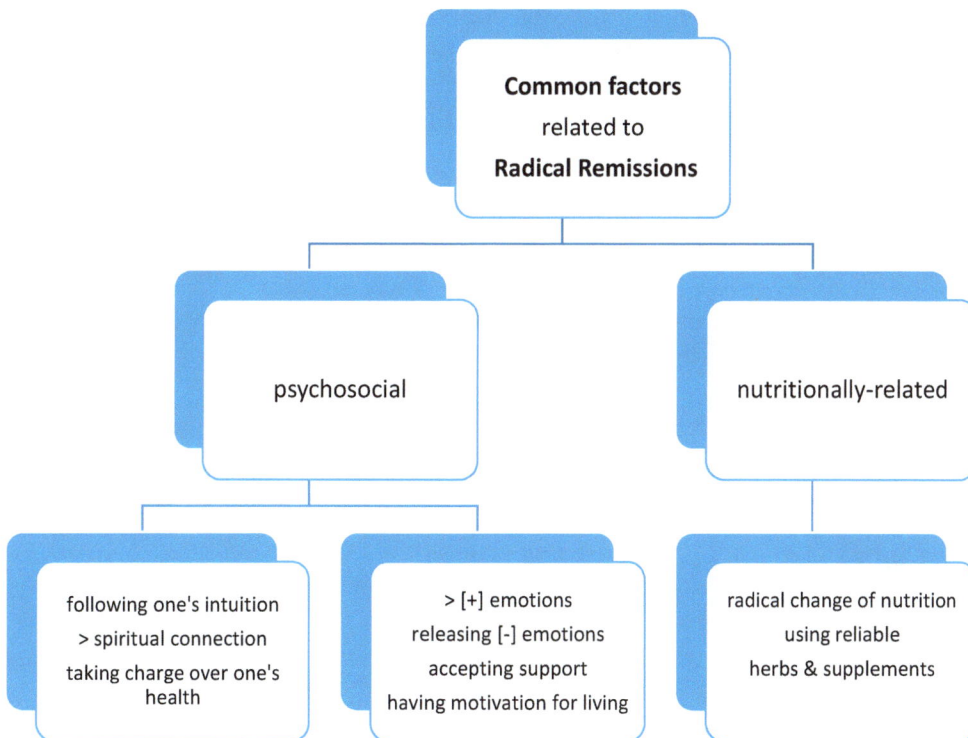

Fig. (1). Common Lifestyle-related Factors Reported in Radical Remission Cases.

Certainly, more research is required to prove that these factors definitely improve the chances of recovery from cancer, in different patient clinical contexts and various populations. For instance, future reports disclosing what exactly the radical remission survivors could do from a research standpoint might show how survivors overcame adverse diagnoses, using some safe interdisciplinary modalities beyond the conventional treatments of surgery, chemotherapy (CHT), radiotherapy (RT), and other "standard" anticancer treatments [3, 5]. With a growing interest in **psycho-oncology** and **evidence-based integrative therapies**, which have been **combined** with **conventional oncology** management, it would be desirable to design an easily accessible, helpful model to support the most vulnerable women with BC, who are interested in this type of noninvasive approach.

Starting from initial case studies, there was no precise database about the patient's management strategies that could have contributed to **extraordinary remissions.** In fact, these patients with unusually favorable recoveries were not formally studied to find out, what exactly they were doing to achieve remissions from cancers, which were known to lead to poor outcomes. Moreover, a majority of such remarkable cancer survivors reported that their physicians did not even ask them about any particular modalities they were using that could potentially contribute to their recoveries [1, 3, 5]. In an attempt to elucidate this subject, three main categories of patients with cancer, who experienced recovery, were suggested (Fig. **2**).

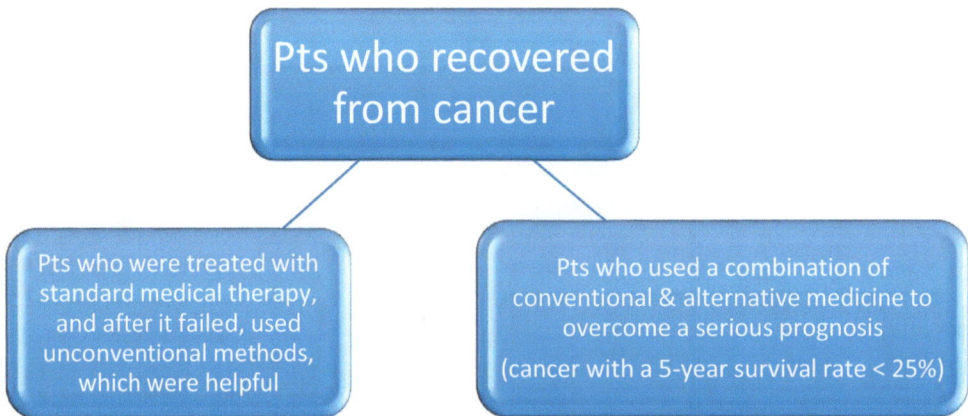

Fig. (2). The Main Categories of Patients with Cancer who Experienced Recovery. Pts, patients.

On the one hand, there is a concern about giving false hopes to patients with advanced malignancies. On the other hand, however, the most remarkable cases of

remissions should be explored, since they may offer a unique learning opportunity about the complex mechanisms of healing. Of course, it should not be ignored that navigating through the patients' expectations is difficult, and therefore, **Radical Remissions** cases need to be discussed with caution, and detailed studying of long-term survivors is a high priority [1, 3, 5].

INDIVIDUAL PATTERNS USED BY SOME PATIENTS WHO EXPERIENCED UNUSUAL RECOVERY FROM CANCER AND TYPICAL REASONS FOR REFUSING CONVENTIONAL ONCOLOGY TREATMENTS

The "**exceptional patients**" with cancer represent survivors, who were diagnosed with advanced stages of cancer (considered incurable by standard medical therapies), and who experienced unexplained survival [6]. Such a phenomenon merits a formal investigation. Interestingly, many of the "**exceptional patients**" often did not use any "magic" or controversial methods to achieve recovery or prolong survival. In contrast, they were often cultivating certain psychological qualities, as well as **internal or external human connections**, effective **patient-doctor communication** patterns, and engagement in the diagnosis and treatment of their malignancy (Fig. **3**) [6]. Moreover, it should be highlighted that many patients, who seek advice about complementary therapies, after they have declined certain conventional oncology treatment options, often have their **particular reasons** to do so [1, 3, 7].

Also, some of them have shared such decisions to refuse standard treatment (totally or partially), while others have not shared these controversial decisions with their treating team. Moreover, several of these patients had never returned to their previous physicians, and thus, they were lost to conventional oncology follow-up. In reality, many of them were just looking for a **second opinion**, meaning for an objective, competent, and emphatic physician, who will listen to them, and with whom they could possibly discuss their difficult, personal decisions [1, 7].

At this point, it is important to realize that some of the typical **reasons for refusing conventional oncology treatment** include concerns about possible adverse effects or complications of standard anticancer treatments (*e.g.*, chemotherapy or radiotherapy), lack of confidence in such treatment effects, hopelessness, helplessness, fear of possible loss of control over life, a decrease of independence or QoL, denial of serious consequences of untreated malignancy, opinions about the futility of anticancer treatments, previous negative experiences (*e.g.*, personal or related to family members or friends), mental disorders, malfunctioning of the health care system, financial limitations, logistic causes (*e.g.*, family or work obligations, long distance to oncology centers), unclear communication with medical team members, and dysfunctional patient-doctor relationship [1, 7, 8].

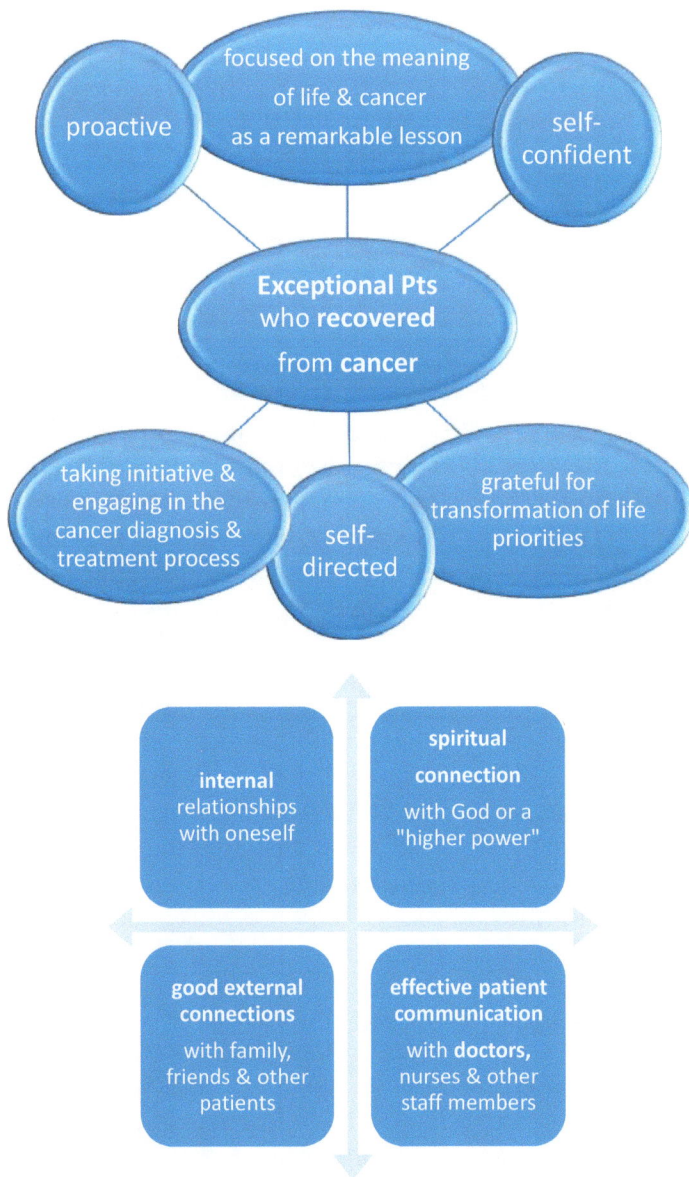

Fig. (3). Distinctive Psychological Characteristics and Examples of Internal and External Connections of Patients Who Recovered from Cancer.

BASIC EXPECTATIONS OF "EXCEPTIONAL" PATIENTS WITH CANCER AND "REVERSIBLE" OBSTACLES FROM THEIR HEALTHCARE PROFESSIONALS

On the one hand, the main decisions that some **"exceptional"** patients often make, reflect predominantly their personal beliefs and values, while the strictly medical recommendations often occupy more distant places on the roadmap of their choices. On the other hand, however, many such patients still have some reasonable **expectations from their healthcare professionals. For instance, they** wish to **keep their relationships with the medical teams**, mainly to have the **reassurance that the healthcare system would not abandon them and** they would not suffer from pain. In addition, they desire to be treated with dignity and have some control over the terminal stages of their life. Whenever necessary, palliative care or hospice services would be provided to them. In the meantime, they would like to enjoy living in the present moment, continue engaging in their regular work, hobbies, or family duties, and participate in meetings with relatives and friends for as long as reasonably possible [1, 8]. In reality, it is challenging for many clinicians to take care of highly independent patients, since they may differ from the typical cases. Due to various reasons, doctors' reactions may not be fully supportive, especially if the patients' choices are unconventional. Of course, physicians understand that patients can make decisions about their own treatment, but when the treatment effects are difficult to predict, many physicians may divide their patients into a category, in which a cure possible, or one, in which it is not possible [1, 8].

Moreover, patients who decline conventional treatment are often called **"noncompliant"** or **"difficult,"** which is stigmatizing. Also, many medical professionals might feel uncomfortable during a confrontation with patients, who chose to go against medical recommendations and are resistant to persuasion. Unfortunately, these circumstances can cause damage to therapeutic relationships and quality of care [1, 8]. It seems that some women, who eventually refused conventional treatments, could have been more prone to accept conventional treatment earlier if they had a better initial experience with their clinicians. For instance, trusted physicians, who were able to deeply understand their concerns, convey hope, educate them about various treatment possibilities, and permit them to take enough time to adjust to their diagnosis, could have influenced their selection of the treatment trajectory. Also, an opportunity to calmly "digest" complex information, prior to choosing any given, standard treatment provides patient comfort and increases therapeutic compliance [1, 7, 8].

THE PILLARS OF EFFECTIVE COMMUNICATION BETWEEN ONCOLOGY PATIENTS AND THEIR PHYSICIANS

In the most optimal scenario, each episode of **communication** between the patient with cancer and the physician or other members of the treatment team should combine the right proportions of **medical advice** and the **patient's personal view** [9, 10]. This is in line with the "**patient-centered care**" model, in which it is necessary to acknowledge the specific role that the **patient's perspective and personal values are essential in the shared decision-making** process. Moreover, effective communication is required to integrate the patients' goals, needs, and values with current medical science, to achieve a well-balanced, patient-friendly, and flexible **treatment plan** [9, 10]. For instance, in the decision-making process, some patients, who initially decline treatment, could later decide to select conventional anticancer treatment options, after receiving clear recommendations, support, and a suitable period of time to analyze the pros and cons of the possible choices. Moreover, clear and honest communication is critical in establishing trust with patients, obtaining information, answering patient questions, recognizing emotions, and guiding or supporting patients in various management-related decisions [9]. In addition, the quality of communication in oncology care may influence both patient and doctor satisfaction, as well as reinforce patient adherence to therapy [10]. Unfortunately, not discussing these therapies during medical visits has often been related to a concern of the physician's disapproval [11]. However, when patients have an impression that their providers are willing to listen to them, are open-minded, interested, and respectful of their opinions, the patients are usually willing to share their experiences with the use of complementary or integrative methods [9, 11].

A **skill set** to **overcome any real and artificial obstacles in communication** between patients with BC and their medical care teams is of great importance. A key component is to learn effective communication techniques to discuss practical aspects of the use of various therapies, and to understand the patient's motivation to engage in these therapies, which may include reducing side effects caused by standard medical treatment, the need for increased emotional support, and improved QoL [9, 11]. In addition, a **successful communication** process requires a calm, open-minded, approach, based on attentive listening, conveying empathy and compassion, and reinforcing hope. In this way, the patients can feel that their choices are respected, even if they make decisions, which are sometimes opposite to the standard medical advice [9].

COMPLEMENTARY AND INTEGRATIVE MEDICINE (CIM) AND INTEGRATIVE ONCOLOGY: BENEFICIAL "LINKS" IN THE CARE OF PATIENTS WITH CANCER

Complementary and integrative medicine (CIM) has recently been recognized as a beneficial domain to support the care of patients with cancer, *via* **managing their somatic, mental, emotional, and spiritual needs, regardless of their prognosis** [10]. In fact, **CIM** plays an important role in relief from physical and emotional suffering and distress. Moreover, the wide spectrum of application of CIM early in the cancer journey, during active therapy, and then, during survivorship or end-of-life periods, reflects many **unmet needs** of such patients, which have not been addressed by conventional medical care [10]. At present, **CIM** plays a more prominent role in oncology care than in the past. Numerous patients afflicted with invasive malignancies, as well as their relatives, caregivers, or friends, are actively searching for professional guidance and straightforward communication with their doctors and other medical team members about the pluses and minuses of possible application of CIM in the management of their cancers, often associated with comorbidities [10, 11]. Similarly, **integrative oncology** reflects a remarkable "chain" connecting conventional oncology with complementary approaches. Many patients with cancer use complementary and alternative therapies during and after conventional cancer treatment. However, these patients are usually reluctant to **discuss such therapies with their oncologists**, who typically don't have time, knowledge, and confidence on how to advise patients on this subject (Fig. **4**) [12]. **Integrative oncology** is a patient-oriented, evidence-based medical field that **uses lifestyle modifications, mind–body practices, and reliable natural products, in coordination with conventional anticancer treatments**. It focuses on safety, scientific evidence, and effective communication to provide appropriate interventions together with standard medical care [12].

THE INTEGRATIVE ONCOLOGY SCHOLARS (IOS) PROGRAM – BRIDGING THE GAP IN THE COMPREHENSIVE CANCER CARE

The **Integrative Oncology Scholars (IOS)** program offers a possibility to augment oncologists' competency in this developing area. It is imperative that oncologists have an access to Integrative Oncology education and training so that they would be able to recommend evidence-based integrative oncology interventions alongside standard anticancer treatments to their patients [13]. The **IOS** course provides to multi-disciplinary teams of oncology providers (*e.g.*, oncologists, nurses, psychologists, therapists, social workers, and pharmacists) in-person sessions and eLearning activities relevant to psychosomatic cancer-associated symptoms, in which integrative oncology interventions can play a significant role, research evidence for different integrative oncology modalities, and communication skills to discuss with confidence various integrative therapies with patients, medical, and complementary healthcare providers [13]. It should be emphasized that **lifestyle modifications** have been shown to have several benefits for patients with cancer [13]. According to recommendations of the **American Cancer Society (ACS),** evidence-based **dietary guidelines** for cancer promote maintaining healthy body weight, consuming fruits, vegetables, whole grains, and legumes, as well as restricting the intake of red and processed meats, sugar, and alcohol [14]. Also, the **National Cancer Institute (NCI)** has provided nutritional guidance to patients, who receive an active oncology treatment, which should be individualized to any given clinical context [15]. In addition, regular **physical activity** during anticancer treatment has been shown to have several psychosomatic benefits (*e.g.*, improved QoL, alleviated symptoms of depression and anxiety, decreased cancer-related fatigue, lymphedema, and chemotherapy-induced peripheral neuropathy, as well as reduced cancer-specific mortality, especially in women with BC) [16]. Optimally, patients should have a pre-exercise assessment and should exercise in a supervised environment. **Mind-body therapies** combine a group of techniques, which influence the mind's interactions with somatic functions, and can elicit a relaxation response [17]. Such therapies illustrate how somatic health conditions and psychological wellness are interconnected [17]. There are several different forms of meditation that have been investigated in patients with cancer, and the best research evidence was gathered with regard to **mindfulness-based stress reduction (MSBR)** and **mindfulness-based cognitive therapy (MBCT),** known as **mindfulness-based interventions (MBI)** [18]. In essence, **mindfulness** means paying attention to the activity of the mind in the present moment. **Mindfulness** helps decrease emotional and physical distress or pain, as well as anxiety, depression, and fear of cancer recurrence [19]. **Yoga**, as a mind–body therapy, combines physical poses with breathing and meditation [20]. Yoga improved the QoL and psychological outcomes [20]. Such therapy should be done under the care of a yoga instructor, who is qualified to work with cancer patients. **Natural products** typically consist of vitamins, minerals, herbs or botanicals, or amino acids [21]. They should be considered strictly in line with the **American Society of Clinical Oncology (ASCO)** and **Society of Integrative Oncology (SIO) guidelines** (Fig. 4) [22]. It should be underscored that the major concerns over using natural or dietary supplements, especially during a course of conventional anticancer therapy include possible interactions with standard oncology treatments (*e.g.*, herb–drug or supplement-drug interactions) [23]. Moreover, in patients undergoing surgery, such products can interfere with blood clotting, anesthetic agents, or other medications [23]. To assure maximal patient safety, oncologists need to precisely communicate with pharmacists.

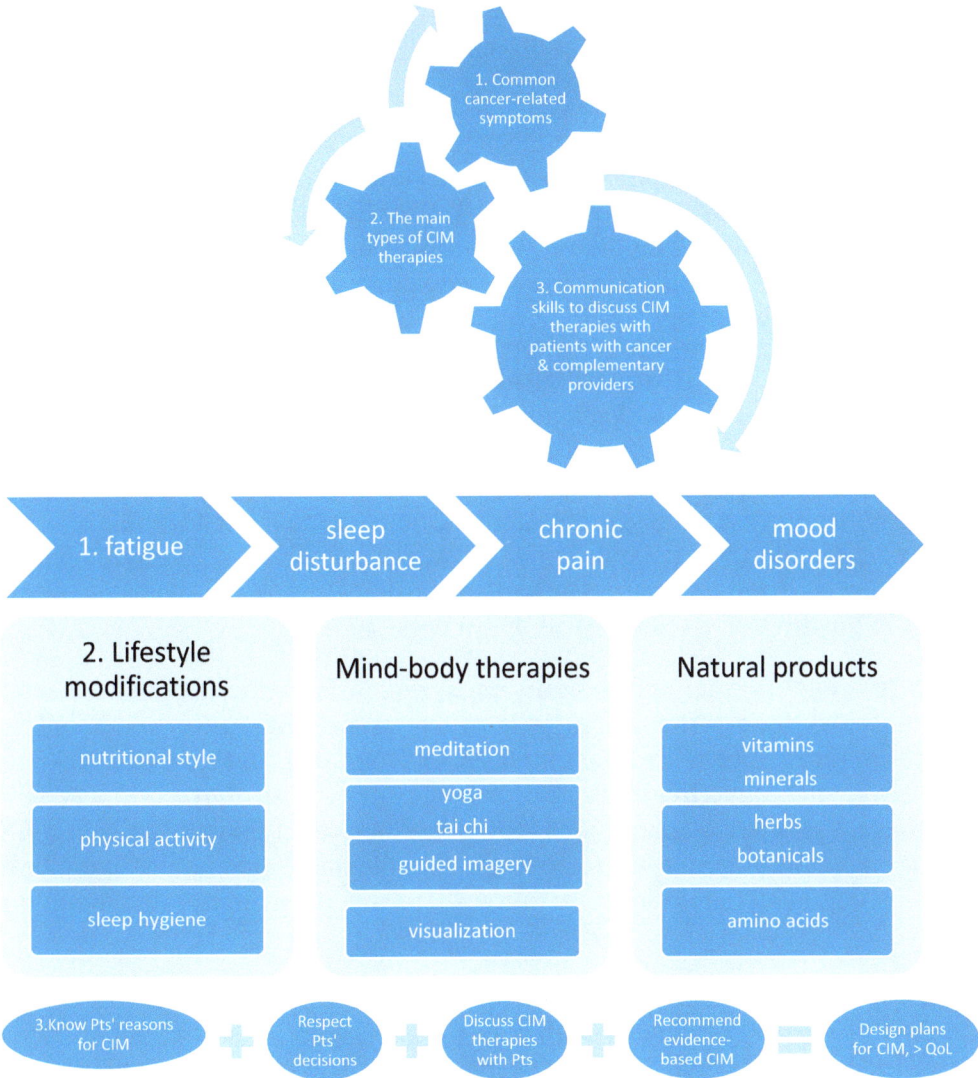

Fig. (4). The Main Topics and Useful Skills Relevant to the Complementary and Integrative Medicine (CIM) Therapies for the Oncology Treatment Teams; QoL, quality of life; Pts, patients.

CONCLUSION

Some patients diagnosed with advanced malignancies, who received a fatal prognosis from their oncologists, were able to defy the odds, and recover. Many of them had used certain therapeutic strategies to prolong their survival, after the failure of established, recommended medical therapies.

Since these "**better than expected**" patient **outcomes** were surprising, but not completely rare, they stimulated a new wave of research, including a recently created **Radical Remission Project**.

This project combines patients with cancer, survivors, their family members, friends, and healthcare professionals (*e.g.*, in form of the online community), and its main objectives are to describe and scientifically verify several radical remission cases. In addition, the project aims to link together the survivors with the current cancer patients to motivate, encourage, and provide hope during the challenging disease journey.

Complementary and **Integrative Medicine** (**CIM**) manages the physical, psychological, emotional, and spiritual needs of patients with cancer, **regardless of their prognosis. CIM** plays an important role in supportive care, during each stage of the cancer trajectory. As more patients with cancer apply **CIM** therapies, oncologists should ask their patients about their exact reasons for the use of such therapies. Also, the cancer treatment team members should be "armed" with the necessary knowledge and **communication** skills, which would help them guide patients in the difficult **decision-making process**.

Integrative oncology is an emerging area, which combines safe and effective complementary therapies together with conventional anticancer treatments in a **patient-centered** model. It is imperative to recommend safe, **evidence-based integrative oncology therapies** and separate them from those options, which don't have sufficient research evidence. In fact, many evidence-based CIM therapies have the potential to improve QoL or alleviate some unpleasant, chronic cancer-related symptoms, not to mention that such approaches are usually cost-effective.

The open, clear, and honest **communication** between patients with cancers (*e.g.*, aggressive subtypes, associated with poor prognosis) and their treatment teams is necessary to confront each stage of the malignancy and to **design a realistic plan** for future therapy. Moreover, quality communication is considered an important skill in oncology care, as one of the factors that affect patient satisfaction, decision-making process, well-being, and adherence to medical advice. Physicians should be confident in discussing **CIM therapies** with patients and recommending evidence-based modalities for their cancer-related symptoms. It has been suggested that oncology healthcare providers expand their knowledge in the field of integrative oncology *via* existing programs or available continuing medical education.

Many **patients who recovered from cancer had something in common**. They decided to:

• Personally take control of their health,

• Follow their intuition,

• Totally change ways of eating,

• Including the use of reliable herbs and supplements;

• In addition, they released suppressed negative emotions,

• Increased positive emotions,

• Embraced support from family, friends, and the medical care team,

• Deepened their spiritual connections,

• Cultivated strong motivations for living;

• They were strongly engaged in the process of diagnosis and treatment,

• Followed recommendations of their doctors (who were willing to listen to them),

• Paid attention to their own intuition.

Cancer has elicited in many patients:

• A sense of courage,

• Change in the philosophy of life,

• Necessary distance to problems,

• Altruistic approach to others.

Also, various safe and effective **Complementary** and **Integrative Medicine (CIM)** or **integrative oncology** interventions (*e.g.*, meditation) allowed many patients to:

• Find internal peace,

• Balance difficult emotional,

• Reduce unpleasant symptoms,

• Accept the extremely difficult cancer-related situation.

Effective communication and addressing the patients' unmet needs are essential for building mutual trust between the patients, their caregivers, or families and the oncology care team members. Even if some patients have initially declined standard oncology care, they can still continue their visits with primary care physicians, and in this way, they are included in the health care system and can count on supportive care services, whenever necessary.

REFERENCES

[1]　Frenkel M. Refusing treatment. Oncologist 2013; 18(5): 634-6.
[http://dx.doi.org/10.1634/theoncologist.2012-0436] [PMID: 23704223]

[2]　Kimball BC, Geller G, Warsame R, *et al.* Looking back, looking forward: The ethical framing of complementary and alternative medicine in oncology over the last 20 years. Oncologist 2018; 23(6): 639-41.
[http://dx.doi.org/10.1634/theoncologist.2017-0518] [PMID: 29523647]

[3]　Frenkel M, Sierpina V, Sapire K. Effects of complementary and integrative medicine on cancer survivorship. Curr Oncol Rep 2015; 17(5): 21.
[http://dx.doi.org/10.1007/s11912-015-0445-1] [PMID: 25749658]

[4]　Deng G, Cassileth B. Integrative oncology: An overview. Am Soc Clin Oncol Educ Book 2014; (34): 233-42.
[http://dx.doi.org/10.14694/EdBook_AM.2014.34.233] [PMID: 24857081]

[5]　The radical remission project. Available at: https://www.RadicalRemission.com(Accessed on: 1 July 2022).

[6]　Frenkel M, Ari SL, Engebretson J, *et al.* Activism among exceptional patients with cancer. Support Care Cancer 2011; 19(8): 1125-32.
[http://dx.doi.org/10.1007/s00520-010-0918-6] [PMID: 20512358]

[7]　King N, Balneaves L, Card C, Nation J, Nguyen T, Carlson L. Surveys of cancer patients and cancer care providers regarding complementary therapy use, communication and information needs. J Altern Complement Med 2014; 20(5): A98-8.
[http://dx.doi.org/10.1089/acm.2014.5259.abstract]

[8]　Frenkel M, Engebretson JC, Gross S, *et al.* Exceptional patients and communication in cancer care—are we missing another survival factor? Support Care Cancer 2016; 24(10): 4249-55.
[http://dx.doi.org/10.1007/s00520-016-3255-6] [PMID: 27169701]

[9]　Frenkel M, Cohen L. Effective communication about the use of complementary and integrative medicine in cancer care. J Altern Complement Med 2014; 20(1): 12-8.
[http://dx.doi.org/10.1089/acm.2012.0533] [PMID: 23863085]

[10]　Frenkel M, Sapire K, Lacey J, Sierpina VS. Integrative medicine: Adjunctive element or essential ingredient in palliative and supportive cancer care? J Altern Complement Med 2020; 26(9): 781-5.
[http://dx.doi.org/10.1089/acm.2019.0316] [PMID: 32924563]

[11]　Davis EL, Oh B, Butow PN, Mullan BA, Clarke S. Cancer patient disclosure and patient-doctor communication of complementary and alternative medicine use: A systematic review. Oncologist 2012; 17(11): 1475-81.
[http://dx.doi.org/10.1634/theoncologist.2012-0223] [PMID: 22933591]

[12]　Karim S, Benn R, Carlson LE, *et al.* Integrative oncology education: An emerging competency for oncology providers. Curr Oncol 2021; 28(1): 853-62.
[http://dx.doi.org/10.3390/curroncol28010084] [PMID: 33578660]

[13]　Zick SM, Czuhajewski C, Fouladbakhsh JM, *et al.* Integrative oncology scholars program: A model for integrative oncology education. J Altern Complement Med 2018; 24(9-10): 1018-22.

[http://dx.doi.org/10.1089/acm.2018.0184] [PMID: 30247974]

[14] American cancer society guideline for diet and physical activity for cancer prevention. Available at: https://acsjournals.onlinelibrary.wiley.com/doi/abs/10.3322/caac.21591 (accessed on: 1 July 2022).

[15] National cancer institute, eating hints: Before, during and after cancer treatment. Available at: https://www.cancer.gov/publications/patient-education/eating-hints (accessed on: 1 July 2022).

[16] Cormie P, Zopf EM, Zhang X, Schmitz KH. The impact of exercise on cancer mortality, recurrence and treatment-related adverse effects. Epidemiol Rev 2017; 39(1): 71-92.
[http://dx.doi.org/10.1093/epirev/mxx007] [PMID: 28453622]

[17] Memorial sloan kettering cancer centre about mind body therapies. Available at: https://www.mskcc.org/cancer-care/diagnosis-treatment/symptom-management/integrative-medicine/mind-body (accessed on: 1 July 2022).

[18] Haller H, Winkler MM, Klose P, Dobos G, Kümmel S, Cramer H. Mindfulness-based interventions for women with breast cancer: An updated systematic review and meta-analysis. Acta Oncol 2017; 56(12): 1665-76.
[http://dx.doi.org/10.1080/0284186X.2017.1342862] [PMID: 28686520]

[19] Cillessen L, Johannsen M, Speckens AEM, Zachariae R. Mindfulness-based interventions for psychological and physical health outcomes in cancer patients and survivors: A systematic review and meta-analysis of randomized controlled trials. Psychooncology 2019; 28(12): 2257-69.
[http://dx.doi.org/10.1002/pon.5214] [PMID: 31464026]

[20] Danhauer SC, Addington EL, Cohen L, *et al.* Yoga for symptom management in oncology: A review of the evidence base and future directions for research. Cancer 2019; 125(12): 1979-89.
[http://dx.doi.org/10.1002/cncr.31979] [PMID: 30933317]

[21] National institutes of health dietary supplements. Available at: https://ods.od.nih.gov/ (accessed on: 1 July 2022).

[22] Lyman GH, Greenlee H, Bohlke K, *et al.* Integrative therapies during and after breast cancer treatment: ASCO endorsement of the SIO clinical practice guideline. J Clin Oncol 2018; 36(25): 2647-55.
[http://dx.doi.org/10.1200/JCO.2018.79.2721] [PMID: 29889605]

[23] Oga EF, Sekine S, Shitara Y, Horie T. Pharmacokinetic herb-drug interactions: Insight into mechanisms and consequences. Eur J Drug Metab Pharmacokinet 2016; 41(2): 93-108.
[http://dx.doi.org/10.1007/s13318-015-0296-z] [PMID: 26311243]

CHAPTER 14

How Can We Redefine Hope and Gratitude to Help Patients with Breast Cancer Build Their "New Life"?

Abstract: There is a need to practically **redefine the future way of life**, among numerous patients with breast cancer (BC). In fact, **spirituality, hope,** and **gratitude** may play a remarkable role in a possible transformation into a **"new life"**. Also, these invisible, positive "forces" recognize patients as individual human beings, which should be connected with their families, caregivers, friends, and medical professionals, as functional "units".

This chapter provides some suggestions for practical approaches to help **design a functional "new life"**, especially for women with aggressive BC (*e.g.*, triple-negative breast cancer (TNBC)). In addition, medical care teams may consider incorporating such supportive modalities into the main therapeutic oncology plan.

Keywords: Breast cancer, Gratitude, Hope, Medical professionals, Patients with cancer, Spirituality.

INTRODUCTION

Many women with **newly diagnosed breast cancer (BC)** or those, who already encountered a disease **crisis** (*e.g.*, due to advanced, recurrent, or **metastatic BC**) often wonder what their life is going to be like during and after anticancer therapies. At that time, they frequently re-evaluate some past experiences and worry about what the future will bring. Some patients are searching for stability or so-called "normal" life. However, they typically experience serious emotional "turbulences" associated with symptoms of **distress, anxiety,** and **depression** relevant to BC.

During the cancer journey, when a **"new reality"** sets in, what was once crucial in life can momentarily change. Some women struggle harder to hang onto who they were, while others are able to simply allow "letting go" and give a chance to the **"new normal"** scenario. This approach often permits them to **discover new meaning in life** that subsequently enables them to move forward, despite experi-

Katarzyna Rygiel

encing many disturbing symptoms or negative emotions. At this point, **mindfulness-based stress reduction (MBSR)**, which offers **mindfulness meditation** to decrease symptoms of **distress, anxiety,** and **depression**, can be extremely helpful in different populations of patients with BC [1]. For instance, according to recent study findings, the psychological symptom reduction reported after the MBSR intervention was clinically significant and meaningful for many patients [1]. In addition, such results have indicated that the reliable improvements on each measurement scale (*e.g.*, worry, depression, anxiety, and distress) can be conveniently assessed and precisely monitored for each involved patient [1].

Many patients with BC grieve the **loss of** the specific "**roles**", they played in life. One of the crucial elements is to help them realize that although BC may occupy a "central" place in their present situation, with time, this can eventually become only a "peripheral" part of their life. This particular view has a remarkable potential to "**open the door**" to new possibilities in the future. At this point, cancer care teams and their patients with BC might be encouraged to know that MBSR alleviates different psychosomatic symptoms, often contributing to meaningful, long-term changes in patients' ways of thinking, feeling, and approaching numerous obstacles related to BC or its therapies [1]. Moreover, women with BC could be reminded of the significance of **hope** and **gratitude** in a daily life struggle to reclaim internal balance and strength to go forward [2].

This chapter outlines some suggestions (according to recent studies) for useful approaches to help **design a functional "new life"**, especially for women with aggressive BC (*e.g.*, triple-negative breast cancer (TNBC)). In addition, medical professionals may consider to incorporate such supportive modalities into the main therapeutic oncology plan.

PRECIOUS "SECRETS" OF LONG-TERM SURVIVORS OF BREAST CANCER

Positive emotions can serve as building blocks for **resilience**, especially at stressful times, like those, experienced by women with BC. Moreover, some positive emotions, such as **gratitude**, may play an adaptive role under such adverse circumstances. Based on a study that examined a group of women with metastatic BC, it has been revealed that grateful responding to received benefits predicted an increased perception of social support (especially in patients sensitive to positive emotions) [2].

Moreover, according to a qualitative study, long-term survivors of BC were "going through" distinct stages of the survival process, such as analyzing the BC diagnosis and its consequences, confronting a possible death, reprioritizing values in life, moving forward, and flashing back (similar to posttraumatic stress disorder (PTSD)).

It should be underscored that several study participants reported that they emerged from their BC experiences with more **gratitude for the gift of life**, a clear sense of self, confidence, and internal power to overcome future health crises. These findings suggest that cancer care team members could incorporate the individual context of a given patient's life to augment the beneficial effects of integrative oncology management [3].

A "FRESH LOOK" AT HOPE, GRATITUDE, AND SPIRITUALITY CONCEPTS IN THE CONTEXT OF PATIENTS WITH BREAST CANCER

Hope and **gratitude** represent an important step in **redefining the future way of life** for numerous women with BC (Fig. **1**) [2, 3]. It should be underscored that cancer care teams are in a unique position to teach their patients with BC to practically apply **hope** and **gratitude** during the most **challenging moments of the cancer care journey**, in agreement with the patient's personal beliefs, family, or social values, and cultural traditions. In fact, despite many sociocultural differences, patients have usually displayed **similar coping mechanisms** [2, 3]. However, their **points of view on cancer-related situations** can be different. Nevertheless, some **universal tools** can be used to aid in surviving many critical situations, and then, practical lessons about **hope** and **gratitude** can **help** them **reclaim a new, functional way of life** [2, 3].

It has been commonly known that patients with BC can use different **coping strategies** for **stress, trauma,** and **adversity.** Unfortunately, some of them are destructive (*e.g.*, alcohol, nicotine, or substance abuse), since they mostly create a temporary illusion, and in reality, augment existing problems or create a harmful "escape" from them. Similarly, denial can go a long way to providing respite from trauma, but cannot resolve difficult, chronic, BC-related problems.

However, some other strategies are productive (*e.g.*, moderate physical exercise, social engagement, or mindfulness meditation), since they are focused on confronting the unavoidable challenges and building resilience to survive cancer itself and its therapies [1 - 3]. In addition, the constructive techniques focused on being hopeful and grateful may also serve as effective **tools for letting go of negative emotions** (*e.g.*, anger, fear, guilt, anxiety, and sadness). Patients who lose their coping skills can often regress into depression, anxiety, and hopelessness. They can lose interest in what was pleasing them in the past, and find out that cancer has "stolen" their joy of life. Moreover, they can lose their sense of identity, which often raises concerns among family members or friends, who, in turn, become frightened of changes, which they see in their suffering relatives. To break this vicious circle, a **new meaning in life** is needed.

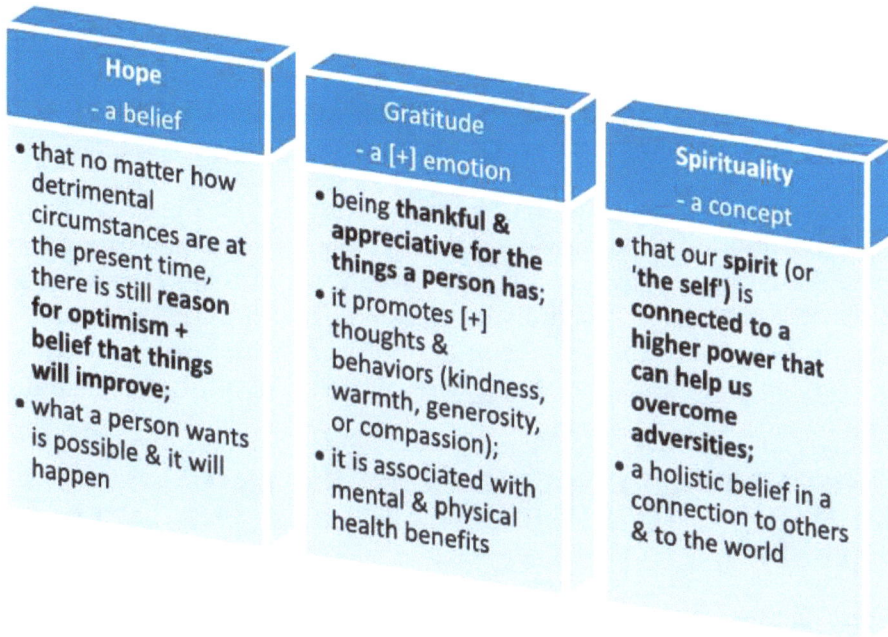

Fig. (1). Practical definitions of Hope, Gratitude, and Spirituality in the context of women with breast cancer.

Gratitude in the Brain: Cerebral Representation of the Gratitude Model

Gratitude is a well-known component of personal well-being and social or family relationships [2]. However, neurocognitive processes that link together certain elements of gratitude still remain unknown.

A recent study, which combined the **functional magnetic resonance imaging (fMRI)** technique and an interactive task to explore how the crucial components of gratitude are encoded in the brain was able to shed some light on presenting a neural model of gratitude [4]. Dynamic modeling of gratitude showed that the neural signals were transmitted to **perigenual anterior cingulate cortex (pgACC)**, suggesting an integrative role of **pgACC** in creating gratitude [4].

Importantly, based on the results of this study, it has been shown that the signals that were passed to **pgACC**, were also related to the degree of gratitude. Revealing such a neural mechanistic background of gratitude may allow integration of the gratitude approach, (as a possible supportive modality) into the comprehensive care for patients with BC [4].

HOW TO DISCOVER A NEW MEANING IN LIFE? – SIMPLE "TAKEAWAYS" FOR PATIENTS WITH BREAST CANCER

Patients with BC as well as their families, caregivers, and friends need supportive guidance, focused on redefining who they are at this critical point, and how to discover new meaning in life ahead. This learning process includes some **transition steps** that can help those, who are most vulnerable to psychophysical trauma caused by BC to move on with life.

In particular, exploring what they are **thankful for** can provide them with necessary respite from the struggle against BC. Moreover, it may contribute to a more positive attitude in different areas, relevant to survival. **Humor** is also an underestimated tool since it can challenge a negative mindset and make others more comfortable with an overwhelming situation, commonly associated with BC. **Prayer**, either religious or universal, can lead to spiritual awakening and consolation [2, 5].

PSYCHOSOMATIC AND SOCIAL EXPERIENCES OF YOUNGER AND OLDER WOMEN WITH BREAST CANCER: A UNIQUE LEARNING OPPORTUNITY

A life-threatening illness, such as breast cancer, especially the TNBC subtype, forces many women to confront a variety of medical, mental, emotional, social, and personal demands. In particular, the experiences related to diagnostic work-up and treatment regimens often result in serious distress. It is widely known that a diagnosis of invasive BC invokes uncertainty that generates many negative emotions, including fear, anger, anxiety, and sadness. TNBC frequently deteriorates a woman's body image, self-esteem, identity, integrity, personal or professional roles, positions, and family or social relationships.

However, despite these commonly experienced challenges, many women still strive to adjust to unpredictable and demanding BC-related circumstances. At this point, family, support groups, cancer care teams, and referrals to specialized services networks are extremely helpful [5]. It should be underscored that knowing the distressing experiences that are present in this population is crucial, since, if left unattended, they can have detrimental physical or psychosocial effects, which influence the quality of life (QoL) of the afflicted women [5].

COMMON DIFFERENCES IN THE PSYCHOSOCIAL PERCEPTIONS OF BREAST CANCER DIAGNOSIS AND THERAPY BETWEEN YOUNGER AND OLDER WOMEN

Usually, **younger women with BC** (*e.g.*, **TNBC**) are at an elevated risk of anxiety and depression in comparison to older women. Moreover, younger women are usually more concerned about their children, work, finances, home, and plans for the future than older women (Fig. **2**). In contrast, older women with BC often suffer from numerous health problems (due to comorbidities), financial difficulties, and isolation from social networks compared to their younger counterparts.

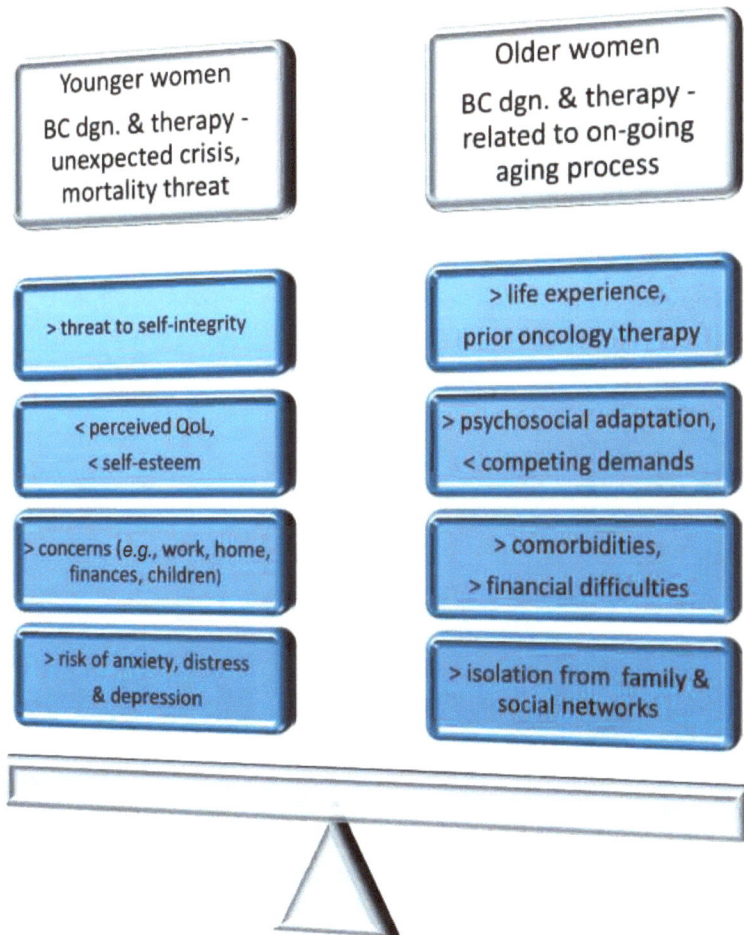

Fig. (2). Common differences in the psychosocial experiences of BC diagnosis and therapy between younger and older women; BC, breast cancer; QoL, quality of life.

Also, psychosocial adaptation can be better in **older women with BC**, since they usually have some past experiences with the medical care teams, (*e.g.*, going through the cancer journey) and are dealing with a relatively small number of competing demands on a daily basis (Fig. **2**) [5]. These factors can contribute to more effective coping and adaption to BC in older women, compared to their younger counterparts [5].

The major concerns for many women for their adjustment to BC, especially at the early stages of the cancer care journey, have been related to personal identity. This is due to the fact that **BC threatens women's self-integrity** and **self-image**. Therefore, in addition to recommended oncology therapies, the **rebuilding of a "new life"** after the BC diagnosis requires generating **new "meaning-making"** based on personal values (Fig. **3**) [5].

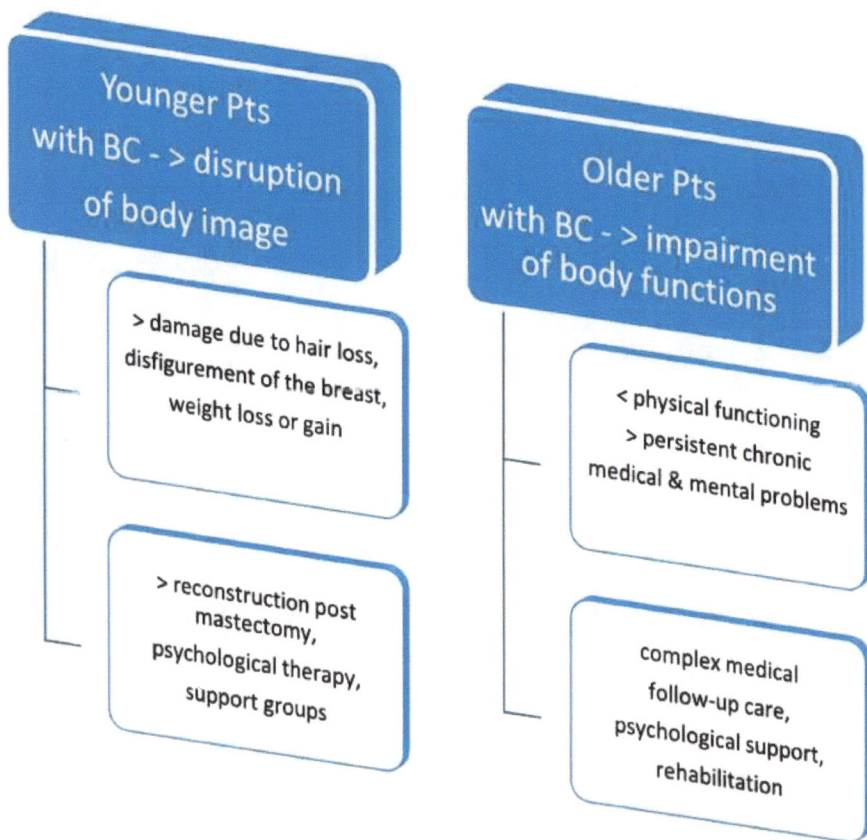

Fig. (3). A comparison between younger and older women in their perceptions and approaches to physical changes due to BC; BC, breast cancer; Pts, patients impairment of body functions.

IMPACT OF THE DIAGNOSIS AND TREATMENT OF BREAST CANCER ON PERSONAL RELATIONSHIPS WITH THE SPOUSE, CHILDREN, AND OLDER PARENTS

It has been known that the patient's diagnosis and treatment of BC can seriously affect their relations with a close circle of people, including spousal relationships, and relationships with children and older parents. The best "case scenario" for **spouses** and **partners** of women with BC would be to flexibly assist with household responsibilities, especially around times of planned therapy (Fig. **4**) [5]. **Children** of women with BC are often negatively impacted by the reduced interactions with their mothers, particularly around surgery, radiotherapy, or chemotherapy regimen. At this point, well-organized child care and interventions, which elevate the mother's mood and augment her motivation to return to her regular duties should improve the family dynamics. **Family relationships** are crucial for both younger and older women with BC because such relationships provide emotional, psychological, and physical support that translates to better health conditions [5].

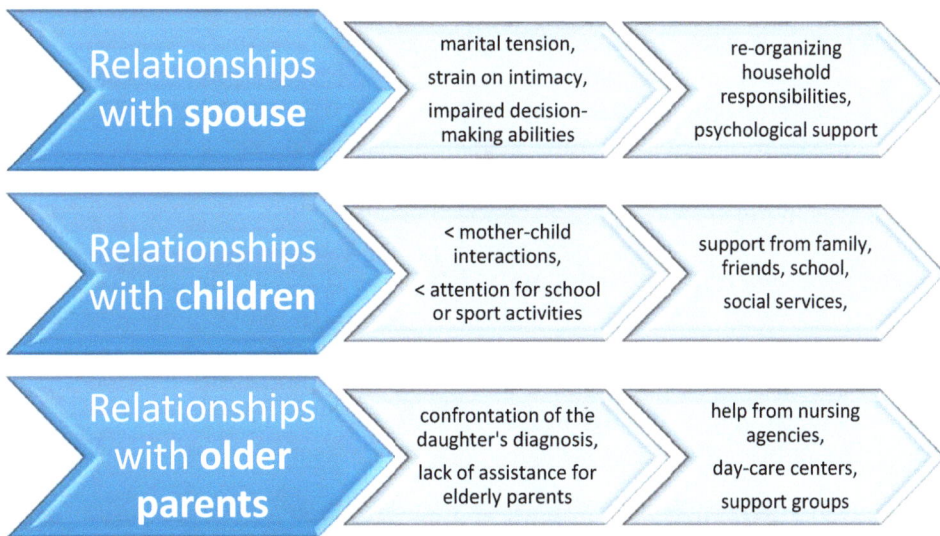

Fig. (4). Commonly encountered problems and suggested solutions in relationships of women with breast cancer with their spouses, children, and older parents.

INVISIBLE "ENEMY" - FEAR OF CANCER RECURRENCE (FCR) AND FEASIBLE INTERVENTIONS TO CONTROL FCR IN THE CARE FOR SURVIVORS OF BREAST CANCER

Looking at life from the perspective of a BC survivor, it appears that incorporating pleasant moments to be aware of every positive circumstance and cherish life with family and friends, whenever possible, are certainly very precious. However, one of the most common threats among many BC survivors is **fear of cancer recurrence (FCR)**, and possible death related to BC. Therefore, **FCR r**emains one of the biggest unmet needs in the BC survivors' population [6]. In an attempt to investigate this problem, a study has evaluated the effects of a brief **gratitude intervention** (a 6-week online gratitude course) on overall **FCR** and death-related FCR, *via* setting meaningful goals for the participants. This study revealed that women in the gratitude intervention group had a reduction in death-related FCR, compared to the control group. Also, such an effect was mediated by meaningful goal pursuit. Furthermore, the gratitude intervention was shown to prevent a decrease in **positive affect (PA)** [7].

CONCLUSION

There are important differences between younger and older women in their perceptions and efforts of restructuring personal identity and " meaning-making" in the face of BC (*e.g.*, its diagnosis and long-term therapy).

The current knowledge about the psychosocial experiences of women with BC in different age groups still remains incomplete and requires further studies, focused on the **unmet needs** of these women. This might allow the implementation of the most appropriate oncology care and support to these populations. Even a brief gratitude intervention can promote well-being and psychological adaptation to BC, by stimulating the pursuit of meaningful goals and decreasing the **fear of cancer recurrence (FCR)**.

Moreover, overwhelmed patients with BC should focus on reinforcing their **positive emotions** in the face of adversity. In addition, when they confront their "old" fears or resistance, which often stem from past traumatic experiences, they need to realize that some degree of **uncertainty is unavoidable**. However, in this process, many women with BC might be able to find **new meaning in life**, in spite of difficult circumstances.

Some feasible **strategies to manage uncertainty** in BC survivors involve being mindful, having effective patient-healthcare provider communication, and handling distress through constructive coping skills. Doctors, nurses, and other medical team members have the unique opportunity to create for their patients an **atmosphere of hope, gratitude, empathy**, and **compassion** that can enhance a healing potential, in addition to the delivery of professional anticancer care.

• **Hope, gratitude,** and **spirituality** may serve as a foundation on which numerous patients with BC can build their "new normal" future.

• **Hope** and **spirituality** can be particularly helpful at the initial step of defining meaning in life.

• After a completed treatment regimen, **gratitude** can aid in transferring meaning into action, for each individual patient.

• **Gratitude** is a positive emotion that enhances high-quality social and family relationships.

REFERENCES

[1]   Hazlett-Stevens H. Clinical significance of stress, depression, anxiety, and worry symptom improvement following mindfulness-based stress reduction.OBM Integr Compliment Med. Reno, NV, USA: University of Nevada 2022; 7: p. (2)022.
[http://dx.doi.org/10.21926/obm.icm.2202022]

[2]   Algoe SB, Stanton AL. Gratitude when it is needed most: Social functions of gratitude in women with metastatic breast cancer. Emotion 2012; 12(1): 163-8.
[http://dx.doi.org/10.1037/a0024024] [PMID: 21707160]

[3]   Carter BJ. Long-term survivors of breast cancer. Cancer Nurs 1993; 16(5): 354-61.
[http://dx.doi.org/10.1097/00002820-199310000-00003] [PMID: 8261383]

[4]   Yu H, Gao X, Zhou Y, Zhou X. Decomposing gratitude: Representation and integration of cognitive antecedents of gratitude in the brain. J Neurosci 2018; 38(21): 4886-98.
[http://dx.doi.org/10.1523/JNEUROSCI.2944-17.2018] [PMID: 29735557]

[5]   Campbell-Enns H, Woodgate R. The psychosocial experiences of women with breast cancer across the lifespan: A systematic review protocol. JBI Database Syst Rev Implement Rep 2015; 13(1): 112-21.
[http://dx.doi.org/10.11124/jbisrir-2015-1795] [PMID: 26447012]

[6]   Dawson G, Madsen L, Dains J. Interventions to manage uncertainty and fear of recurrence in female breast cancer survivors: A review of the literature. Clin J Oncol Nurs 2016; 20(6): E155-61.
[http://dx.doi.org/10.1188/16.CJON.E155-E161] [PMID: 27857253]

[7]   Otto AK, Szczesny EC, Soriano EC, Laurenceau JP, Siegel SD. Effects of a randomized gratitude intervention on death-related fear of recurrence in breast cancer survivors. Health Psychol 2016; 35(12): 1320-8.
[http://dx.doi.org/10.1037/hea0000400] [PMID: 27513475]

CHAPTER 15

The Self-kindness Component of Mindfulness Meditation: A Helpful Strategy to Enhance Emotion Regulation and Reduce the Depression and Distress Symptoms in Women with Breast Cancer

Abstract: It has been demonstrated that one of the components of **mindfulness meditation,** called **self-kindness,** plays a prominent role in **alleviating distress perception,** and **reducing depressive symptoms,** especially among **younger women with breast cancer (BC),** who represent a particularly vulnerable patient population, often struggling not only with a serious illness but also with numerous family and work-related obligations.

This chapter will describe in detail **self-kindness** as a technique to help **ease distress, anxiety,** and **depressive feelings,** as well as **enhance resilience** and establish objective health-related expectations or goals for **patients with cancer,** including women with an aggressive subtype of BC, such as **triple-negative breast cancer (TNBC).**

Keywords: Anxiety, Distress, Depression, Emotion regulation, Mindfulness meditation, Mindful awareness practice (MAP), Mindfulness-based interventions (MBI), Resilience, Rumination, Self-kindness.

INTRODUCTION

The essence of **mindfulness** is the practice of **focusing attention** on the "**here and now**" and accepting whatever arises in the awareness, with curiosity, and without judgment. However, some mechanisms for effective interventions, which can be translated into daily practice, still need to be elucidated in more detail.

A recent study examined some **emotion regulation strategies,** as factors that influence the effects of **mindfulness meditation** among young women, undergoing treatment for BC, in whom risks of psychological distress and depression are considered high. In fact, degrees of perceived **distress or depression** at **breast cancer (BC)** diagnosis, and then, during many critical moments of the BC progression, or in the treatment process are usually higher in younger females, than in their older counterparts [1]. This is pertinent to **patients with triple-negative breast cancer (TNBC)**, who often receive a diagnosis of this aggressive malignancy at a younger age.

It has been noted that **Mindfulness-Based Interventions (MBI)** can decrease psychological distress and depressive symptoms in patients with cancer, cancer survivors, and many other populations (*e.g.*, patients with chronic psychophysical diseases) [2, 3]. **It seems that** women with TNBC would be a good target population for **MBI**, and in particular, for the selected, "patient-friendly" components, such as the **self-kindness** approach, which could be translated into a daily routine.

This chapter will describe in detail s**elf-kindness** as a technique to help **ease distress, anxiety,** and **depressive feelings,** as well as **enhance resilience** and establish realistic health-related expectations and goals for **patients with cancer,** including women suffering from **TNBC**.

THE SELF-KINDNESS – A BASIC COMPONENT OF MINDFULNESS MEDITATION THAT CAN IMPROVE EMOTION REGULATION, DECREASE DISTRESS PERCEPTION AND INCREASE RESILIENCE

Self-kindness, as an **emotion regulation strategy**, can play a unique role in reducing distress in younger women with BC [3, 4]. Although **self-kindness** still requires further studies, to assess its effects in different age groups of women with BC, it is considered a safe, feasible, and beneficial approach, and thus, it appears suitable for **women with BC** (*e.g.*, TNBC), who are frequently in the younger age category [5].

It has been suggested that **Mindfulness-Based Interventions (MBI)** reduce distress *via* better **emotion regulation.** Moreover, **MBI** can "operate" through the "channels", by which it is possible to change the patterns of experiencing and expressing emotions [3, 4]. Notably, impaired emotion regulation has been connected to higher degrees of perceived distress [3, 4] and depression [3 - 5]. This can have particularly deteriorating consequences in patients with TNBC. In a recent clinical study, two contrasting **emotion regulation** processes, namely: **self-kindness** and **rumination,** were addressed by using a standardized intervention, in the form of the **Mindful Awareness Practice (MAP)** [6]. The study results have shown that the **MAP** reduced the feelings of perceived distress and depressive symptoms in a younger group of BC survivors [5 - 7].

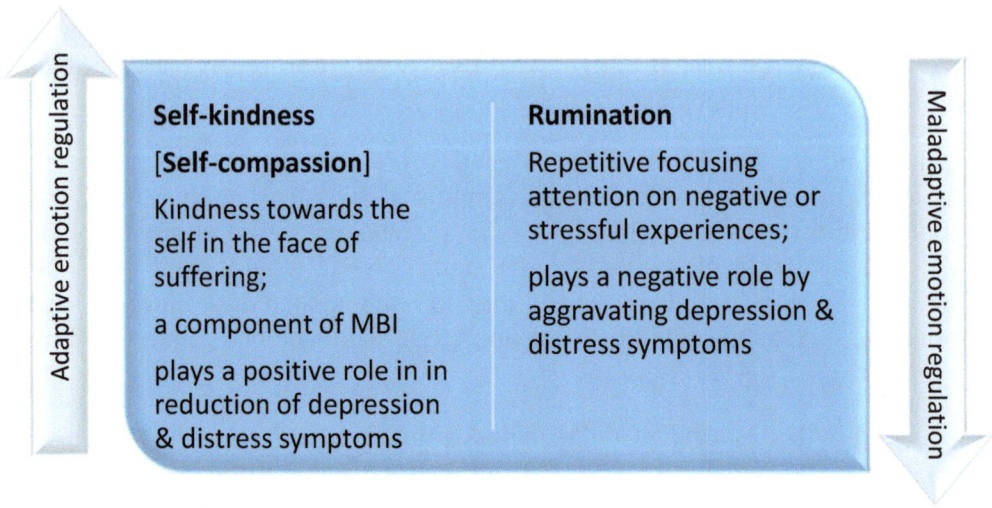

Fig. (1). The main characteristics of two emotion regulation processes linked to depression and distress - self-kindness and rumination; MBI, Mindfulness-Based Interventions.

These encouraging study findings would merit further exploration and possible implementation, as one of the supportive care options, for women suffering from TNBC.

TWO OPPOSITE DIRECTIONS OF THE EMOTION REGULATION - SELF-KINDNESS STRATEGY AND RUMINATION PROCESS

In brief, **self-kindness** is an **adaptive emotion regulation strategy**, which includes the generation of **kindness towards the self in the face of personal suffering** (Fig. **1**) [8]. **Self-kindness (**or **self-compassion)** is one of the components of a multi-dimensional construct, related to lowering the negative impact of depressive symptoms on the psychosomatic condition [8]. As an illustration of this view, in a study focused on depression, it was reported that directing kind thoughts toward the self was equally effective to a cognitive reappraisal, for a successful decrease of a negative mood, in the depressed participants [9].

In opposition to that, **rumination** is a maladaptive emotion regulation process that includes passive, repetitive **focusing attention** on the causes and consequences of **negative or stressful experiences** (Fig. **1**). Rumination often predicts the onset of depression and the persistence of its symptoms [10]. Unfortunately, women who are diagnosed with BC are also more prone to **depression,** often associated with insomnia, anxiety disorders, or other mental problems [10].

BC and the relevant uncertainty of the future, as well as the fear of the subsequent courses of anticancer therapies, can seriously upset many aspects of the life of the afflicted women. It should be underscored that clinical depression is not only a psychological disorder, but also a disease that can deteriorate the organism on many physical levels (*e.g.*, due to weakening of the immune defenses, changing hormonal regulation system, and increasing the production of pro-inflammatory cytokines). Moreover, frequent mood changes can cause non-adherence to therapies, or may adversely interfere with the response to treatment, accelerating the unfavorable BC progression [10].

In line with that, **MBI**, such as **MAP**, involves simple exercises, which allow women to do the intentional **"step back" to avoid entanglement with automatic distressing thoughts,** and in this way, **refrain from rumination**. It has been reported that MBI reduces rumination in cancer survivors and individuals with mood disorders [11]. Therefore, encouraging early detection and management of mental health problems can help patients better cope with BC, its therapies, and their adverse consequences.

THE COMBINATION OF ATTENTION, SENSE OF SELF, BEHAVIOR, AND MOTIVATION – A BUSY "INTERSECTION" WHERE THE "TRAFFIC" CAN BE CONTROLLED BY THE SELF-KINDNESS APPROACH

Importantly, **the MBI** includes some patient-friendly concepts, educational techniques or exercises that promote kindness directed towards the self, namely **self-kindness (or self-compassion)** (Fig. **2**) [6]. **MBI** can increase the **self-compassion** and has also been shown to reduce some symptoms of depression and perceived distress [6, 12].

Since the **increases in self-kindness** and the **decreases in rumination** are connected with mindfulness, the big challenge is to effectively teach the MBI to patients with the most aggressive cancers, such as TNBC. At this point, a reasonable solution may be a **six-week mindfulness training practice** (*e.g.*, designed to reduce perceived distress and depressive symptoms by enhancing self-kindness and decreasing rumination) [6, 12].

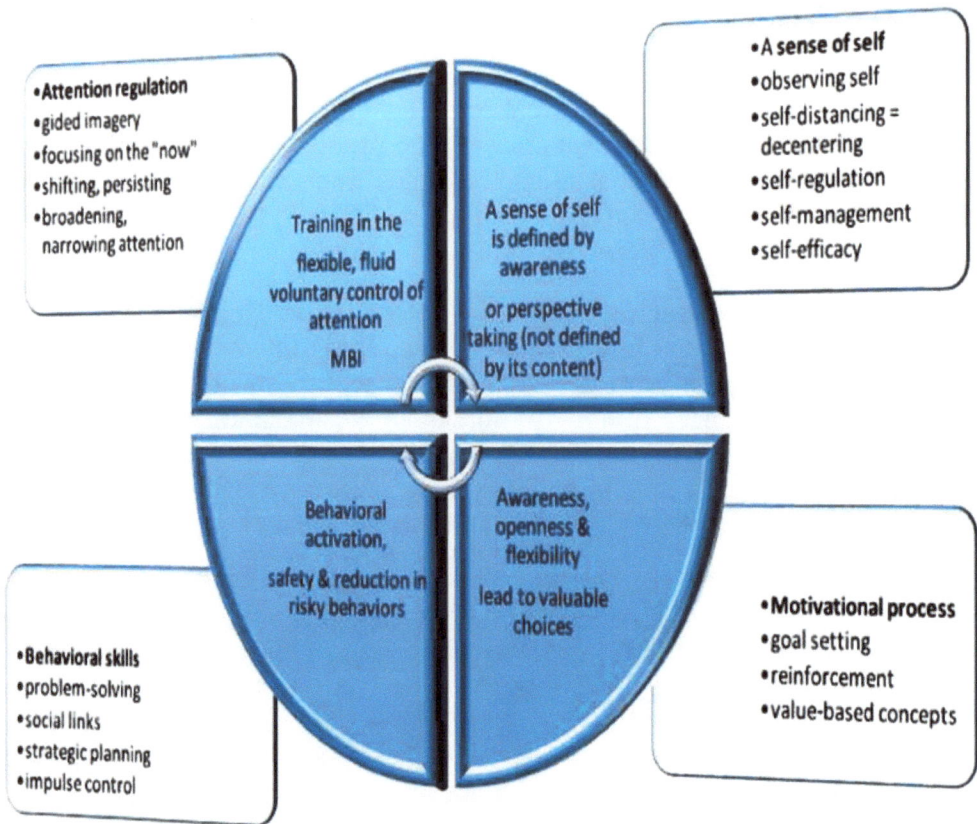

Fig. (2). A combination of processes of change in the attention, sense of self, behavior, and motivation, which can be modified by the self-kindness, mindfulness meditation, or behavioral therapy approaches; MBI, Mindfulness-Based Interventions.

CONCLUSION

Self-kindness is an adaptive emotion regulation process. It should be highlighted that **self-kindness** can influence the **reduction of depressive symptoms,** and perceived distress **feelings (**independently from the decrease in rumination), after applying the **mindfulness** intervention. Moreover, the effects of self-kindness on the perceived distress **symptoms** are in line with research connecting **positive emotions** with increased **resilience to stress.**

It has been demonstrated that **self-kindness** plays a key role in reducing distress among younger BC survivors. In addition, **emotion regulation** can naturally fluctuate over time, so that some women may initially rely on the interventions to reduce rumination. Fortunately, MBI may also have delayed, positive effects on the perceived distress. In the future, analyses of larger populations, including different age groups of patients with BC are required to confirm these findings.

• **Self-kindness** is not only simple to apply but also superior to many other supportive therapeutic approaches.

• **Increased self-kindness** and **decreased rumination** can contribute to the **decline in perceived distress** and **depression** symptoms. This is critically important to the medical care and QoL of many women with TNBC.

• A woman with TNBC can be more comfortable just by following the natural self-kindness attitude, cultivating positive emotions, and having a calm mind to effectively control her distress or anxiety.

• An increased hope, self-confidence, and sense of security may gradually diminish feelings of anxiety, distress, depression, and worry among several women with TNBC.

REFERENCES

[1]   Champion VL, Wagner LI, Monahan PO, *et al.* Comparison of younger and older breast cancer survivors and age-matched controls on specific and overall quality of life domains. Cancer 2014; 120(15): 2237-46.
[http://dx.doi.org/10.1002/cncr.28737] [PMID: 24891116]

[2]   Goyal M, Singh S, Sibinga EMS, *et al.* Meditation programs for psychological stress and well-being: A systematic review and meta-analysis. JAMA Intern Med 2014; 174(3): 357-68.
[http://dx.doi.org/10.1001/jamainternmed.2013.13018] [PMID: 24395196]

[3]   Carlson LE. Mindfulness-based interventions for coping with cancer. Ann N Y Acad Sci 2016; 1373(1): 5-12.
[http://dx.doi.org/10.1111/nyas.13029] [PMID: 26963792]

[4]   Miller JT, Verhaeghen P. Mind full of kindness: Self-awareness, self-regulation, and self-transcendence as vehicles for compassion. BMC Psychol 2022; 10(1): 188.
[http://dx.doi.org/10.1186/s40359-022-00888-4] [PMID: 35906630]

[5]   Bower JE, Partridge AH, Wolff AC, *et al.* Targeting depressive symptoms in younger breast cancer survivors: The pathways to wellness randomized controlled trial of mindfulness meditation and survivorship education. J Clin Oncol 2021; 39(31): 3473-84.
[http://dx.doi.org/10.1200/JCO.21.00279] [PMID: 34406839]

[6]   Boyle CC, Stanton AL, Ganz PA, Crespi CM, Bower JE. Improvements in emotion regulation following mindfulness meditation: Effects on depressive symptoms and perceived stress in younger breast cancer survivors. J Consult Clin Psychol 2017; 85(4): 397-402.
[http://dx.doi.org/10.1037/ccp0000186] [PMID: 28230391]

[7]   Bower JE, Crosswell AD, Stanton AL, *et al.* Mindfulness meditation for younger breast cancer survivors: A randomized controlled trial. Cancer 2015; 121(8): 1231-40.
[http://dx.doi.org/10.1002/cncr.29194] [PMID: 25537522]

[8]   Pinto-Gouveia J, Duarte C, Matos M, Fráguas S. The protective role of self-compassion in relation to psychopathology symptoms and quality of life in chronic and in cancer patients. Clin Psychol Psychother 2014; 21(4): 311-23.
[http://dx.doi.org/10.1002/cpp.1838] [PMID: 23526623]

[9]   Diedrich A, Grant M, Hofmann SG, Hiller W, Berking M. Self-compassion as an emotion regulation strategy in major depressive disorder. Behav Res Ther 2014; 58: 43-51.
[http://dx.doi.org/10.1016/j.brat.2014.05.006] [PMID: 24929927]

[10]   Nolen-Hoeksema S, Wisco BE, Lyubomirsky S. Rethinking rumination. Perspect Psychol Sci 2008; 3(5): 400-24.
[http://dx.doi.org/10.1111/j.1745-6924.2008.00088.x] [PMID: 26158958]

[11]   Labelle LE, Campbell TS, Carlson LE. Mindfulness-based stress reduction in oncology: Evaluating mindfulness and rumination as mediators of change in depressive symptoms. Mindfulness 2010; 1(1): 28-40.
[http://dx.doi.org/10.1007/s12671-010-0005-6]

[12]   Gu J, Strauss C, Bond R, Cavanagh K. How do mindfulness-based cognitive therapy and mindfulness-based stress reduction improve mental health and wellbeing? A systematic review and meta-analysis of mediation studies. Clin Psychol Rev 2015; 37: 1-12.
[http://dx.doi.org/10.1016/j.cpr.2015.01.006] [PMID: 25689576]

CHAPTER 16

Compassion-Focused Therapy (CFT): Introducing a Process-based System of Psychotherapy to Help Patients with Breast Cancer

Abstract: Compassion-focused therapy (CFT) integrates techniques from cognitive-behavioral therapy with concepts from psychology and neuroscience. The main objective of **CFT** is to use compassionate mind training to help individuals develop and maintain the experiences of inner warmth and stability, through the cultivation of compassion (including **self-compassion**).

This chapter will describe in detail **self-compassion** as a technique to help ease distress, anxiety, or depressive feelings, as well as enhance resilience and establish objective health-related expectations and goals for patients with serious chronic diseases, such as cancer, including triple-negative breast cancer (TNBC).

Keywords: Behavioral practices, Compassion-focused therapy (CFT), Negative emotions, Psychoeducation, Self-compassion.

INTRODUCTION

Compassion is an important derivative of the **biopsychosocial** process of care, which was developed to assure protection, safety, and support of the most vulnerable patients [1].

Moreover, **compassion** can offer encouragement and guidance for learning how to regulate threatening emotions, which are overwhelming or destructive [1]. In this constantly evolving **process** of psychotherapy, one of the main universal components is **Compassion-Focused Therapy (CFT)**, which is a system that integrates techniques from cognitive-behavioral therapy with concepts from psychology, and neuroscience [1]. The main purpose of **CFT** is to use compassionate cognitive training to help individuals develop and maintain the experiences of inner warmth or safety, through the cultivation of an attitude of compassion (including self-compassion) [2].

Katarzyna Rygiel

Such a concept of **compassion**, as an **innovative therapeutic option**, is based on internal **wisdom** and **courage that might characterize many** patients with cancer or other serious, chronic diseases. Moreover, compassion is viewed as a **constellation** of different **abilities, insights, motivations,** and **competencies,** which can be flexibly applied as potential **therapeutic modalities** for many types of psychosomatic problems [1, 2].

CFT can be delivered as a practical educational **course**, during which a **functional analysis** of common **safety behaviors** used by many patients can be conducted [2]. This **analysis** can subsequently be compared to the functional model of caring behavior and compassion. During this **process,** finding some specific points for a potential **compassionate self-correction** may serve as a very helpful solution to many difficult problems, which are often encountered by chronically ill patients (*e.g.*, including those with advanced or metastatic triple-negative breast cancer (TNBC) and its comorbidities).

In addition to the usual caring, which provides protection and support, **compassion** offers some unique ways of **regulating negative emotions**. Most importantly, it should be underscored that negative emotions often contribute to the patient's psychosomatic destabilization. As a counterbalance to that, the compassionate style of reasoning, imagining, and acting can be learned, exercised, and possibly introduced into a daily routine. Therefore, it would be beneficial to teach, guide, and encourage patients to use these simple techniques, as a part of the multidisciplinary supportive therapy.

This chapter will describe **self-compassion** as a technique to help ease distress, anxiety, or depressive feelings, enhance resilience, and establish realistic health-related expectations and goals for patients with serious chronic diseases, such as cancer, including TNBC.

A CONCEPT OF COMPASSION AS AN INNOVATIVE THERAPEUTIC MODALITY USING BEHAVIORAL APPROACHES - POSSIBLE BENEFITS OF CFT FOR THE PATIENTS WITH BREAST CANCER

The CFT can help patients **depersonalize** and **decenter from their inner experiences**, which are undesirable. At this point, it would be useful for patients to recognize that they naturally have a particular type of consciousness, which is free of content [2]. The content is usually created from genetic predispositions and social or environmental exposures that are, in fact, random experiences of consciousness. Moreover, such knowledge and insights can play a crucial role in reducing many destructive effects of suffering from isolation, distress, despair, marginalization, shame, or irrational self-criticism, among many vulnerable patients with breast cancer (BC) [2].

Furthermore, subsequent **empathy training** can help such patients recognize that they may unintentionally arrive at some "unnecessary" states of suffering (for themselves or others, like caregivers or family members). Therefore, teaching them how to "reorganize" their internal "software" can possibly help them find some "hidden obstacles" within themselves so that they can override them, to be able to function at a more acceptable or comfortable level. Also, it should be highlighted that **CFT** may help patients recognize that practicing several forms of **mindfulness** can increase their sensitivity to different states of mind [2]. This, in turn, may allow them to be aware of specific motives and emotions that they experience during their disease and therapy journey. Furthermore, **mindfulness** is one of the pillars of CFT, which can help detect when exactly one should **switch the attention, thoughts, emotions, and motives away from the unhelpful or unacceptable, toward the most helpful or acceptable patterns** (Fig. **1**) [2, 3].

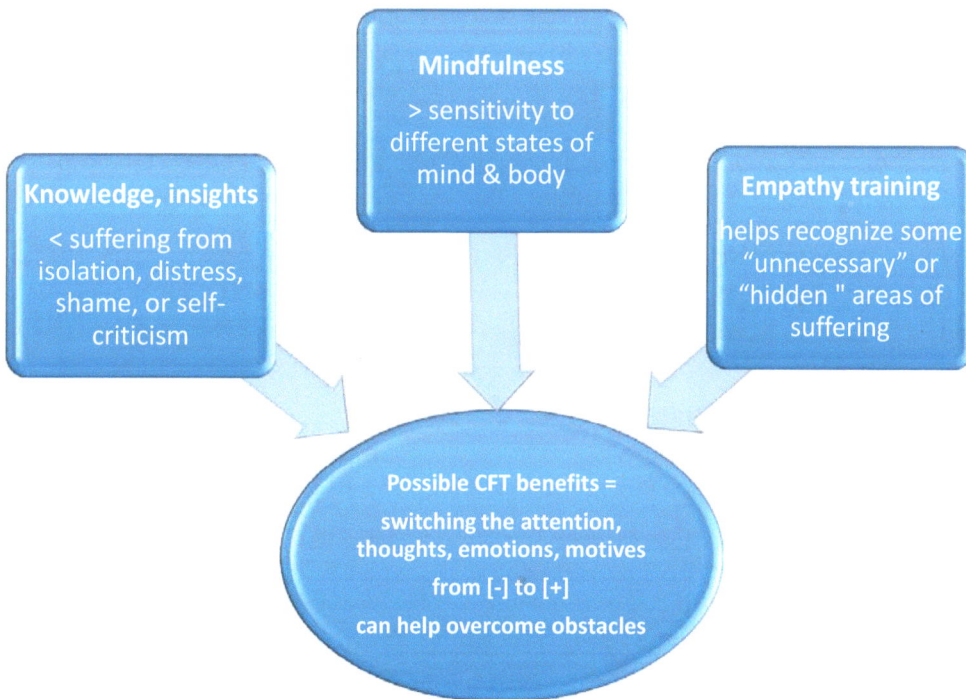

Fig. (1). Possible benefits of CFT for patients with breast cancer; CFT, Compassion-Focused Therapy.

ACCESSIBLE TECHNIQUES FOR ENHANCING THE BIDIRECTIONAL MIND AND BODY CONNECTIONS

Concurrently, the **CFT** may allow patients to refine their mental awareness and abilities to distinguish between complicated motives, dynamic emotions, and traditional beliefs, which may play a significant role, among many women with BC. This awareness is the origin of **wisdom, psychosomatic integration,** and **compassionate behavior** [3].

Furthermore, mental awareness is deeply associated with somatic awareness. As a consequence, the CFT provides useful directions on **how to use the body to be able to more effectively support the mind.** Some available techniques to calm down the mind and body include, for instance influencing the vagal nerve tone, *via* breathing exercises or by using certain body postures and physical exercises [2]. In addition, composing well-balanced nutritional meals, as well as de-escalating threats, and augmenting positive emotions also contribute to the reduction of distress, anxiety, and discomfort.

It should be underscored that the **CFT** offers patients a range of **mind and body training practices** that include **breathing techniques, meditation, visualization,** and other therapeutic skills such as **writing or journaling, acting or role-playing,** using easily–accessible objects or images to help differentiate feelings. In addition, patients can learn how to apply various forms of **art, music,** and **dance**, depending on a given patient preference (Fig. **2**) [2]. These therapeutic activities can help reduce distress and bring relaxation, which are very important for integrating patient support with the main anticancer plan of care.

A DIFFERENT PERSPECTIVE ON POSSIBLE "REPROGRAMMING" NEGATIVE EMOTIONS: A PSYCHOEDUCATION AND BEHAVIORAL PRACTICES FOR IMPROVEMENT OF THE PATIENTS' FUNCTIONING

Importantly, the **CFT** helps patients reflect on what is really meaningful to them. For different ethnic minority groups of patients with complex medical histories (*e.g.*, including serious, chronic diseases, like BC, as well as psychological trauma, violence, or social injustice), an intense therapeutic action aimed at anxiety, fear, and irrational resistance is necessary for **processing negative emotions or distrust**, and **"reprogramming"** them successfully by the afflicted patients [3, 4]. Furthermore, it is crucial to recognize that many **emotional blockages** (*e.g.*, fear, avoidance, or resistance) represent, in fact, only "artificial" obstacles. Interestingly, the CFT considers the sensation of fear as **"intuitive protection"** that needs to be accurately interpreted, to serve in some critical situations, as a reasonable protective approach in the face of real harm [2, 3]. Also, it should be noted that **guided discovery** can help refine a deep understanding of the complex nature of the mind and compassion. Consequently, a combination of **psychoeducation** and **behavioral practices**, in which the professional therapeutic relationships, between the engaged patients and their therapists, are maintained may allow CFT to effectively work with difficult emotions. In this way, **the patients are motivated to be real partners with the therapeutic team** members, during their journey. Furthermore, such engaged patients can actively be "in charge" of many emotional and behavioral aspects of their disease, therapy, and general functioning [3, 4].

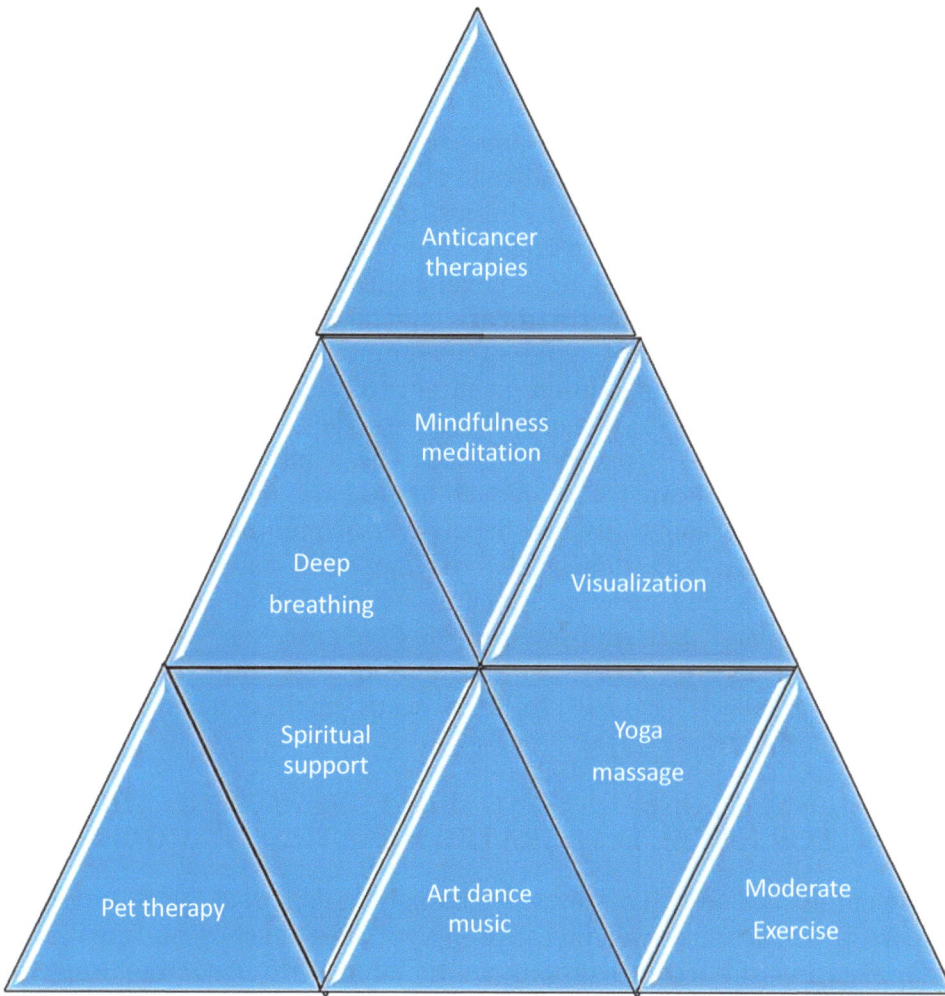

Fig. (2). Examples of therapeutic activities that can help reduce distress and bring relaxation.

CHALLENGES IN INTRODUCING NOVEL INTEGRATED CARE MODELS - CONSIDERING THE USE OF HORIZON SCANNING METHODOLOGIES

According to the World Health Organization **(WHO)**, **integrated care** is defined as an **approach to strengthening people-centered health systems** *via* **promoting the delivery of quality services**, which are **based on the multidimensional needs** of the populations and individual persons. These services should be provided by coordinated multidisciplinary teams of professionals [5]. However, in "real life", such a theoretical approach is very difficult to achieve in clinical practice, due to numerous obstacles. Fortunately, a potentially helpful solution to this challenge may be offered by **horizon scanning methodologies**, which can identify and prioritize innovations, at the early stages of their development. These **methodologies** have been examined for a possible application in healthcare planning (*e.g.*, novel healthcare interventions, *etc.*) [5]. It should be underscored that **integrated care** may take many forms, and this term itself can also include various types of integration (*e.g.*, service integration, clinical integration, *etc.*). In addition, in **integrated care,** it is very difficult to successfully develop new healthcare delivery models, mostly because of the absence of established concepts, procedures, and structures for the multidimensional type of care [5]. Moreover, **healthcare providers** with different professional expertise and skills can have diverse opinions about prioritizing medical needs, goals, and dimensions of integrated care, which are most important to deliver, and exact procedures, which should be used for these purposes [5]. Similarly, **patients with various chronic, serious, or incurable diseases** *(e.g.*, metastatic TNBC with comorbidities), often complicated by socioeconomic problems, also have different needs, goals, and expectations with regard to healthcare services [5].

ENABLING AND CONSTRAINING FACTORS TO THE HORIZON SCANNING FOR NOVEL INTEGRATED HEALTHCARE MODELS

In an attempt to shed some light on some complex topics relevant to **integrated healthcare**, a recent study, was investigating possible **barriers and facilitators to the application of horizon scanning methodologies**, for **detecting integrated healthcare delivery models**, from the perspective of medical personnel This analysis was conducted in accordance with the **Capability, Opportunity and Motivation model of Behavior (COM-B)** and other relevant theoretical frameworks [5].

Offering new options for the development of **integrated healthcare** has been challenging, mostly because of the lack of universal definitions and concepts of integrated care, as well as the multidisciplinary nature of integrated care. Regardless of that, **horizon scanning** may offer a potential structured strategy to detect future innovative and feasible ways of healthcare concepts.

In particular, the recent study, addressing these ideas, was aimed to examine perceptions of determinants for adopting **horizon scanning in the context of the development of integrated healthcare models** [5]. The findings of this study might serve as valuable lessons, which can potentially help in the development of interventions targeting barriers and promoting facilitators to adopt horizon scanning **methodologies** for assessing novel healthcare delivery models [5].

Hopefully, further studies could explore in detail the horizon scanning as a tool for addressing the emerging integrated healthcare models, since developing and implementing innovative services, procedures, and processes in the healthcare system can potentially improve population health status, including some disadvantageous groups of patients (*e.g.*, women with metastatic TNBC).

CONCLUSION

Compassionate mind training can be used to help people develop experiences of inner warmth, and peace, *via* compassion and self-compassion."

In summary, modern research is showing how compassion can alter a whole spectrum of neurophysiological connections, in both patients and their caregivers. Recently, the findings of some studies have enriched a traditional view of how **compassion** and **empathy-based care** may contribute **to emotion regulation** and **desirable behavioral changes**, even in the face of serious, chronic diseases with poor prognosis patients (*e.g.*, women with metastatic TNBC).

Compassion-Focused Therapy (CFT) is an example of the modern style of psychotherapy, which applies various **cognitive, behavioral, and educational techniques.** Moreover, the **CFT** represents **a process therapy**, encompassing **mindfulness, compassion, psychoeducational,** and **behavioral techniques,** which have been already validated, in different medical, mental, psychological, and social contexts.

For different ethnic minority groups of patients with complex medical histories (*e.g.*, including serious, chronic diseases, like TNBC, as well as psychological trauma, violence, or social injustice), the interventions aimed at serious anxiety, fear, and irrational resistance are necessary for successful **processing of negative emotions or distrust**, and **"reprogramming"** them by the afflicted patients.

Furthermore, it is crucial to recognize that, in fact, many **emotional blockages** (*e.g.*, fear, avoidance, or resistance) represent, only "artificial" obstacles, and patients should be empowered to overcome them.

It is expected that the patient outcomes would improve, upon a deeper understanding of the nature of the human mind and possible translation of compassionate behaviors and emphatic approaches to daily care, among the most vulnerable patients (*e.g.*, women with advanced or metastatic TNBC).

In addition, novel **horizon scanning methodologies** can be useful for identifying, assessing, and prioritizing innovations in healthcare delivery models, at their early stages, to help meet the complex medical and personal needs, including some disadvantaged ethnic minority groups of patients.

• **Compassion and mindfulness** as the main pillars of **Compassion-Focused Therapy (CFT)**, which can help detect when exactly one should **switch the attention, thoughts, and emotions away from the unhelpful or unacceptable, and toward the helpful or acceptable patterns.**

• The **CFT** offers a range of **mind and body training practices to** patients that include breathing techniques, visualization, meditation, behavioral practices, and other therapeutic skills such as writing or journaling, acting or role-playing, using simple and easily–accessible objects or images to help differentiate feelings, as well as applying various forms of art, music, and dance, as supportive methods of care.

• The **CFT** helps patients reflect on what is really meaningful in their life.

REFERENCES

[1]   Gilbert P. Compassion: From its evolution to a psychotherapy. Front Psychol 2020; 11: 586161.
        [http://dx.doi.org/10.3389/fpsyg.2020.586161] [PMID: 33362650]

[2]   Gilbert P. Explorations into the nature and function of compassion. Curr Opin Psychol 2019; 28: 108-14.
        [http://dx.doi.org/10.1016/j.copsyc.2018.12.002] [PMID: 30639833]

[3]   Mascaro JS, Florian MP, Ash MJ, *et al.* Ways of knowing compassion: How do we come to know, understand, and measure compassion when we see it? Front Psychol 2020; 11: 547241.
        [http://dx.doi.org/10.3389/fpsyg.2020.547241] [PMID: 33132956]

[4]   Mongrain M, Keltner D, Kirby J. Editorial: Expanding the science of compassion. Front Psychol 2021; 12: 745799.
        [http://dx.doi.org/10.3389/fpsyg.2021.745799] [PMID: 34589036]

[5]   Nuth Waggestad-Stoa M, Traina G, Feiring E. Barriers and facilitators to adopting horizon scanning to identify novel integrated care models: A qualitative interview study. BMJ Innov 2022; 8(2): 65-71.
        [http://dx.doi.org/10.1136/bmjinnov-2021-000804]

CHAPTER 17

How Can Medical Professionals Maintain Compassion for Their Patients with Breast Cancer?

Abstract: Compassion in the medical field differs from its traditional meaning in daily life. In medicine, **compassion includes a desire to understand an individual's suffering, together with a wish to relieve it**. In essence, **compassion** offers a unique concept, according to which, the modern science of compassion can be practically applied to suffering people, in many circumstances. This is particularly important for some vulnerable groups of patients (*e.g.*, ethnic minorities), such as women with **breast cancer (BC)** (*e.g.*, in advanced or metastatic stages, with comorbidities and socioeconomic problems).

This chapter presents some suggestions (based on recent research reports) for helpful **strategies that medical professionals can use** daily, **to help maintain compassion** for their patients with serious diseases, including some aggressive **cancers** (*e.g.*, Triple-Negative Breast Cancer (TNBC)).

Keywords: Breast cancer (BC), Compassion, Empathy, Medical professionals, Patients with cancer, Sustainable compassion training (SCT), Transactional model of compassion (TMC).

INTRODUCTION

Compassion is one of the most important **ingredients of healthcare**, certainly desired by patients and their families. Unfortunately, in the past, research was mainly focused on **compassion fatigue** or **burnout**, and not on the **beneficial role of maintaining compassion for patients** by the medical teams in charge of their care [1]. In medicine, **compassion includes a desire to understand an individual's suffering, together with a sincere wish to relieve it** [2]. Naturally, compassion involves awareness and sensitivity to recognize physical or emotional suffering, feeling for the suffering person, tolerating some degree of discomfort (relevant to another individual's suffering), as well as motivation to actively relieve suffering [3].

The desire to alleviate suffering is the main attribute that differentiates compassion from empathy or sympathy [2, 3]. Simply put, **empathy** is the capacity to understand or feel what another person is experiencing. That means the ability to place oneself in another's position. Empathy includes a range of cognitive, emotional, and social processes, mostly concerned with understanding others, and thus, different types of empathy can be distinguished (Fig. **1**).

This chapter presents some suggestions (based on recent research reports) for helpful **strategies that medical professionals can use** daily, **to help maintain compassion** for their patients with serious diseases, including **cancer** *(e.g.,* Triple-Negative Breast Cancer (TNBC)).

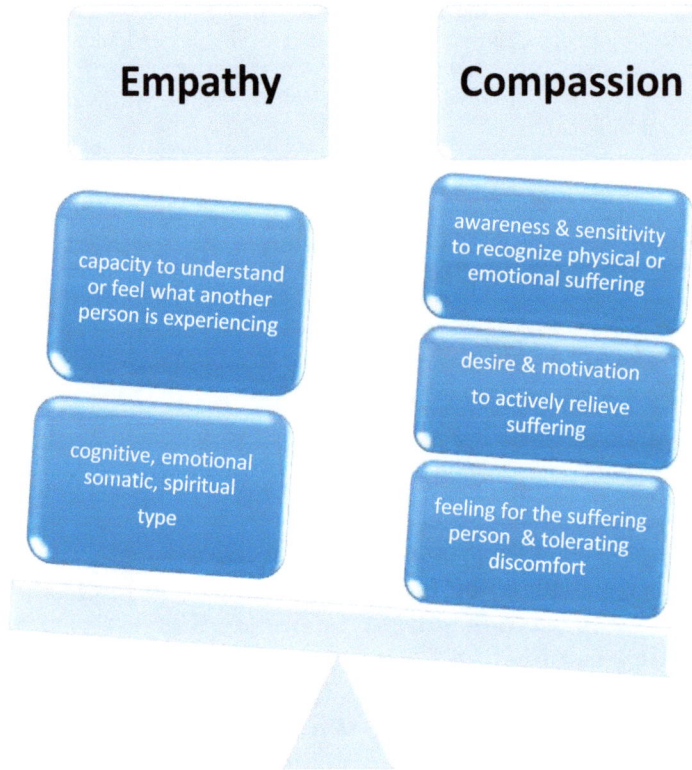

Fig. (1). A comparison of compassion and empathy.

WHY COMPASSION AND EMPATHY ARE SO CRUCIAL TO DELIVERING THE HIGH-QUALITY HEALTHCARE?

In an attempt to answer this question, some basic facts need to be considered, as follows:

1). **Compassion** and **empathy** are extremely important, due to their documented **correlations with beneficial patient outcomes** (*e.g.*, decreased anxiety), increased patient satisfaction, reinforced patient-doctor relationships, decreased **posttraumatic stress disorder (PTSD)** after medical emergencies or disasters, and improved overall health outcomes [4].

2). **Compassion** is associated with **positive consequences for physicians** or nurses (*e.g.*, greater work satisfaction or patient retention), and financial compensation, not to mention economic advantages for health care systems, due to fewer medical errors or malpractice lawsuits [5].

3). **Compassion** among physicians can **counterbalance** some harmful **stress-related reactions** [5].

Therefore, based on this evidence, compassion is a professional duty of physicians and nurses, and also, one of the patient's rights [6]. Moreover, this is an essential component for effective healthcare delivery in any setting. Therefore, discussing some feasible **strategies** that medical professionals can use to maintain **compassion** in the healthcare environment would be beneficial to the patients and to their medical providers [4, 6].

HOW THE HEALTHCARE PROFESSIONALS COULD MAINTAIN THEIR COMPASSION OR EMPATHY IN A DAILY PRACTICE?

According to a recent small study, focused on mental health, conducted among the nursing personnel and patients under their care, it was reported that **asking patients questions** and **reflecting on their individual difficulties** were the most commonly documented strategies when trying to apply an **empathic or compassionate approach** into daily medical practice [7]. Furthermore, psychological writings indicate that **mindfulness meditation**, **self-compassion**, and **connecting with patients** can help establish empathic, trustworthy relationships [8, 9].

It should be highlighted that **empathy** can offer a helpful **"window" to compassion**. However, there are some subtle differences between these two terms, mostly with regard to certain healthcare structures or contexts. Nevertheless, the **way how healthcare professionals maintain their compassion or empathy**, and which strategies are the most effective in particular circumstances, still remain unknown and deserve exploration in further clinical studies.

LESSONS LEARNED FROM STUDIES OF MEDICAL PROFESSIONALS ABOUT THEIR STRATEGIES FOR MAINTAINING COMPASSION AND EMPATHY FOR PATIENTS

In a recent study, medical professionals were asked questions about how they maintained compassion for their patients. An analysis of their answers suggested that the compassion-maintaining strategies were usually concentrated in specific fields, and most professionals were seeking to maintain **compassionate** care **for their patients,** using internal strategies [4]. Of course, it is conceivable that the use of particular strategies is related to working in different clinical environments, in which these strategies are easily accessible (*e.g.*, brief walks to improve the mood and concentration of the mind or relieve muscle tension would be more feasible, when professional duties are scheduled in more organized or predictable ways when a reliable cross-coverage by another staff member is available, and a facility location is suited for safe walking or exercising) [4]. Certainly, in the future, long-term, large-scale, multicenter studies on how compassion can be maintained over time, especially for patients with serious, chronic diseases are merited.

THE TRANSACTIONAL MODEL OF COMPASSION (TMC): AN IMPORTANT PROCESS TO ENHANCE COMPASSION SKILLS

To shed new light on some nuances relevant to **compassion**, it is helpful to evaluate some approaches, used by many experienced and respectful medical professionals. These data may offer some valuable **educational "tools" to train new members of medical teams on how to practically develop and maintain compassion** in daily clinical practice. Current research in this area has been focused on simple and effective interventions that might be smoothly introduced in many healthcare settings. For instance, the **Transactional Model of Compassion (TMC)** considers **compassion as a dynamic process**, affected by a combination of components derived from the physicians and nurses, patients and their family members, clinical circumstances, and environmental or institutional factors (Fig. **2**) [1, 10]. Data obtained *via* **TMC** indicate that the common barriers to compassion in a given setting may change in a predictable manner, depending on the specific characteristics of various medical fields [10]. Notably, it may be possible to overcome many of such predictable barriers with some coordinated efforts focused on education and experience [11].

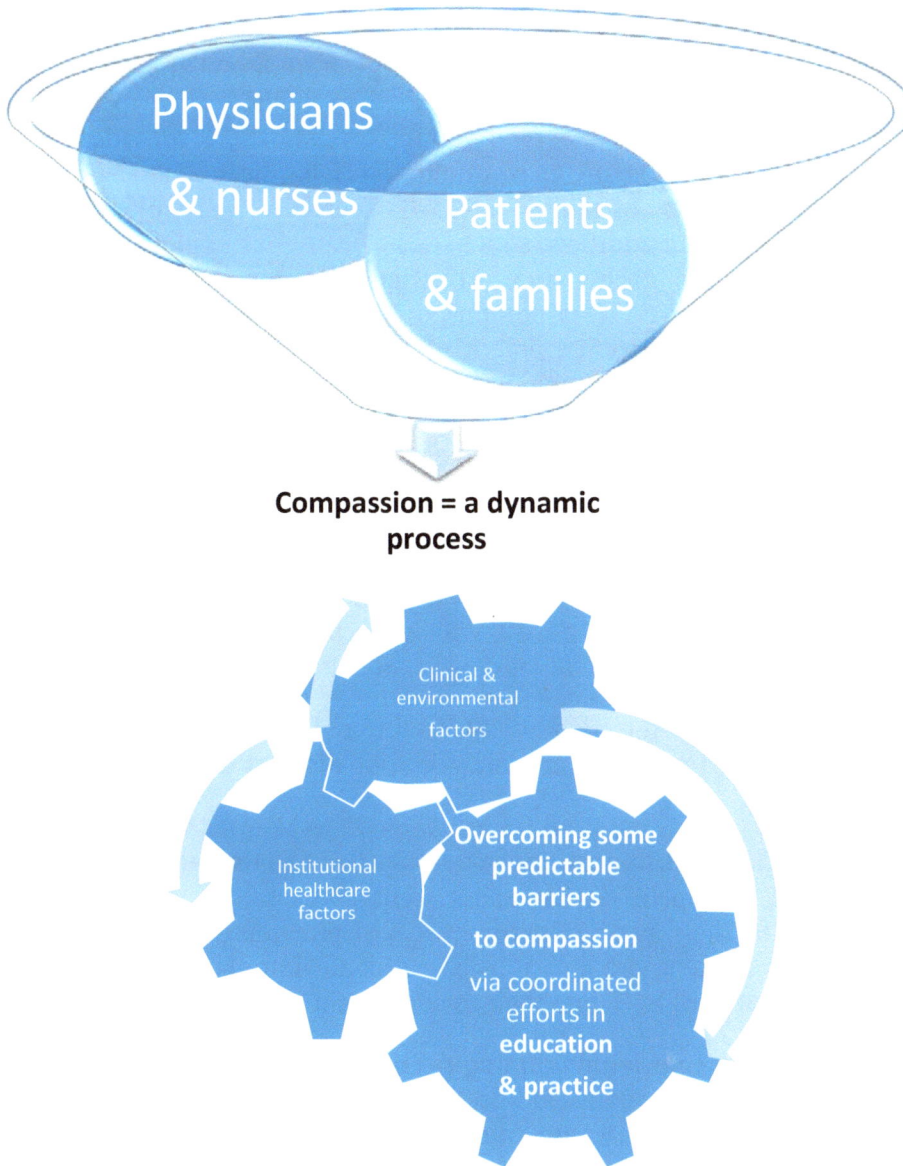

Fig. (2). The Transactional Model of Compassion (TMC).

SUSTAINABLE COMPASSION TRAINING (SCT): A POTENTIAL STRATEGY TO BE USED BY MEDICAL PRACTITIONERS

Sustainable Compassion Training (SCT), which combines **mindfulness and compassion** training, facilitates the care for self and others (that is especially important for patients with serious diseases, like BC with comorbidities, and their caregivers). In particular, **SCT** uses **meditation** to fulfill the **complex psychosomatic needs** of the participants [12]. In short, **SCT** consists of **meditation practices** (that were adapted from the tradition of Buddhism) and modern **psychological approaches**, in the areas of medical care, mental health, educational support, social work, *etc* [12]. In this way, **SCT** provides a unique **blend of spiritual and scientific components. SCT** has been practiced in various settings, including groups of individuals, who search for particular qualities of care with compassion. In addition, some scientific studies explore the effects of **meditation training to gather new knowledge about the potential of the human mind** [12]. The **SCT** is composed of the **receptive, deepening, and inclusive mode** of contemplative practice [12]. Moreover, each of these modes contains **meditation practices**, which are interconnected. The **receptive** mode helps practitioners find access to qualities of compassion, safety, acceptance, and wisdom. Similarly, the **deepening** mode helps them settle in those qualities, with relaxation and inner peace, which have healing potential for the mind and body. Likewise, the **inclusive** mode helps them connect awareness to fulfill different needs with a compassionate attitude. Based on these modes of practice, the **meditations for cultivating empathy and compassion** are aimed to create solidarity with other persons in a way, which can be free of compassion fatigue, empathic distress, physical, mental, or emotional exhaustion, and burnout [12].

Some important **characteristics** of **SCT** differ **from other contemporary meditation-training programs** and include four **distinct components** (Fig. **3**), listed below.

1). **Accommodation of different, more personalized goals for the participants**, *via* constructing an open secular space. This is achieved by allowing the participants to find their own, individual ways of practicing patterns. Moreover, this permits them to incorporate various backgrounds into the meditation practice and to map the pattern of SCT into their own perspectives or beliefs [12].

2). **An accent on the relational starting point of meditation**, which means that SCT begins with receiving care *via* building a relational field, which serves as a secure base for practical learning of the caring abilities, which subsequently should be extended to others. Also, practitioners may be guided by examples of more experienced practitioners, who accomplished reasonable solutions to their problems [12].

3). **Opportunities for practitioners to be present to all thoughts and feelings** in the environment of deep **awareness**, in which the difficult feelings and thoughts can be relaxed, healed, or released. In line with SCT, caring capacities are innate properties of the mind (rather than a skill that must be created). This view is in agreement with some perspectives on care and compassion, which have contributed to survival in the past [12].

4). **Liberation within suffering** is available based on the concept that all emotions are constructed, and thus empty at their core. Therefore, liberation can occur with experiential insight into the emptiness of emotions, in unity with awareness. In this concept, "destructive" emotions are distorted expressions of awareness that precede them. Freedom from destructive emotions (*e.g.*, delusion, greed, or hatred) is available within the emotions themselves. This view can empower the practitioner "to be with suffering" in a way that provides the holding environment for difficult emotions to neutralize them. This, in turn, may lead to self-liberation. Such a **self-liberation** of emotions is distinct from meditation programs, which promote self-compassion (*e.g.*, by bringing kindness to one's emotions) [12].

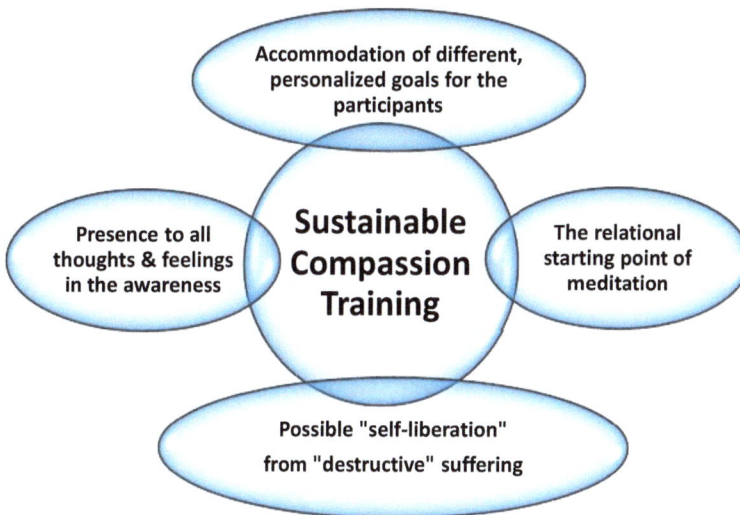

Fig. (3). Components of the Sustainable Compassion Training (SCT).

NAVIGATING THROUGH THE MAIN STRATEGIES FOR COMPASSION IN THE PATIENT CARE – HELPFUL DIRECTIONS TO CONSIDER FOR MEDICAL PROFESSIONALS

Since **compassion** is essential to safe and effective clinical management and psychological benefits for the patients, medical staff, and the entire healthcare system, it is crucial to invent, teach, and provide a friendly atmosphere, in which medical professionals could apply these strategies to maintain compassion for their patients [13].

These **strategies** can be more **internally** or **externally focused**. They may usually include a blend of approaches, which are focused on the self (*e.g.*, self-care and self-management, as well as strategies that specifically involve changing the way the individuals think about themselves, their professional roles, and the specific life circumstances of their patients) *vs.* those, concerned mostly with the suffering patients [14].

In addition, some strategies can be viewed as "**immediate**" (*e.g.*, for emergency use, in some acute medical problems or dramatic situations) *vs.* others that can serve as "**long-term**" (*e.g.*, for chronic or palliative care, in emotionally or physically exhausting situations) and reflect universal **self-maintenance strategies**.

Although many of these strategies can be subjectively perceived as helpful for maintaining compassion, additional studies are needed to investigate, if such strategies will really translate into a patient's perception of improved medical care. Moreover, in further research on compassion in medicine, empirical studies assessing the efficacy of certain interventions, such as **mindfulness**, which is **connected with compassionate feelings and behaviors** would be merited [10]. Hopefully, this may allow the introduction of some compassion-enhancing techniques into medical education, professional training, and clinical practice.

THE IMPORTANCE OF APPLYING PROCESS-BASED INTERVENTIONS TO THE CLINICAL/CANCER CARE TEAMS FIRST, AND THEN, TO THEIR PATIENTS

It should be highlighted that, most optimally, the **process-based interventions** require some transition period to be applied to the medical practitioners first, before introducing them to their patients (Fig. **4**) [15]. Since these novel **process-based interventions** are mostly experiential, there is a reasonable belief that one cannot teach, what one cannot do. In addition, such techniques are frequently based on natural psychological processes, which in some cancer-related circumstances, still need to be explored in more detail [15]. Nevertheless, the main purpose of the novel **interventions** is to detect and possibly rearrange some adverse psychological processes, and then, substitute them with beneficial ones.

For instance, in **mindfulness-based cognitive therapy (MBCT)** and in **acceptance and commitment therapy (ACT)**, mindfulness practice is a common denominator for both the patients and their therapists [15]. In essence, mindfulness addresses topics of values and meaning-making, as well as emotional openness and perspective-taking. In this way, the patients and the therapists can be mutually engaged in the ongoing psychological processes of change [15].

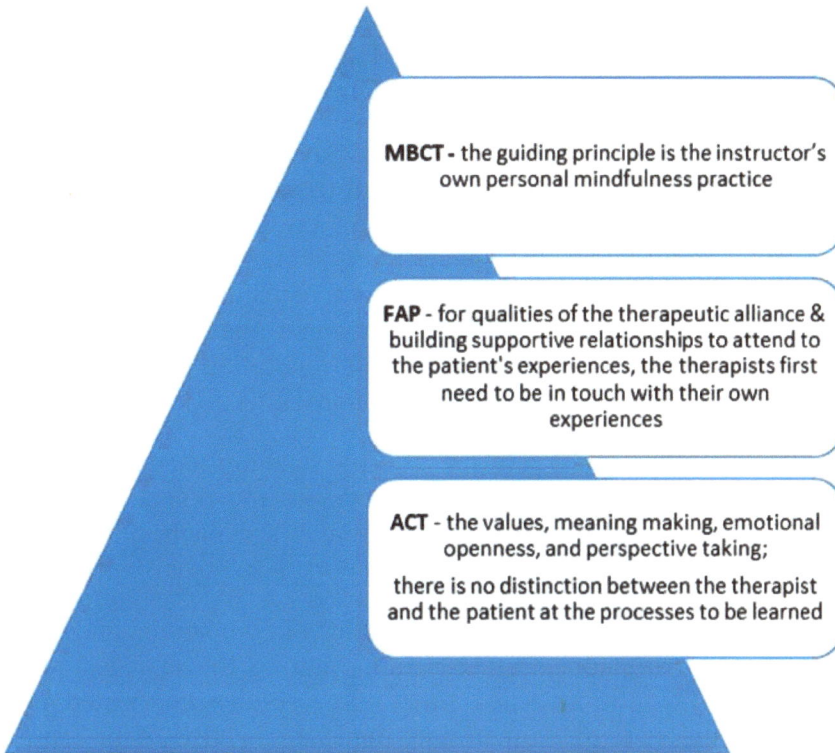

Fig. (4). Selected, patient-centered, **process-based interventions;** MBCT, mindfulness-based cognitive therapy; FAP, functional analytic psychotherapy; ACT, acceptance and commitment therapy.

Similarly, **functional analytic psychotherapy (FAP)** addresses the therapeutic alliance, and some options on how to use them, to establish close, supportive relationships between patients and their care teams [15]. In particular, the application of **FAP** linked with an empirical approach, based on continuous evaluation of a patient's clinical parameters and psychological factors illustrates a **process-based strategy,** which can be a useful component, in addition to the usual therapeutic approach [15]. Moreover, the **process-based interventions** focused on patient's-specific processes of change are **superior to the standard** ones, since they include the influence of psychological variables, in addition to cancer-related symptoms only [15].

CONCLUSION

Compassion (understanding an individual's suffering, and a strong desire to relieve it) and empathy are important to deliver high-quality healthcare, which is correlated with beneficial patient outcomes (*e.g.*, decreased anxiety, increased

QoL, and reinforced patient-doctor relationships). In addition, maintaining **compassion** and empathy in daily practice has **positive consequences for physicians,** nurses, or other medical practitioners (*e.g.*, greater work satisfaction or patient retention, and reduction of some harmful stress-related reactions).

In particular, **self-focused strategies**, used by some medical professionals (*e.g.*, **self-care interventions**), can be very helpful to maintain quality care for their patients, as well as a positive atmosphere for co-workers, caregivers, and the healthcare environment. The **Transactional Model of Compassion (TMC)** considers compassion as a dynamic process, affected by a combination of components derived from the physicians and nurses, patients (or their families), clinical circumstances, and environmental or institutional factors. **TMC** is an important process that can enhance compassion skills.

Sustainable Compassion Training (SCT) encompasses mindfulness and compassion training to facilitate the care for self and others. SCT consists of meditation practices and modern psychological approaches, in the areas of medical care, mental health, educational support, and social work.

In summary, prompt access to the innate abilities of compassion and care (for self and others) could bring long-lasting results, among the engaged patients and teams of medical practitioners. In the future, studies conducted on various populations of patients (*e.g.*, women with metastatic TNBC, with comorbidities, from different ethnic groups) and their medical teams are needed. Simultaneously, research on the strategies, which may **sustain compassion** over time, among **medical professionals**, would be beneficial for the patients, and the entire healthcare system. Also, determining the main factors that may interfere with compassion in health care contexts, and focusing on overcoming barriers to comp-assionate and emphatic patient care should be explored in clinical studies, in the future.

• **Compassion** expressed by medical professionals for their suffering patients is an important ingredient in their outcomes, especially in cases of chronic and serious diseases (*e.g.*, advanced or metastatic TNBC with comorbidities).

• Simple and friendly techniques, such as **asking patients questions** and **reflecting on their difficulties** are the most common **empathic and compassionate approaches** in medical practice.

• **Self-compassion** means bringing kindness to one's emotions, which can be especially important for patients with serious diseases (like TNBC with comorbidities) and their caregivers.

• **Sustainable Compassion Training (SCT)** can include **personalized goals for the** participants, by allowing them to find their own, individual way of practice, which includes their own perspectives or beliefs about the meditation practice. In addition, practice is guided by experienced practitioners, who have found reasonable solutions to their problems.

REFERENCES

[1]   Fernando AT III, Consedine NS. Beyond compassion fatigue: The transactional model of physician compassion. J Pain Symptom Manage 2014; 48(2): 289-98.
[http://dx.doi.org/10.1016/j.jpainsymman.2013.09.014] [PMID: 24417804]

[2]   Sinclair S, Norris JM, McConnell SJ, *et al.* Compassion: A scoping review of the healthcare literature. BMC Palliat Care 2016; 15(1): 6.
[http://dx.doi.org/10.1186/s12904-016-0080-0] [PMID: 26786417]

[3]   Strauss C, Lever Taylor B, Gu J, *et al.* What is compassion and how can we measure it? A review of definitions and measures. Clin Psychol Rev 2016; 47: 15-27.
[http://dx.doi.org/10.1016/j.cpr.2016.05.004] [PMID: 27267346]

[4]   Baguley SI, Dev V, Fernando AT, Consedine NS. How do health professionals maintain compassion over time? Insights from a study of compassion in health. Front Psychol 2020; 11: 564554.
[http://dx.doi.org/10.3389/fpsyg.2020.564554] [PMID: 33447247]

[5]   Trzeciak S, Roberts BW, Mazzarelli AJ. Compassionomics: Hypothesis and experimental approach. Med Hypotheses 2017; 107: 92-7.
[http://dx.doi.org/10.1016/j.mehy.2017.08.015] [PMID: 28915973]

[6]   Bramley L, Matiti M. How does it really feel to be in my shoes? Patients' experiences of compassion within nursing care and their perceptions of developing compassionate nurses. J Clin Nurs 2014; 23(19-20): 2790-9.
[http://dx.doi.org/10.1111/jocn.12537] [PMID: 24479676]

[7]   Gerace A, Oster C, O'Kane D, Hayman CL, Muir-Cochrane E. Empathic processes during nurse-consumer conflict situations in psychiatric inpatient units: A qualitative study. Int J Ment Health Nurs 2018; 27(1): 92-105.
[http://dx.doi.org/10.1111/inm.12298] [PMID: 28019705]

[8]   Block-Lerner J, Adair C, Plumb JC, Rhatigan DL, Orsillo SM. The case for mindfulness-based approaches in the cultivation of empathy: Does nonjudgmental, present-moment awareness increase capacity for perspective-taking and empathic concern? J Marital Fam Ther 2007; 33(4): 501-16.
[http://dx.doi.org/10.1111/j.1752-0606.2007.00034.x] [PMID: 17935532]

[9]   Fulton CL. Self-compassion as a mediator of mindfulness and compassion for others. Couns Values 2018; 63(1): 45-56.
[http://dx.doi.org/10.1002/cvj.12072]

[10] Fernando AT, Skinner K, Consedine NS. Increasing compassion in medical decision-making: Can a brief mindfulness intervention help? Mindfulness 2017; 8(2): 276-85.
[http://dx.doi.org/10.1007/s12671-016-0598-5]

[11] Dev V, Fernando AT III, Kirby JN, Consedine NS. Variation in the barriers to compassion across healthcare training and disciplines: A cross-sectional study of doctors, nurses, and medical students. Int J Nurs Stud 2019; 90: 1-10.
[http://dx.doi.org/10.1016/j.ijnurstu.2018.09.015] [PMID: 30476724]

[12] Condon P, Makransky J. Sustainable compassion training: Integrating meditation theory with psychological science. Front Psychol 2020; 11: 2249.
[http://dx.doi.org/10.3389/fpsyg.2020.02249] [PMID: 33041897]

[13]   Frampton SB, Guastello S, Lepore M. Compassion as the foundation of patient-centered care: The importance of compassion in action. J Comp Eff Res 2013; 2(5): 443-55.
[http://dx.doi.org/10.2217/cer.13.54] [PMID: 24236742]

[14]   Sanchez-Reilly S, Morrison L, Carey E, *et al.* Caring for oneself to care for others: Physicians and their self-care. J Support Oncol 2013; 11(2): 75-81.
[http://dx.doi.org/10.12788/j.suponc.0003] [PMID: 23967495]

[15]   Hayes SC, Hofmann SG. *Third-wave* cognitive and behavioral therapies and the emergence of a process-based approach to intervention in psychiatry. W Psychiatry 2021; 20(3): 363-75.
[http://dx.doi.org/10.1002/wps.20884] [PMID: 34505370]

APPENDIX

METASTATIC BREAST CANCER

This **appendix** provides practical information, definitions of professional medical terminology, and **lists of common questions** about **metastatic BC, its diagnosis, and multidisciplinary therapy,** to help patients effectively communicate with their medical providers and caregivers.

The main purpose of this **appendix** is to educate and empower women suffering from BC to be able to openly **discuss their goals, needs, expectations,** and **concerns** before selecting the most optimal **treatment or supportive care options** for their individual clinical and personal context (based on the main reference: https://www.nccn.org/patientresources/patient-resources/metastatic-breast-cancer-2020).

HIGHLIGHTS FOR PATIENTS WITH BREAST CANCER TO REMEMBER & PRACTICAL QUESTIONS TO ASK

Where does Breast Cancer (BC) Start?

Breast cancer (BC) starts in the cells of the breast

• Almost all BCs are carcinomas (cancers originating from the cells, which line the inner or outer surfaces of the body).

• Cancer cells behave differently than normal cells (*e.g.*, unlike healthy cells, cancer cells can spread and form tumors (metastases) in other body parts).

Origins of BC:

1. Ductal BC

Starts in the cells that line the milk ducts (tubes that carry milk from the lobules of the breast to the nipple; the most common type of BC.

2. Lobular BC

Starts in the lobules (milk glands) of the breast (Fig. **1**).

How does BC Spread in the Body?

Primary BC, or primary tumor – is a local mass formed by cancer cells.

Invasive BC – is the one that has spread from the milk ducts or lobules into the surrounding breast tissue or nearby lymph nodes (LN).

Metastatic BC – is a cancer that has spread from the primary breast tumor into other parts of the body.

In this process, cancer cells break away from the primary tumor and travel through blood or lymph vessels to distant areas. Once in other sites, cancer cells may form secondary tumors (metastases) (Fig. **2**).

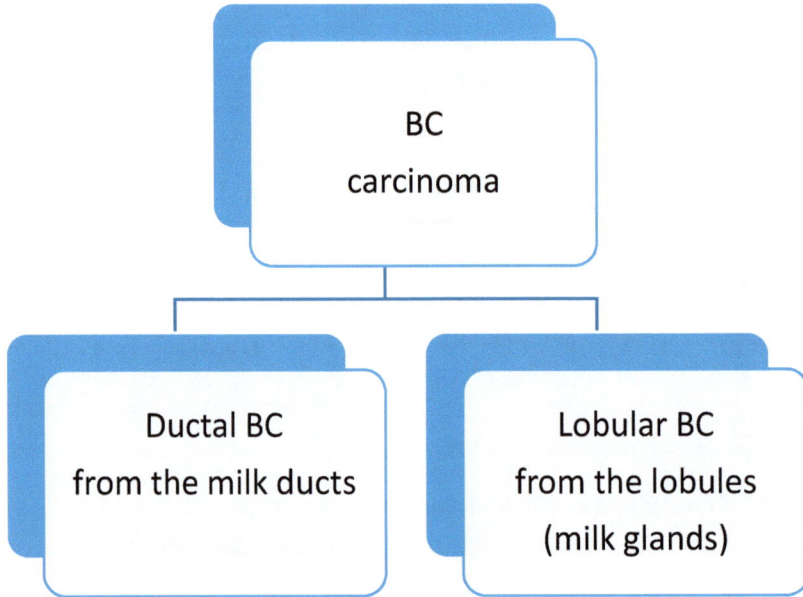

Fig. (1). Origins of breast cancer (BC).

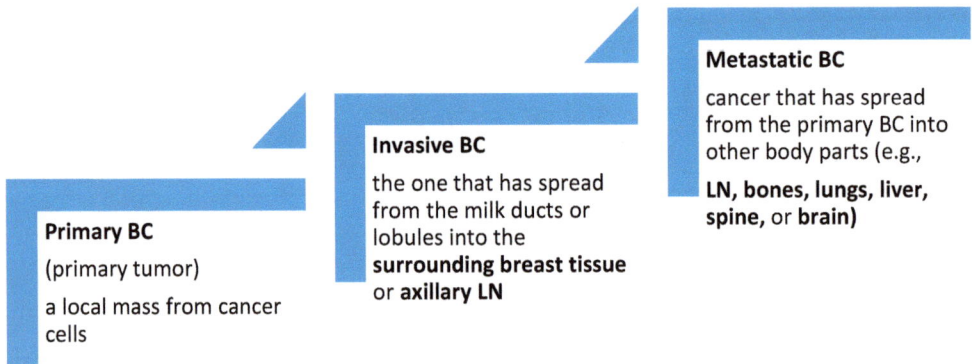

Fig. (2). Spread of breast cancer (BC). LN, lymph nodes.

Cancer that has spread to a nearby body part, such as the axillary lymph nodes, is called a **local metastasis**. It might be referred to as a **local/regional disease, invasive,** or **locally advanced.**

Cancer that has spread to a body part far from the primary tumor is called **distant metastasis**. BC can metastasize to the **bones, lungs, liver, spine,** or **brain**.

HOW DO YOU CHOOSE AN OPTIMAL TREATMENT PLAN FOR A WOMAN WITH TRIPLE-NEGATIVE BREAST CANCER (TNBC)?

In general, choosing a treatment plan that is optimal for a given woman with BC requires (in addition to standard diagnostic medical work-up) **testing for estrogen, progesterone**, and **HER2 (ER, PR,** and **HER2) receptors** since these important components of hormonal and molecular signalization pathways contribute to the growth and spread of BC.

In the case of **TNBC,** receptors for estrogen, progesterone, and HER2 are not found, meaning that the BC cells have tested negative for estrogen hormone, progesterone hormone, and HER2 receptors. Therefore, since there are:

• No estrogen or progesterone **hormone receptors (HR)**, **endocrine therapy (ET) is not an option,**

• No HER2 receptors, **anti-HER2-targeted therapy is not an option**.

As a result, without any of these receptors, TNBC is more challenging to treat, and usually, **systemic therapy** is used, including multiple lines, which are given:

• Until TNBC progression occurs or

• Unacceptable toxic effects develop (that create serious health risks for a patient).

Usually, TNBC

• Has a more **aggressive behavior,**

• Is more **likely to metastasize,** and

• Often returns after treatment - **resistance** develops when TNBC stops responding to therapy.

In consequence, selecting a treatment plan that is most appropriate for a given woman with TNBC is difficult, and requires continuous, effective communication, and cooperation between a patient and her Treatment Team members.

What is the Role of Monitoring in Patients with TNBC?

The main goal of monitoring is to determine whether or not treatment provides benefits (keeping BC stable), what adverse effects are present, and how effective is their control (*e.g.,* watching for symptoms caused by BC, including pain from bone metastases).

Monitoring usually includes

• physical exams.

• laboratory blood tests.

• radiology imaging scans, and

• tumor, lymph nodes', or tissue testing (*e.g.*, biopsy).

Monitoring has been used to determine if BC is responding to treatment, or if it is resistant, and progressing.

For instance, if the bone disease is present, a patient often needs to be treated with preparations of calcium, vitamin D, and either denosumab, zoledronic acid, or pamidronate.

Also, a stomatology consultation prior to starting any of the bone-targeted agents is recommended. If an anticancer treatment is not helping any more, and it is making a patient feel worse, then it might be the moment to consider its termination, while continuing palliative and supportive care.

What are some Recommended or Preferred Options in the Systemic Therapy for HER2-negative BC?

Recommended or preferred options in the systemic therapy for **HER2-negative BC** often include different combinations of pharmacotherapy agents (Tables **1** and **2**).

Table 1. Recommended or preferred options in the systemic therapy for **HER2-negative BC**.

Recommended Pharmacotherapy Options	Pharmacotherapy Agents
Anthracyclines	doxorubicin or liposomal doxorubicin
Taxanes	paclitaxel
Anti-metabolites	capecitabine or gemcitabine
Microtubule inhibitors	vinorelbine or eribulin
For *BRCA1* or *BRCA2* mutations - PARP inhibitors	olaparib or talazoparib
For *BRCA1* or *BRCA2* mutation - platinum agents	carboplatin or cisplatin
For NTRK fusion	larotrectinib or entrectinib
For MSI-H/dMMR	pembrolizumab
For PD-L1 expression of more than 1% - ICI	atezolizumab + albumin-bound paclitaxel
Other options	Cyclophosphamide
	Docetaxel
	Albumin-bound paclitaxel
	Epirubicin
	Ixabepilone

Table 2. Additional combinations therapies used in some cases of **HER2-negative BC**.

Combination Therapy	Pharmacotherapy Agents
AC	doxorubicin + cyclophosphamide
EC	epirubicin + cyclophosphamide
CMF	cyclophosphamide + methotrexate + fluorouracil
GT	gemcitabine + paclitaxel
Other options	gemcitabine + carboplatin
	paclitaxel + bevacizumab
	carboplatin + paclitaxel or albumin-bound paclitaxel
	docetaxel + capecitabine

Multiple lines of systemic therapy are often given until BC progression or unacceptable toxicity (a serious risk to a woman's overall health) occurs.

How BC Progression can be Manifested?

BC progression can be manifested by various symptoms experienced by patients and changes or new abnormal findings documented by different tests (Fig. **3**).

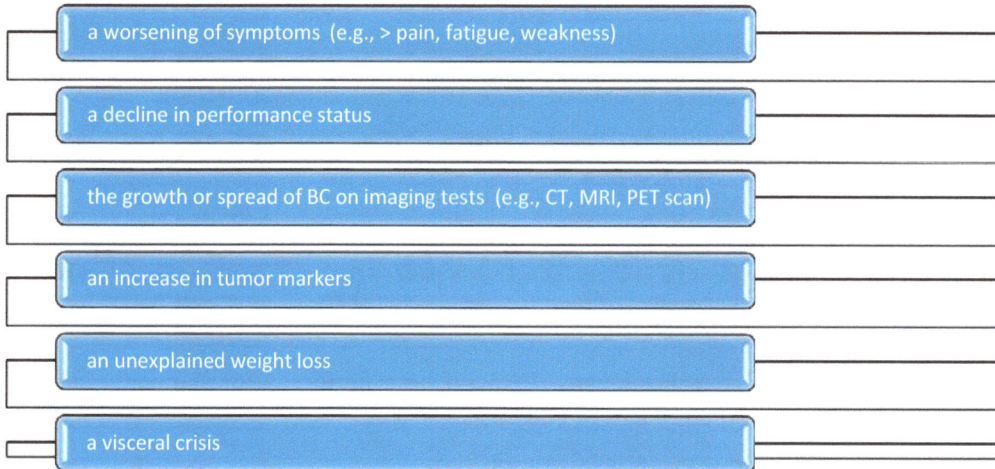

- a worsening of symptoms (e.g., > pain, fatigue, weakness)
- a decline in performance status
- the growth or spread of BC on imaging tests (e.g., CT, MRI, PET scan)
- an increase in tumor markers
- an unexplained weight loss
- a visceral crisis

Fig. (3). Examples of subjective and objective manifestations of BC progression. BC, breast cancer; CT, MRI, PET.

WHAT ARE THE MAIN TOPICS THAT A PATIENT WITH BC AND HER PHYSICIAN NEED TO DISCUSS BEFORE CONSIDERING AN APPLICATION OF THE NEW LINE OF SYSTEMIC THERAPY?

Before a new line of systemic therapy is applied, a patient with BC and her physician need to discuss the patient's individual condition from her personal point of view, in agreement with medical recommendations for her management (Fig. **4**).

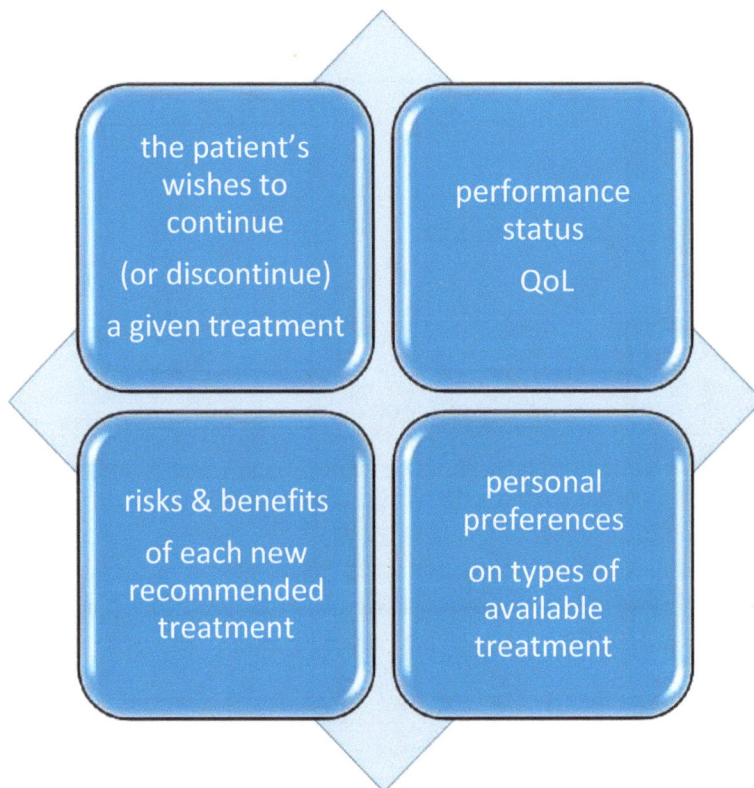

Fig. (4). Points to consider before a new line of systemic therapy for BC is applied, during a discussion between a patient and her physician. BC, breast cancer; QoL, quality of life.

After multiple lines of systemic therapy, it might be time to consider stopping systemic therapy and focusing on supportive care, especially when

• the possible adverse effects (AE) of continuing with another line of systemic therapy would most probably outweigh the benefits.

• a patient strongly prefers palliative care.

What are the most Important Steps in Shared Decision-making?

In shared decision-making, a patient and her doctor share medical information, analyze the diagnostic and therapeutic options and agree on a certain treatment plan (Fig. **5**).

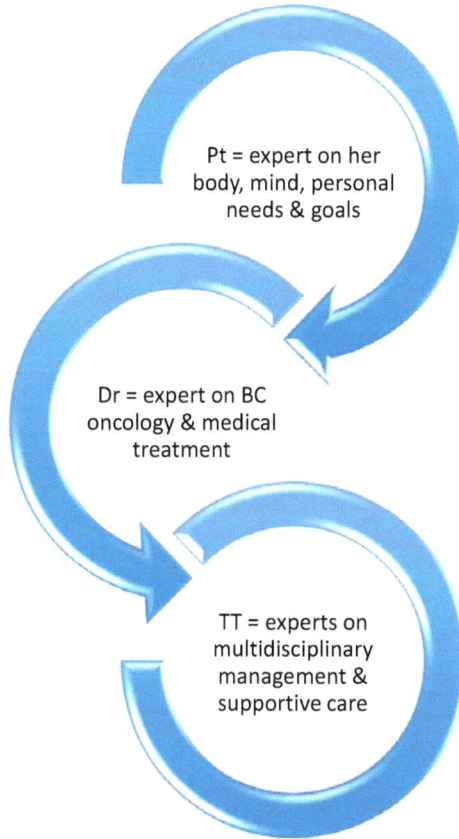

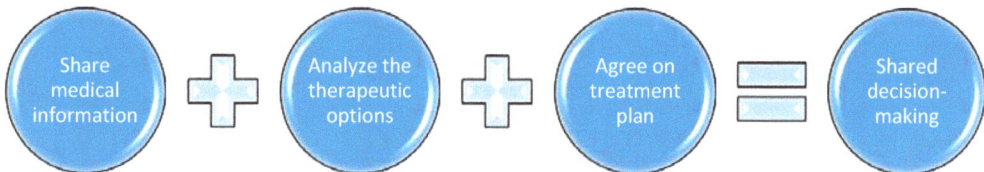

Fig. (5). Shared decision-making between a patient with BC and her doctor. BC, breast cancer; Pt, patient; Dr, doctor; TT, therapeutic team.

Such decisions should consist of an exchange between a patient's personal needs and her doctor's professional medical expertise.

WHICH FACTORS USUALLY PLAY A ROLE IN THE PERSONAL OR SHARED DECISION-MAKING OF PATIENTS WITH BC?

A patient's opinions, beliefs, and feelings about different types of therapies, their complications, side effects, and their impact on daily functioning are usually very important in personal or shared decision-making (Fig. **6**).

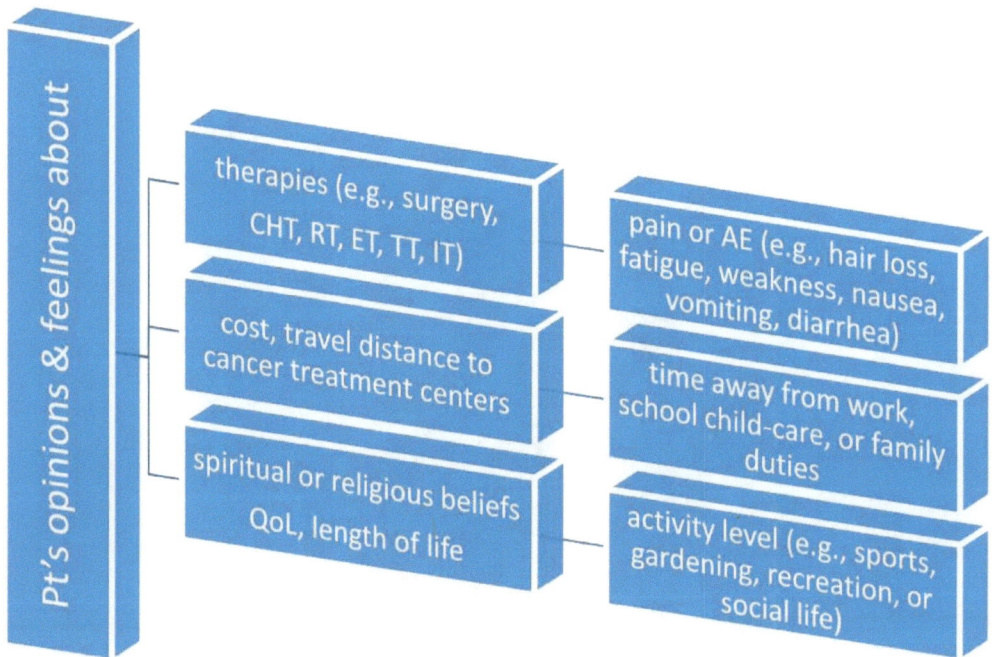

Fig. (6). Common factors which can play a role in personal or shared decision-making. AE, adverse effects; CHT, chemotherapy; RT, radiotherapy; ET, endocrine therapy; TT, target therapy; IT, immunotherapy; QoL, quality of life;.

It's important for every woman with BC to feel comfortable with the anticancer treatment of her choice. This starts with having an open conversation between a patient and her doctor. During this honest conversation, a woman should not be afraid to clearly express what she expects or wants from a particular anticancer treatment approach (Fig. **7**).

IN WHICH WAY A SECOND OPINION CAN BE HELPFUL FOR A WOMAN DIAGNOSED WITH BC?

It is natural and appropriate to wish to begin anticancer immediately. However, it may be prudent to have another oncology expert review a patient's clinical scenario and test results, in order to express an independent professional, second opinion in the form of a proposed treatment plan.

Preparation for the second opinion involves

• verification rules on second opinions with an insurance company.

• copies of all medical records to be sent for a second opinion.

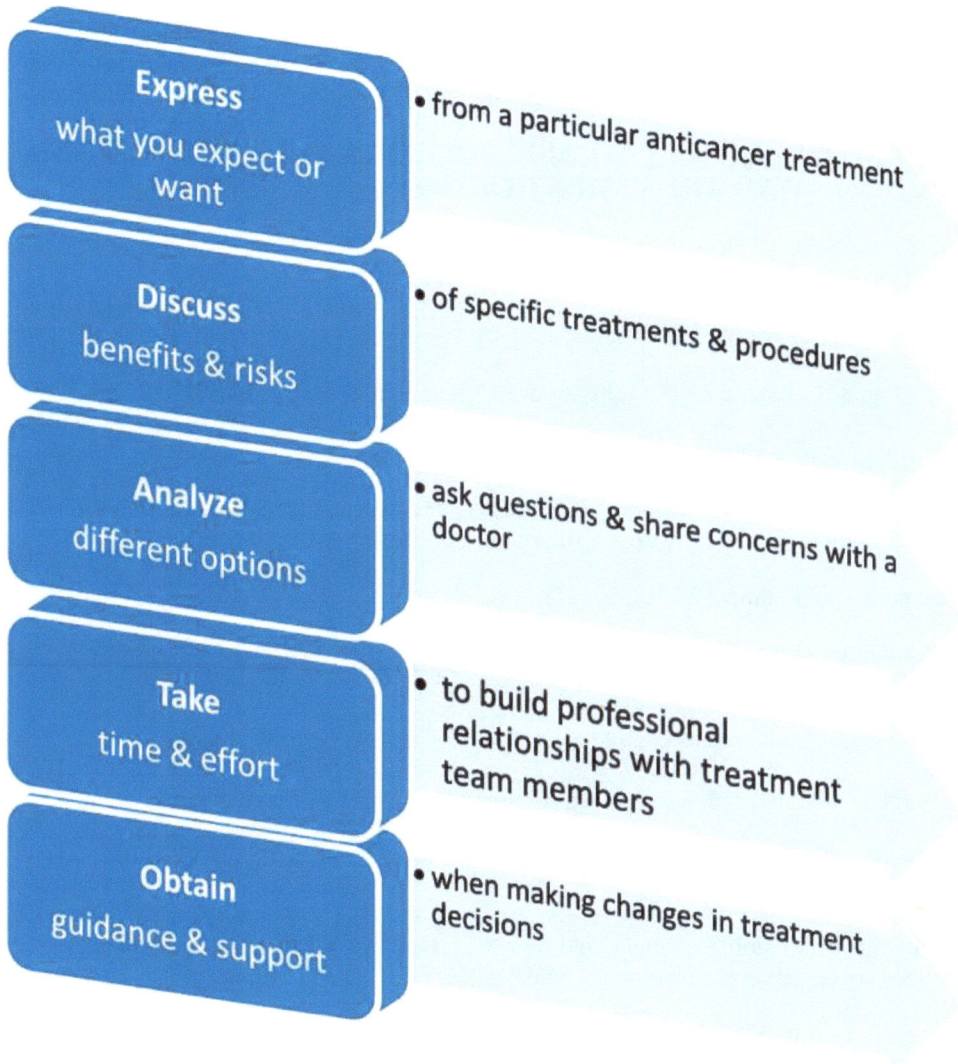

Express
what you expect or want
• from a particular anticancer treatment

Discuss
benefits & risks
• of specific treatments & procedures

Analyze
different options
• ask questions & share concerns with a doctor

Take
time & effort
• to build professional relationships with treatment team members

Obtain
guidance & support
• when making changes in treatment decisions

Fig. (7). EDATO – an approach to shared decision-making while discussing any anticancer treatment option.

WHAT ARE THE MAIN BENEFITS OF ATTENDING SUPPORT GROUPS?

Support groups are useful since they usually involve a broad spectrum of patients at different stages of anticancer treatment (*e.g.*, from women newly diagnosed with BC to the ones who completed treatment). This allows us to ask many "burning" questions and exchange experiences in a friendly and stimulating atmosphere.

If a given hospital, cancer treatment center, or community doesn't offer support groups for patients with BC, such services can be available on the websites (listed under references).

POSSIBLE QUESTIONS TO ASK DOCTORS ABOUT BC DIAGNOSIS, PROGNOSIS, AND TREATMENT OPTIONS

Helpful for making treatment decisions, considering a patient's goals and expectations from various treatments.

1. General questions about BC diagnosis & prognosis (Fig. **8**).

2. "Decalogue" of practical questions about BC treatment options (Fig. **9**).

3. Specific questions about various treatments for BC (Fig. **10**).

AE, adverse effects; RT, radiation therapy; CHT, chemo therapy; ET, endocrine therapy; TT, target therapy; IT, immune therapy; QoL, quality of life;

4. Questions about clinical trials (Fig. **11**).

5. Questions about the side effects of BC treatment (Fig. **12**).

• Making treatment decisions is a patient's choice, on the basis of professional medical recommendations, in an individual clinical & personal context.

• It should be kept in mind that supportive care will always be provided.

• The therapeutic modalities for patients with invasive or metastatic BC are often complex and diversified.

• Usually, the evaluation, treatment, and follow-up recommendations in the standard oncology guidelines are based on the results of clinical trials.

• However, to optimize the treatment of BC (*e.g.*, maximize cure or minimize toxicity), participation in prospective clinical trials will allow patients in different clinical situations to receive the most appropriate anticancer treatment.

• This might also contribute to better treatment outcomes in the future.

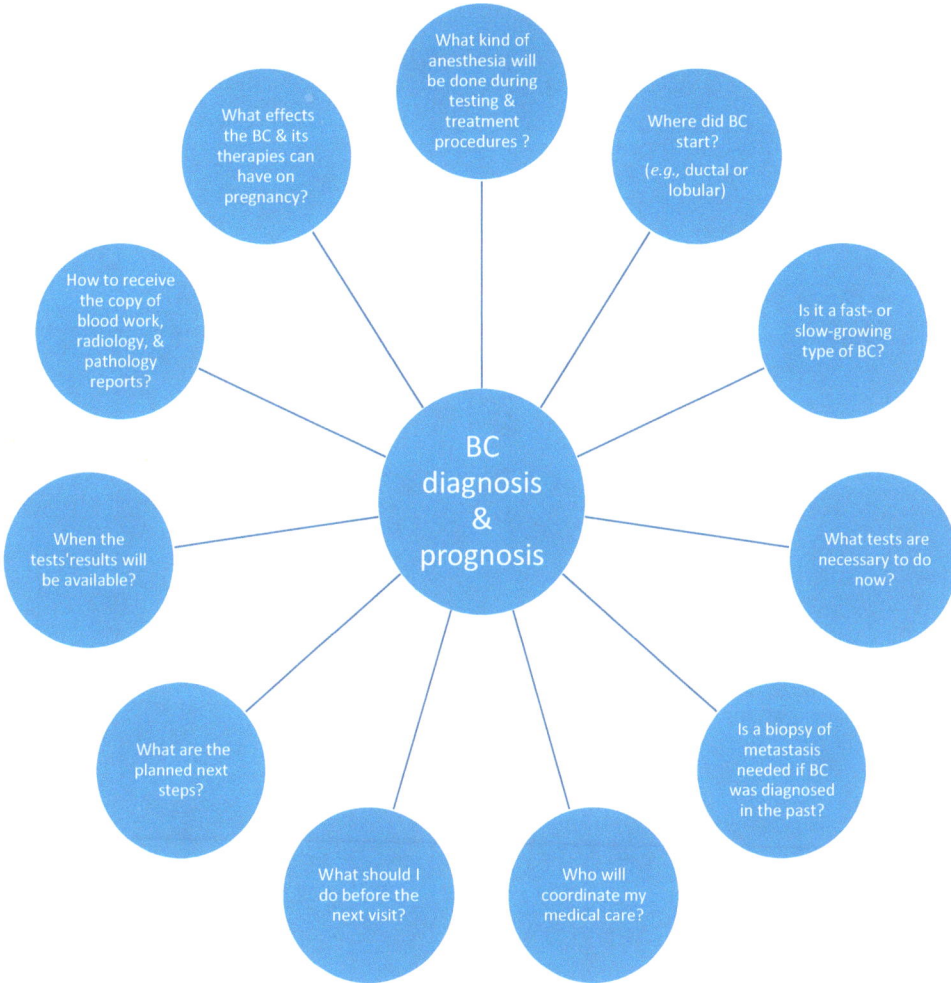

Fig. (8). Helpful general questions to ask about BC diagnosis & prognosis. BC, breast cancer.

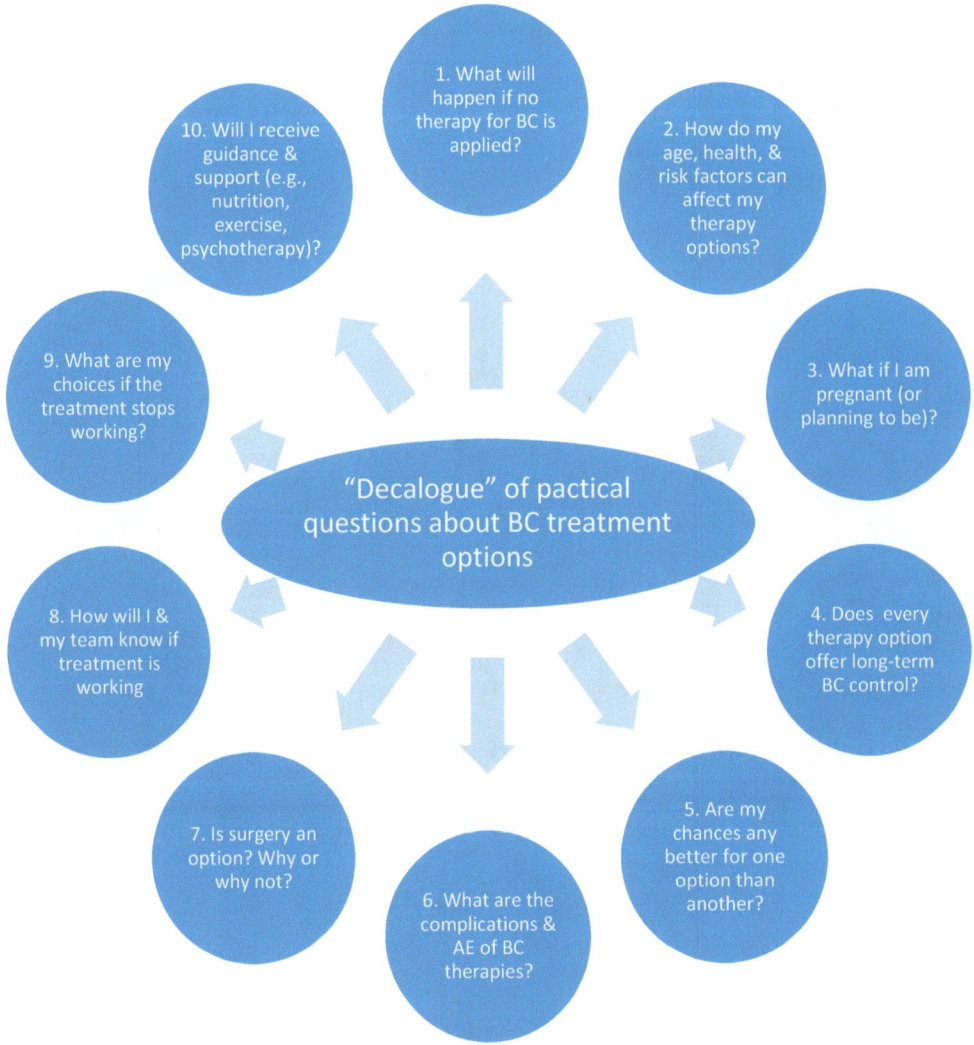

Fig. (9). Practical questions to ask about possible BC treatment options. BC, breast cancer.

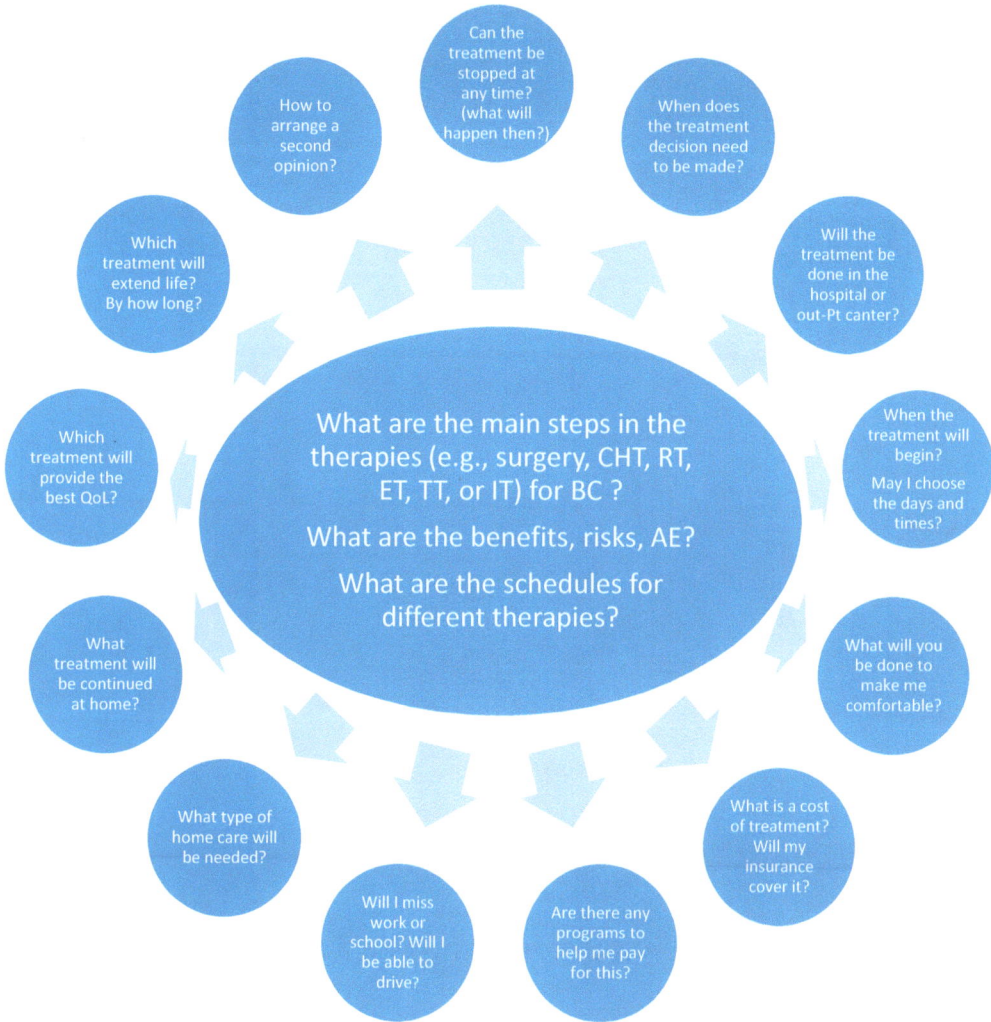

Fig. (10). Specific questions to ask about various treatments for BC. BC, breast cancer.

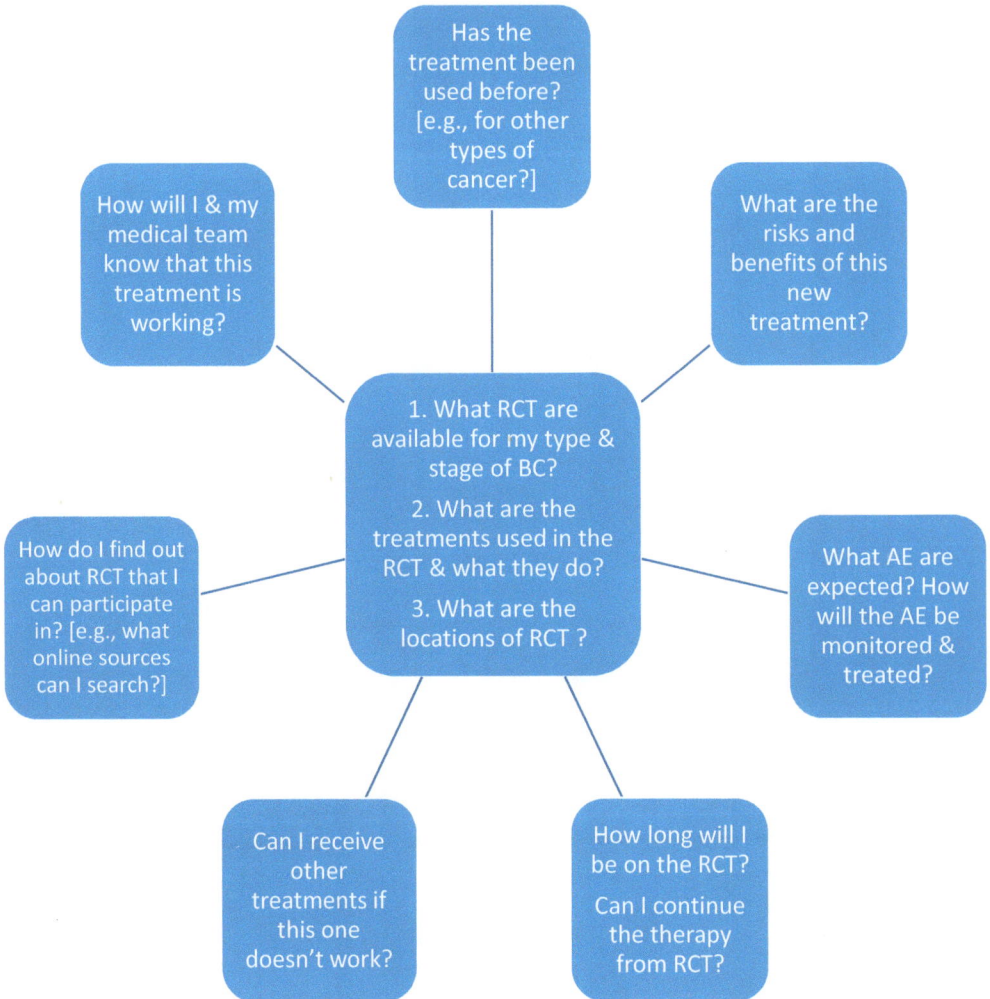

Fig. (11). Questions to ask about clinical trials. RCT, randomized control trial; BC, breast cancer; AE, adverse effects;.

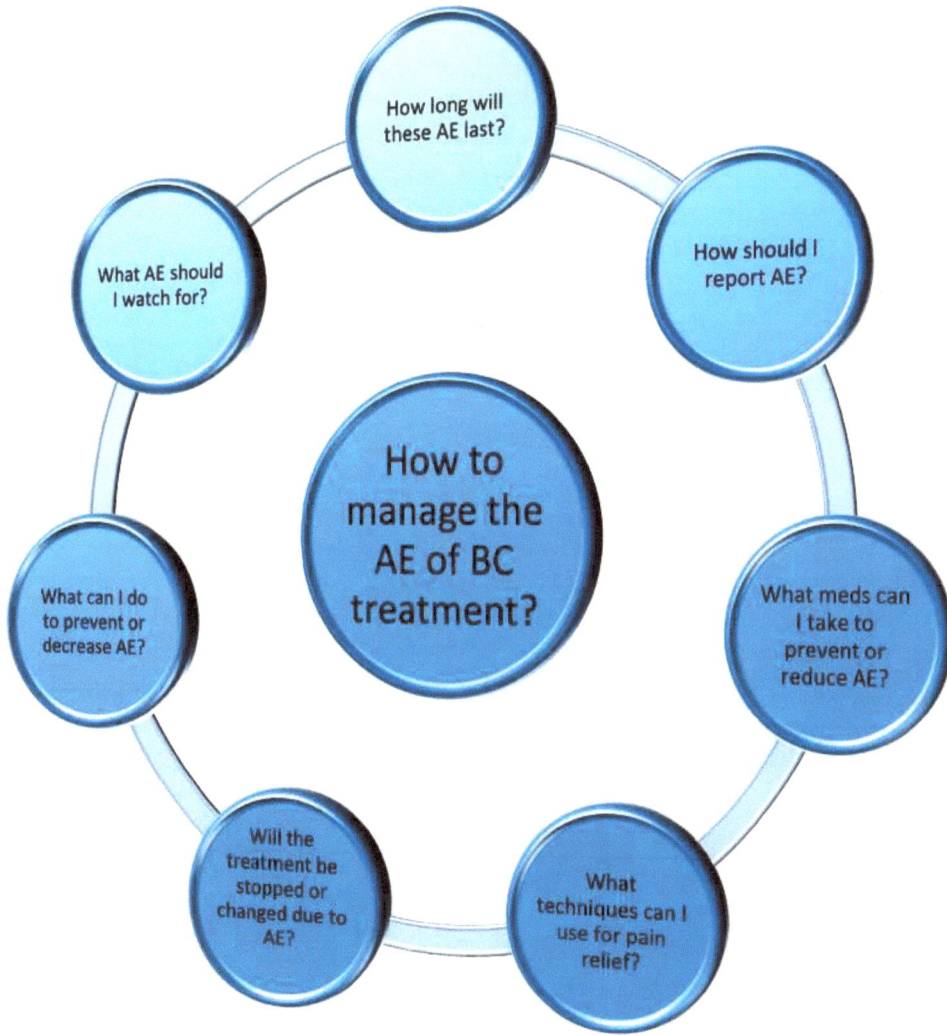

Fig. (12). Questions to ask about side effects of BC treatment; AE, adverse effects; BC, breast cancer; meds, medications;.

REFERENCES & RESOURCES

www.cancer.org/treatment/understanding-your-diagnosis/what-is-cancer.html

www.cancer.org/cancer/breast-cancer/non-cancerous-breast-conditions.html

www.cancer.org/cancer/breast-cancer/understanding-a-breast-cancer diagnosis/breast-cance-
-hormone-receptor-status.html

www.cancer.org/cancer/breast-cancer/understanding-a-breast-cancer diagnosis/breast-cance--her2-status.html

www.cancer.org/cancer/breast-cancer/understanding-a-breast-cancer diagnosis/breast-cance--grades.html

American Cancer Society – www.cancer.org/cancer/breast-cancer

Breast Cancer Alliance – www.breastcanceralliance.org

Breastcancer.org - breastcancer.org

Breast Cancer Trials - breastcancertrials.org

DiepCFoundation - diepcfoundation.org

FORCE: Facing Our Risk of Cancer Empowered - facingourrisk.org

Living Beyond Breast Cancer (LBBC) - lbbc.org

National Cancer Institute (NCI) - cancer.gov/types/breast

Sharsheret - sharsheret.org

Young Survival Coalition (YSC) - youngsurvival.org

Information for Finding a Clinical Trial

• Search the National Institutes of Health (NIH) database for clinical trials

(*e.g.*, whom to contact, and how to enroll).

Look for an open clinical trial for your specific type of cancer - Go to ClinicalTrials.gov.

• The National Cancer Institute's Cancer Information Service (CIS) provides up-to-date information on clinical trials (call 1.800.4.CANCER (800.422.6237) or go to cancer.gov.)

HELPFUL MEDICAL TERMINOLOGY

Aromatase Inhibitor (AI) - a medication that lowers the level of hormone estrogen in the body.

Axillary Lymph Node (ALN) - a lymph node located near the armpit.

Bilateral oophorectomy - a surgical procedure that removes both ovaries.

Biopsy - removal of small amounts of tissue or fluid to be tested for disease (*e.g.*, BC).

Cancer stage - rating of the growth and spread of neoplastic tumors.

Carcinoma - cancer that starts in cells that form the lining of organs and structures in the body.

Clinical trial – a research study on a test or treatment to evaluate its safety (*e.g.*, any possible side effects) and efficacy (*e.g.*, how well it works for the treatment of disease, such as BC).

Complete Blood Count (CBC) - a lab test that includes the numbers of blood cells (BC) (*e.g.*, WBC – white BC, or leukocytes, RBC – red BC, or erythrocytes, and platelets)

Computed Tomography (CT) –an imaging radiology test that uses x-rays from many angles to make a picture of the inside of the body organs and tissues.

Connective tissue - supporting and binding tissue that surrounds other organs and tissues.

Contrast - a substance put into the body to make clearer pictures during imaging tests.

Duct - a tube in the breast that drains breast milk.

Endocrine Therapy (ET) or Hormone Therapy (HT) - a treatment that stops making or inhibits the action of hormones in the body.

Estrogen (E) - a hormone that develops female body traits (*e.g.*, breast).

Estrogen Receptor (ER) - a protein inside of cells that binds with estrogen.

Fertility - the ability to become pregnant and have a child.

Genetic counseling – a discussion with a medical expert about the risk for a disease (*e.g.*, TNBC) caused by changes in genes (*e.g.*, *BRCA1/2*).

Hereditary breast cancer - Breast cancer (BC) that was likely caused by abnormal genes passed down from mother to daughter.

Hormone – a chemical in the body that activates cells or organs.

Hormone Receptor–negative (HR-) cancer - cancer cells that don't use hormones to grow or spread.

Hormone Receptor–positive (HR+) cancer - cancer cells that use hormones to grow or spread.

Human Epidermal Growth Factor Receptor 2 (HER2) - a protein on the edge of a cell that sends signals for the cell to grow.

Immunohistochemistry (IHC) - a lab test of cancer cells to find specific cell traits involved in abnormal cell growth.

Invasive breast cancer - cancer cells have grown into the supporting tissue of the breast.

Kinase inhibitor – an anticancer agent that blocks the transfer of phosphates.

Liver function test - a test that measures chemicals made or processed by the liver.

Lobule - a gland in the breast that makes breast milk.

Luteinizing Hormone-Releasing Hormone (LHRH) - a hormone in the brain that helps control the production of estrogen by the ovaries.

Lymph - a clear body fluid that contains white blood cells.

Lymph Node (LN) – a small clusters of specialized disease-fighting cells located throughout the body.

Magnetic Resonance Imaging (MRI) - a test that uses radio waves and powerful magnets to make pictures of the internal organs and tissues of the body.

Medical oncologist - a doctor who's an expert in anticancer pharmacologic therapies.

Menopause - the interval of time in a woman's lifecycle, when menstrual periods end.

Metastasis - the spread of cancer beyond the breast and nearby lymph nodes to distant sites like bone, lung, liver, or brain.

Mutation - an abnormal change in the genetic instructions in cells for making new cells and controlling their behavior.

Noninvasive breast cancer - cancer cells have not grown into the supporting tissue of the breast.

Ovarian ablation – a group of methods used to stop the ovaries from making hormones.

Ovarian suppression - a group of methods used to lower the amount of hormones produced by the ovaries.

Pathologist - a doctor who's an expert in testing cells and tissue to find disease.

Performance status - a rating of general health.

Premenopause - the state of having regular menstrual periods.

Positron Emission Tomography (PET) – the use of radioactive material to see the shape and function of different body parts.

Postmenopause - the state of the end of menstrual periods.

Primary tumor - the first mass of cancer cells in the body.

Progesterone – a female hormone that is involved in sexual development, menstrual periods, and pregnancy.

Prognosis - the expected pattern and outcome of a disease based on laboratory and radiology tests.

Radiation Therapy (RT) - the use of high-energy rays to destroy cancer cells.

Selective Estrogen Receptor Down-Regulator (SERD) - anticancer agent that blocks the effect of estrogen.

Selective Estrogen Receptor Modulators (SERM) - anticancer agent that blocks the effect of estrogen.

Side effect or Adverse effect (AE) - an unhealthy physical or emotional response to treatment.

Supportive care – a treatment for the symptoms or health conditions caused by cancer or cancer therapy.

Systemic therapy – a treatment of cancer throughout the body.

Triple-Negative Breast Cancer (TNBC) – a breast cancer that is not hormone-positive or HER2-positive.

SUBJECT INDEX

A

Acid 81
  arachidonic 81
  eicosapentaenoic 81
Actions 80, 201
  intense therapeutic 201
  pro-inflammatory cytokine's 80
Acute myeloid leukemia 31
ADP-ribose 5, 11, 31, 54, 56, 59, 65, 66, 67, 104
Agents 9, 31, 61, 84, 164, 175
  anesthetic 175
  anti-HER2 61
  anti-infective 31
  chemotherapeutic 84
  environmental toxic 9
  genomically-targeted 164
  organohalogenated 9
Aggressive malignancy 27, 192
AKT inhibitors 34
Alanine transaminase 31
Analyses 27, 39, 41, 57, 156, 161, 196, 199, 203, 209
  protein expression 57
Angiotensin-converting enzyme (ACE) 85, 86, 88, 89
  inhibitors (ACEIs) 85, 88, 89
Angiotensin receptor 85, 86, 87, 88, 89
  blockers (ARBs) 85, 88, 89
  neprilysin inhibitor (ARNIs) 86, 87
Anthracyclines 24, 27
Antibody drug conjugate (ADCs) 22, 25, 27, 33, 35, 54, 56, 58, 59, 65, 66, 67, 71, 73, 74
Anticancer therapies 83, 84, 175
  cardiotoxic 83, 84
  conventional 175
Aspartate transaminase 31
Autonomic nervous system 118, 119, 120, 121, 122, 123

B

Basal-like immune activated (BLIA) 23
BDNF gene 81
Bone metastases 45
Brain 31, 81, 85
  derived neurotrophic factor (BDNF) 81
  metastasis 31
  natriuretic peptide (BNP) 85
BRCA 62, 67, 73, 103
  gene mutation 62, 67, 73
  somatic 103
BRCA-mutated 66, 67
  cell death 67
  HER2-negative metastatic breast cancer 66
BRCA mutations 10, 55, 62, 65, 67, 68, 74
  somatic 55, 67, 68, 74
BRCA2 7, 11, 55, 62, 66, 74, 156, 162
  gene mutations 66
  genes 7, 55, 162
  mutations 11, 62, 74, 156
Breast 5, 7, 9, 11, 15, 33, 78
  cancer gene 5, 7, 11
  magnetic resonance imaging 15
  tissue 9
  tumors 33, 78

C

Cancer 7, 26, 27, 33, 55, 62, 97, 156, 158, 164, 166, 168, 177, 194, 206, 214
  aggressive 27, 164, 166, 168, 194, 206
  epithelial 33
  lung 156
  ovarian 7, 55, 62
  progression 97
  refractory 158
  related symptoms 177, 214
  stem cell (CSC) 26
Carcinogenesis 158
Cardiac 82, 83, 84, 85, 86, 88, 89, 92
  arrhythmias 82, 83

dysfunction 83
magnetic resonance (CMR) 83, 84, 86, 88, 89
muscle fibers 85
resynchronization therapy (CRT) 86, 88
risk stratification 92
Cardiogenic shock 87
Cardiomyocytes 85
Cardiooncologist 88
Cardiopulmonary fitness 90
Cardiotoxicity 82, 83, 84, 86, 87, 88, 89, 90, 92
developing 82
profiles 83
therapy-induced 92
Cardiovascular diseases 8, 10, 11, 79, 85, 88, 124
Central nervous system (CNS) 58, 120
Cerebrospinal fluid 40
Chemotherapy 23, 43, 44, 54, 56, 59, 65, 66, 77, 78, 79, 80, 82, 88, 89, 156, 169, 170
adjuvant 23
standard cytotoxic 156
traditional 54
Chest X-ray 88
Chronic diseases 78, 85, 129, 130, 135, 198, 199, 201, 204, 209
Clarithromycin 30
CNS metastases 58
Cognitive 77, 78, 81, 82, 143, 145, 146, 151
defusion 143, 145, 146, 151
dysfunction 77, 78, 81, 82
Comparison 29, 215
of pembrolizumab 29
sustain 215
Compassion 129, 130, 136, 206, 211
fatigue 206, 211
meditation 129, 130, 136
Complementary 82, 114, 166, 167, 170, 174, 176, 177, 178
and integrative medicine (CIM) 82, 166, 167, 174, 176, 177, 178
therapies 114, 170
Complete responses 11, 26, 48, 69, 103, 104, 159
pathologic 11, 69
pathological 26, 48, 103, 104
Constipation 114
Conventional oncology management 169
Coronary heart disease (CHD) 82, 83, 85, 122

Corticosteroids 28, 29
Cyclin-dependent kinase (CDK) 44, 58

D

Damage, mitochondrial 80
Damaged DNA repair machinery 35
Death 86, 161
cardiac 86
tumor cell 161
Depression 77, 78, 81, 175, 181, 182, 183, 186, 191, 192, 193, 194, 196
Deprivation, chronic estrogen 61
Diabetes mellitus 23
Diagnosis, metastatic 59
Diarrhea 28, 29, 30, 31
Diseases 28, 29, 68, 83, 87, 88, 109, 132, 133, 135, 140, 149, 162, 192
chronic psychophysical 192
coronary artery 88
interstitial lung 28, 29
kidney 87
malignant 109, 149
mental 132, 135
metastatic 68
neoplastic 162
neurological 133
peripheral vascular 83
psychosomatic 140
Disorders 23, 83, 109, 114, 124, 131, 140, 170, 194
gastrointestinal 124
mental 109, 140, 170
metabolic 23
neuropsychiatric 131
psychiatric 114
thromboembolic 83
Distress thermometer (DT) 108, 111, 112, 115
DNA 40, 55, 161
damage response (DDR) 55
methylation 161
mutations 161
DNA breaks 8, 32, 67
double-stranded 67
irreparable 32
repairing 8
single-strand 67
DNA repair 62, 162
deficits 62
pathways 162

Dyslipidemia 10

E

Echocardiography 83, 84, 89
Effective communication techniques 173
Effects 85, 124
  compromising anticancer 85
  mental health 124
Electrolytes 31, 86
Endocrine-disrupting chemicals (EDC) 9
Endothelial dysfunction 90
Epidermal growth factor receptor 5, 25
ERI tumor material 155
Estrogen stimulation 61
Expression, protein 57

F

Factors 2, 8, 12, 14, 15, 23, 25, 31, 34, 57, 60,
    81, 99, 161, 162, 164, 169, 177, 187,
    191
  anti-vascular endothelial growth 34
  brain-derived neurotrophic 81
  dietary 14
  economic 99
  environmental 23, 162
  genetic 81, 162
  socio-environmental 2
  socio-epidemiological 161, 164
  transcription 25
Failure, ovarian 82
Fatigue 28, 29, 30, 31, 68, 79, 81, 90, 124,
    136, 175
  decreased cancer-related 175
Fatty acid desaturase 81
FDA-approved 42, 55
  DNA damage response 55
  test 42
  therapies 42
Financial 186, 208
  compensation 208
  difficulties 186
FISH- amplification 73
Functional 129, 131, 150, 184, 214
  analytic psychotherapy (FAP) 150, 214
  magnetic resonance imaging 129, 131, 184

G

Gemcitabine 30, 67, 69
  doublet therapy 69
Gene(s) 2, 4, 7, 25, 32, 42, 92, 105
  driver 105
  mutations 7
  tumor suppressor 4, 25, 32
Genetic 7, 32, 42, 45, 48, 74, 81, 82, 91, 161
  alterations 42, 161
  biomarkers 91
  mutations 7, 32, 45, 48, 74
  polymorphisms 81, 82
Germline 31, 32, 33, 35, 56, 67, 69, 74, 103,
    104
  BRCA1 74
  harbored 33
Germline BRCA 32, 67, 70, 74
  mutations 67, 70
Germline mutations 55, 66, 67, 156
  pathogenic BRCA1 156
Gestational diabetes 23
Glycated hemoglobin 88
Glycoprotein 33, 56
  transmembrane 56
Growth 32, 33, 56
  malignant cell 32
  regulating cellular 56
  stimulating signal 33
Guideline-directed medical therapy (GDMT)
    86, 88

H

Headache 28, 29, 30
Healing processes 119
Health 8, 15, 59, 109, 114, 115, 129, 130, 175,
    178, 183, 194, 208, 211, 215
  conditions, somatic 175
  crises 183
  insurance 8, 15
  mental 208, 211, 215
  problems, mental 130, 194
  services, mental 114, 115
Healthcare 1, 10, 98, 99, 172, 203, 204, 206,
    212, 215
  disparities 1
  integrated 203, 204
  services 203

system 98, 99, 172, 204, 212, 215
Heart disease 83, 85, 129
    coronary 83, 85
Heart failure (HF) 82, 83, 84, 85, 86, 87, 88,
    92
Hemochromatosis 86
Hemodynamic compromise 87
Hepatic metastases 58, 60
HER2 45, 61, 71, 72
    gene amplification 71
    heterogeneity 72
    immunohistochemistry 72
    intratumoral heterogeneity 71
    mutations 45
    protein overexpression 71
    signaling pathways 61
    targeted therapy 61
Heterogeneity 15, 59, 60, 102, 103
    genetic 60
    intratumor 59, 60, 102
Hormone 9, 80
    melatonin 80
    replacement therapy 9
Human epidermal growth factor receptor 1, 2,
    4, 5, 22, 24, 39, 42, 53, 54, 56, 65, 66,
    102, 104
Hypertension, pulmonary 83

I

Immune 28, 29, 34
    mediated pneumonitis 28, 29
    tumor surveillance system 34
Immunohistochemistry 27, 72
Immunomodulatory 3, 4, 5, 23, 25, 103
Immunotherapy 11, 65, 66, 68, 69, 70, 73, 74,
    77, 78, 91
Inflammatory cytokines 85
Inhibitors 39, 42, 55, 56
    aromatase 39, 42, 55
    tyrosine kinase 56
Injury, cardiomyocyte 85
Insomnia 81, 122, 124, 193
Insulin resistance dysglycemia 10
Integrative oncology management 183

L

Ligand-binding domain (LBD) 26

Liver metastases 58
Luminal androgen receptor (LAR) 5, 23, 25,
    26, 103
Lymphedema 77, 78, 80, 81, 91, 175

M

Machine learning 134
Magnetic resonance imaging (MRI) 15, 83,
    113, 129, 131, 184
Malignant tumor dynamics 40
Mammalian target 34, 58
Mammography 9
Medicine, personalized 77, 91, 96, 97, 101,
    105, 157
Menopause 12, 82
    chemotherapy-induced 82
Meta-cognitive therapy (MCT) 142, 143
Metabolic 2, 10, 23
    comorbidities 2
    complications 10
    dysfunctions 23
    syndrome 10, 23
Metabolism 8, 81
    fatty acid 81
    lipid 8
Metabolomics 96, 97, 100
Metals, heavy 10, 15
Metastasis 2, 58
Metastatic lesions 43, 54, 60, 61
Mindfulness-based 139, 142, 143, 151, 175,
    182, 213, 214
    cognitive therapy (MBCT) 139, 142, 143,
        151, 175, 213, 214
    stress reduction (MBSR) 175, 182
Monoclonal antibody 56
Monotherapy 32, 74
Multifactorial risk factors 6
Multigene assays 60
Mutations 33, 39, 40, 44, 56, 61, 104
    activating 33, 56, 61
    genomic 39, 40
    pathogenic 44
    somatic 104
Myelodysplastic syndromes 31
Myocardial 84, 85, 86, 88
    fibrosis 84
    infarction 85, 88
Myocarditis 86

N

Neuropathy 80, 92
  refractory 80
Neutropenia 28, 29, 30, 31
Neutropenic fever 31
Nucleotide polymorphisms, single 82

O

Olaparib 32, 67, 68
  monotherapy 32
  therapy 67, 68
Oncology care, palliative 166, 167
Oxidative-stress-associated mitochondrial
    dysfunction 80

P

Parasympathetic nervous system (PNS) 118,
    120, 121, 125, 126, 130
Peripheral 77, 78, 80, 83, 92, 175
  neuropathy (PN) 77, 78, 80, 92, 175
  vascular disease (PVD) 83
Personalized 40, 48
  ctDNA assay 48
  oncology management 40
Pneumonitis 30
Polymerase 5, 11, 31, 44, 54, 56, 59, 65, 66,
    67, 103, 104
  chain reaction 44
  enzyme poly adenosine diphosphate-ribose
    103
Progesterone production 82
Protein(s) 5, 7, 31, 33, 56, 58
  kinase 5, 31, 33, 56, 58
  tumor suppressor 7
Psychological disorder 194

Q

Quadruple-negative breast cancer (QNBC) 22,
    23, 24, 25, 27, 34, 35

R

Rehabilitation 13, 89, 92
  cardiac 92

therapists 92
Relapse, metastatic 48
Repair DNA damages 7, 11, 67, 161
Risk, cardiac 92

S

Single nucleotide polymorphisms (SNPs) 82
Soil pollutions 10, 15
Stress 90, 101, 108, 118, 119, 120, 121, 123,
    124, 136, 183, 195
  chronic 101, 121
  management techniques 119
  oxidative 90
  related damages 124
Stroke, ischemic 88
Symptoms 82, 122, 182
  gastrointestinal 122
  gynecologic 82
  menopausal 82
  psychosomatic 182

T

Therapies, gene-targeted 158
Topoisomerase 33, 56, 71
Toxic effects 90
Transcription factor (TF) 25
Transcriptomics 60, 96, 97, 100
Tumor(s) 26, 33, 40, 45, 57, 66, 67, 71, 74,
    158, 161
  biopsies 45, 57, 158
  driving signaling networks 33
  growth 26
  infiltrating lymphocytes 66, 74
  malignant 40, 67
  microenvironment 71, 161
  mutations 45
  profiling 158
Tumor heterogeneity 40, 53, 54, 59, 60, 62,
    162
  genetic 60
  malignant breast 62
Tumorigenesis 55
Tumorigenicity 60

V

Vascular endothelial growth factor (VEGF) 34

Vomiting 28, 29, 30, 31

W

Women's healthy eating and living (WHEL)
    13

www.ingramcontent.com/pod-product-compliance
Lightning Source LLC
Chambersburg PA
CBHW050822220326
41598CB00006B/291